Biotechnology and Biopharmaceutical Manufacturing, Processing, and Preservation

**Drug Manufacturing
Technology Series**

Volume 2

Edited by
Kenneth E. Avis
Vincent L. Wu

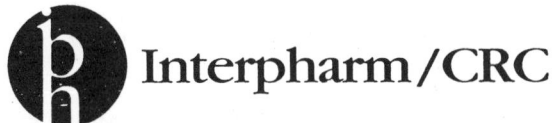 Interpharm/CRC

Boca Raton   London   New York   Washington, D.C.

FIRST INDIAN REPRINT 2009

Library of Congress Cataloging-in-Publication Data

Biotechnology and biopharmaceutical manufacturing, processing, and
preservation / Kenneth E. Avis,Vincent L. Wu, editors.
     p. cm.—(Drug manufacturing technology series : v. 2)
Includes bibliographical references and index.
ISBN 1-57491-016-7 (hbk.)
    1. Biochemical engineering. 2. Protein drugs—Storage.
3. Protein drugs—Preservation. 4. Pharmaceutical biotechnology.
    I. Avis, Kenneth E., 1918- . II. Wu, Vincent L.   III. Series.
TP248.3.P76 1996
615′.10—dc20   96-12623

Visit the CRC Press Web site at www.crcpress.com

© 1996 by CRC Press LLC
Interpharm is an imprint of CRC Press

No claim to original U.S. Government works
International Standard Book Number 10: 1-57491-016-7
International Standard Book Number 13: 978-1-57491-016-2
Library of Congress Card Number 96-12623
Printed and bound in India by Replika Press Pvt. Ltd.

FOR SALE IN SOUTH ASIA ONLY

CONTENTS

3. Process Design Considerations for Large-Scale Chromatography of Biomolecules 61

Richard Wisniewski
Egisto Boschetti
Alois Jungbauer

4. Lyophilization of Protein Pharmaceuticals 199

John F. Carpenter
Byeong S. Chang

FOREWORD

The *Drug Manufacturing Technology Series* of applied reference books was launched with the release of *Sterile Pharmaceutical Products: Process Engineering Applications,* as Volume 1, in November 1995. The goal of providing a reference that will assist chemists, biologists, engineers, pharmacists, and other practitioners in solving problems associated with the manufacture of high quality pharmaceutical products is continued in this second volume. While the first volume focused on process engineering issues, this volume focuses on the issues associated with the processing and preservation of biotechnological products, and is a logical companion to Volume 1. There is no doubt that biopharmaceutical processing depends on sound engineering practices.

As mentioned in the Foreword to Volume 1, the lack of practical information on how to perform many aspects of high quality pharmaceutical processing in a handy reference book form has led to the development of this series. The theoretical principles for the development of pharmaceutical dosage forms of drugs has been published extensively; however, the great body of experiential knowledge in the field lies largely untapped. To correct this deficiency, the *Drug Manufacturing Technology Series* is being developed.

It is clear that neither of these two volumes has exhausted the topics that must be covered in their respective areas. Therefore, as might be expected, additional volumes are being developed to incorporate both engineering and biotechnological aspects of product preparation. Because the processing of biotechnological products is an emerging discipline, and because many aspects of large-scale manufacturing are in the developmental stage, particular emphasis is needed in these areas of practice, including some of the unique characteristics of quality assurance for such pharmaceutical products. Therefore an effort will be made to satisfy these additional needs in forthcoming volumes.

One of the shortcomings encountered in any series of books, even though there is a recognizable relationship among them, is a means of linking the information in the series. To solve this problem, a Key Concept Index is being developed to help the user find key concepts in the various volumes. This will greatly increase the utility of the entire series. Therefore, this index will be expanded with each subsequent volume, and will be provided with each book. The *Drug Manufacturing Technology Series* Key Concept Cross-Reference Index will be separate from the detailed subject index of each volume.

The excitement that I feel in playing a role in producing this practical technology in written form will be experienced and shared by you, the user, only if you find the contents truly beneficial, thus making your job more enjoyable and productive, and giving you a role on the cutting edge of advancing technology. To this end I shall continue to commit myself.

Kenneth E. Avis
March 1996

1

INTRODUCTION

Kenneth E. Avis

The University of Tennessee

Vincent L. Wu

Genentech, Inc.

Pharmaceutical products of biological origin, such as vaccines, have been known and utilized in therapy for human patients for many years. Only recently, products of biological origin with more definable composition and highly specific therapeutic effects have been developed. Normally, these products are administered to human patients by injection and must, therefore, meet all of the requirements for sterile parenteral products. Further, these products normally contain specific proteins and are identified as biotechnology products or, alternatively, as biopharmaceutical products. They are subject to the characteristic stability problems encountered with protein molecules. Therefore, purifying, compounding, processing, and preservation technologies essential for these biomolecules must be developed; these processes are quite distinctive from those for other sterile pharmaceutical products.

This book has been written to meet a need for practical information to aid researchers and scientists responsible for developing and implementing the unique technologies required for the large-scale preparation of sterile biotechnology products in accord with good manufacturing practices. Although not intended as an exhaustive treatise, this book emphasizes the pertinent technologies uniquely applicable to the large-scale preservation and processing of aqueous biopharmaceutical products. Because of product stability limitations, appropriate design and planning of process campaigning for multiple products is essential for efficient manufacturing operations. This book will identify unique ways in which efficient process campaigning is possible; it will also reveal aspects of appropriate facility design as well as certain economic considerations.

The design of process campaigning for aqueous biopharmaceutical products is dictated by their stability constraints. One of the most effective means of preserving biomolecules in aqueous systems for a limited, but often extended, period of time is freezing. However, freezing and subsequent thawing for further processing places significant stress on the protein molecules. Therefore, the bulk freezing and thawing of large volumes of in-process biopharmaceuticals must be designed and controlled very carefully. In chapter two of this book, Wisniewski and Wu discuss the requirements for this unique process. There are many advantages to storing an in-process protein product in a single, large container while awaiting further processing. However, significant factors that must be controlled in order to achieve a successful outcome of such processing include processing time, temperature and solute distribution in the solid and liquid phases, pH change, convectional and density stratification effects, and the possibility of recrystallization. Process considerations for achieving a successful outcome are the subjects of this chapter. The authors provide sufficient theoretical background information to substantiate the design requirements for the process. They also include considerations for the design and use of equipment, including details of the critical freezing and thawing steps to be performed. An extensive bibliography of 122 literature references is also provided.

An essential requirement for the safe and effective use of therapeutic proteins is very high product purity. In chapter three Wisniewski, Boschetti, and Jungbauer discuss process development, process design, and the design and operation concepts of the chromatographic method used to achieve the required high product purity on a large scale. Liquid chromatography has proven to be the optimal purification technique not only to achieve high product purity on a large scale but also to provide efficient productivity, process reliability, and robustness at a minimal cost. These criteria distinguish industrial chromatography from laboratory-scale preparative techniques where separation resolution is more prominent. The authors provide an exceptionally detailed and thorough description of chromatographic media, system hardware and other components, and system integration and performance. Sufficient theoretical concepts are presented to provide the background and substantiation for process development, scale-up, and optimization of the process. This very thorough chapter also contains an extensive bibliography (240 references) that reviews the subject matter.

The fourth chapter in this book is an exposé of the principles and the application of these principles to the preservation of protein molecules by the process of lyophilization (freeze-drying). Carpenter and Chang present a lucid and detailed account of the use of lyophilization as a means for removing water from a protein preparation in order to achieve long-term stability during packing, shipping, and storage prior to administration of the product to a human patient. However, the authors point out that without proper insight into the lyophilization process and how it affects proteins, it is not a simple task to remove water by freeze-drying without damaging the protein. Further, not only must the specific conditions for optimum protein stability be determined and established, but the appropriate nonspecific stabilizing additives required for the formulation must be determined. These subjects are thoroughly developed by the authors in this chapter. Organizationally, the authors first discuss the economical design of a lyophilization cycle that results in the desired cake properties and residual moisture. They next consider how to design formulations that stabilize proteins during both freezing and drying, including the mechanisms for stabilization by additives. The final section consists of a discussion of the optimization of formulations for long-term storage with a focus on the impact of physical properties of the dried solid on protein stability. A literature review of 90 references concludes the chapter.

Achieving and maintaining the sterility and overall purity of parenteral products is a continuing focus of effort in good manufacturing practices by the pharmaceutical industry. One of the newer process methods utilized to improve the sterility assurance levels of aseptic processing is blow-fill-seal (b/f/s) technology. Essentially, the b/f/s process utilizes in-line machinery that forms a plastic container, fills it, and then seals it within a relatively small enclosure, with the critical environmental exposure operations protected with HEPA–filtered laminar flow air. In chapter five Wu and Leo present a case study in the qualification and use of a b/f/s system for the processing of a biopharmaceutical product. Issues reviewed include facility design, sterility assurance, validation, and the operational performance of the system. The authors point out that most of the issues explored are not limited to biotechnology products, but are applicable to pharmaceutical products in general. Specific concerns for the use of the system with sensitive protein products include assessment of heat imparted to the product, extractables from plastics, and product stability. A list of 7 literature references is provided.

In chapter six Hughes discusses an integrated approach for designing a pharmaceutical production facility for multiple products. The author states that the rationale for a multiproduct facility rather than one dedicated to a single product includes the following factors:

- The relatively small projected market for many new products

- The worldwide pressure to reduce costs for therapeutic agents

- New manufacturing technologies and equipment that have improved process control

- Advances in analytical techniques that have enhanced characterization of product in-process steps and the identification of contaminants and impurities

In this context the author aims to clarify the principle concerns of multiproduct processing, present the prevailing industry and regulatory viewpoints, suggest an integrated facility design development strategy, and review general biotechnology facility design requirements with an emphasis on the desirable features to include in a multiproduct facility. A list of 17 literature references is also given.

The final chapter, written by Wheelwright, provides an insight into economic and cost factors relative to engineering aspects of biotechnological processing. The author has divided the chapter into four main areas. The author begins by reviewing background factors and definitions. He then discusses the costs associated with development and its impact on later costs. This is followed by a description of facilities costs, including design and construction, and inherent considerations of operating costs. The author states that a vigilant evaluation of those factors that impact costs, especially future costs, at early stages of the development and planning process will have a significant impact on minimizing the cost as well as minimizing the time required to bring a new product to market. A comparison of fundamental questions, such as a dedicated plant versus a shared plant, new construction versus renovation, the number of purification steps versus process yield, and acceptable risk versus payback, allows quantification of economic return and maximization of value to investors. A list of 19 references concludes the chapter.

It is anticipated that the theoretical and practical information presented will make this book a highly useful tool for those involved in the large-scale processing and preservation of sterile biotechnological products. Since the topics covered are not exhaustive, additional topics will be covered in future books in the *Drug Manufacturing Technology Series.*

2

LARGE–SCALE FREEZING AND THAWING OF BIOPHARMACEUTICAL PRODUCTS

Richard Wisniewski

NASA Ames Research Center

Vincent Wu

Genentech, Inc.

Protein products often have limited stability in the liquid state, yet may need to be stored for extended periods of time—for example, prior to lyophilization. Depending on the stability and storage period desired, biological products are often stored at 5°C, below -70°C, or as lyophilized product. The ability to freeze a bulk protein solution, and thereby hold it under stable conditions, offers significant economic and manufacturing advantages.

Freezing and thawing large volumes of bulk protein product has become an essential step in the manufacture of biopharmaceuticals at Genentech, Inc. The ability to freeze a product and hold it stable for extended periods of time provides flexibility for the manufacturing process and plays a key role in maximizing the productivity of multiproduct facilities for cell culture, purification, and filling and finishing. The process of freezing bulk product, followed by thawing at a later time, allows cell culture and purification activities to be conducted in a campaign mode: Production facilities focus on the manufacture of one product to build its inventory, while frozen bulk inventory of other products provides a steady supply of various products to the filling and finishing facilities. Figure 2.1 illustrates various steps in a typical biopharmaceutical manufacturing process where freezing hold steps may be implemented. Bulk material may be frozen in a concentrated form after final purification steps to minimize vessel storage requirements.

Figure 2.1. Bulk product may be frozen and stored after key process steps to provide manufacturing flexibility and to facilitate campaigning of multiproduct facilities. Savings in operating costs are realized when lots are pooled to produce larger and fewer final batches, thus reducing quality control expense and manufacturing labor.

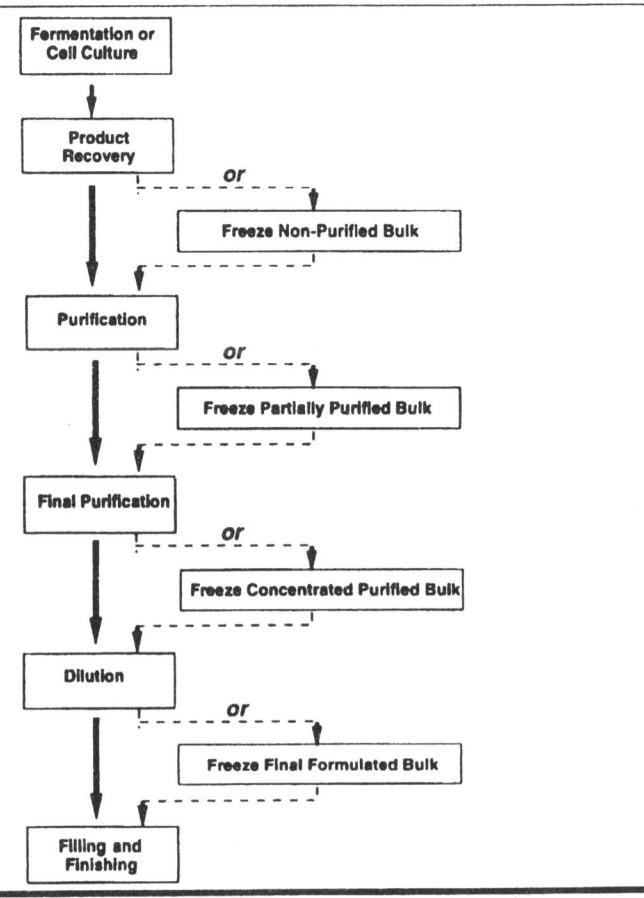

Once a frozen bulk inventory is established, an option exists of pooling multiple batches to produce larger lot sizes. There are significant savings realized by pooling product to produce larger and fewer batches of filled vials since the number of required quality control tests are reduced. Quality control costs for biotechnology products are a considerable part of the cost of goods. For example, quality control testing for the filled vial, not including quality control testing for the bulk product, is estimated to be in the range of 12–20 percent of the total cost of goods. However, the largest savings offered by the freezing and thawing process is realized due to the reduced capital investment in the construction of expensive facilities, since running the plant in a campaign mode and building a frozen bulk inventory may preclude the need for dedicated production facilities to produce a constant supply of bulk product. The ability to build a large inventory of frozen bulk product also makes it possible to provide adequate supply for the introductory market launch of a biotechnology product.

The use of a specially designed, stainless steel, portable freeze-thaw vessel, sized to the batch, was found to be suitable for the sterile storage and handling of bulk protein product at Genentech. Product transfer and filtration into a stainless steel portable vessel is consistent with current good pharmaceutical manufacturing operations. There are many advantages in storing product in a single, large container. Dividing the batch into multiple, smaller volumes may increase the possibility of product contamination, add operational steps, require additional quality control testing, and require careful batch tracking procedures to avoid product mixup from multiple batches. The stainless steel vessels lend themselves to clean-in-place (CIP) and steam-in-place (SIP) procedures, and provide a robust containment system for frozen shipment of large quantities of protein product to manufacturing partners with filling and finishing operations in the U.S., Europe, and Asia.

A number of factors must be considered when protein products are to undergo a freeze-thaw process. For example, the product must not be allowed to change its physicochemical characteristics nor lose its biological activity during the freezing or thawing processing steps. The processing steps must avoid causing detrimental changes, such as product precipitation, permanent denaturation, oxidation, or multimer formation (Agarwal and Sohal 1994; Manning et al. 1989; Wang and Hanson 1988). These factors become especially important when one is designing large scale freeze-thaw systems for protein products.

Due to the large liquid volumes involved, the factors that become important in the successful outcome for freezing proteins are processing time, temperature and solute distribution in the solid and liquid phases, pH change, convectional and density stratification effects, and a possibility of ice recrystallization. Due to long product phase change times, such as those resulting from transition from the liquid state through multiphase solidification to a low temperature solid, interactions among solutes and between ice and solutes must be well understood.

This chapter describes the principles and process design considerations for freezing and thawing protein solutions on a large scale. Freeze-thaw systems designed to handle bulk product volumes greater than 100 L have been used for several years at Genentech, Inc., as a method for preserving formulated and preformulated bulk parenteral biopharmaceutical products.

The section entitled "Freezing" discusses the thermodynamics of protein denaturation and the stability of proteins as described by changes in Gibbs free energy. The importance of promoting dendritic ice growth during freezing to provide a more uniform distribution of solutes is discussed. The need to minimize convection during freezing to reduce cryoconcentration effects is emphasized, followed by a review of recent literature on the interaction of solutes with the ice-liquid interface and the influence of proteins and small molecules on ice crystal growth.

Process design principles for thawing and the use of forced convection provided by recirculation of the solution to improve heat transfer, and to provide homogeneity of the melting solution, are described in "Thawing." Approaches to freeze-thaw development, including the use of a pilot-scale freeze-thaw vessel, and an approach to the analysis of the distribution of frozen solutes in a vessel to determine cryoconcentration effects is presented in "Freeze-Thaw Process Development."

"Large-Scale Freezing and Thawing of Biopharmaceuticals" outlines design and process control considerations for freezing and thawing in a jacketed, portable, stainless steel vessel with an internal heat exchanger. Formulation considerations are then presented for freezing bulk product. Heat transfer principles that take into account natural convection, diffusion, and the shape of the solid-liquid interface are reviewed in "Heat and Mass Transfer."

"Vessel Design" discusses a jacketed, freeze-thaw container that utilizes internal heat transfer surfaces with fins to divide the vessel volume into compartments, to reduce freezing and thawing time, to reduce cryoconcentration effects, and to provide directional freezing from the bottom of the vessel upward.

The elements of a mechanical-based refrigeration system for freezing and thawing that circulates heat exchange medium to the freeze vessel jacket and internal heat exchange surfaces are presented in "Freeze-Thaw Refrigeration System." Use of silicone fluid as a heat exchange medium and the use of liquid nitrogen as a refrigerant are also discussed.

Considerations for product storage and shipping in an insulated shipping container are presented in "Product Storage and Shipping." A brief overview on a sampling scheme prior to and after freezing product is presented in "Product Release and Sampling." The next section outlines stability considerations and an approach for qualifying multiple freeze-thaw cycles. The final section addresses approaches to the validation of freezing and thawing processes based on time and temperature criteria.

FREEZING

Thermodynamics of Protein Cold Denaturation

Prior to subjecting protein product to freezing and thawing, one must consider the possibility of protein cold or heat denaturation during the freezing and thawing processes, although usually the cold denaturation process is reversible (Azuaga et al. 1992; Biringer and Fink 1988). The presence of solutes may affect protein structure at low temperatures and the solutes may have stabilizing or destabilizing effects (Arakawa and Timasheff 1982 a and b; Arakawa et al. 1991; Carpenter and Crowe 1988; Carpenter et al. 1991). Diller (1992) included a thorough review of low temperature processes in biological systems with and without phase change. Parts of that work are relevant to the large-scale freeze and thaw processes of cell suspensions and biological molecules. Other references pertinent to freezing and storing protein solutions are works on the effects of low temperatures on enzymes by Douzou (1980) and Fink (1986) and on food proteins by Fennema (1982).

During the freeze/thaw process it is important that the protein be maintained in its native state, since there is a possibility of cold or heat denaturation during the freezing and thawing steps. The protein may have two distinct states—native and denatured—and the transition between these two states may be described by changes in enthalpy (ΔH), entropy (ΔS) and Gibbs free energy (ΔG):

$$\Delta G = \Delta H - T\Delta S$$

Using temperature as a variable, the enthalpy of transition may be determined by accurate calorimetry methods by measuring temperature changes. Changes in protein state involve energy absorption or release that can be measured (e.g., energy determined from areas of absorption peaks). Protein denaturation is associated with an increase in heat capacity (Privalov 1989).

Gibbs free energy change is associated with the work required to disrupt the structure of proteins and is used to describe protein stability. The Gibbs free energy is temperature dependent; it has a parabolic shape with a maximum at a temperature that varies depending on the protein. The maximum stability of a protein at its native state temperature (T_s) occurs when the entropy difference of the native and denatured state is zero, at which point stability depends on the enthalpy differences between the native and denatured states. At temperature values above and below T_s, the Gibbs free energy decreases and protein stability decreases as well. The shape of the Gibbs free energy curve suggests that both high and low temperature denaturation are possible thermodynamically. The difference is that during heat denaturation the heat is absorbed (increase in enthalpy and entropy), while cold denaturation involves heat release (decrease in entropy and enthalpy). The cold denaturation of protein is not always easy to demonstrate experimentally since the declining part of the Gibbs free energy curve below T_s may be below 0°C, and thus is in the frozen state for aqueous solutions. Nevertheless, the cold denaturation of proteins has been confirmed in numerous experiments (Franks et al. 1988; Griko 1989; Griko and Privalov 1992; Griko and Kutyshenko 1994; Privalov 1990).

The difference in the Gibbs free energy between the native and denatured states of proteins is small (5–20 kcal/mol), or less than $1/10$ kT per residue where k is Boltzmann's constant (Dill 1990).

Values of heat capacity change, enthalpy and entropy changes, and resulting Gibbs free energy changes can be estimated for globular proteins if the buried apolar and polar surface areas of the protein molecules are known (Murphy and Freire 1992). Estimated values are close to experimental data. Therefore, one may estimate the thermodynamic properties and Gibbs free energy prior to calorimetric studies. For example, for myoglobin the values (calculated and experimental) are as follows:

- Change in heat capacity: 2.5 and 2.6 kcal/°Kmol

- Change in enthalpy: 107 and 101 kcal/mol

- Change in entropy: 307 and 282 cal/°Kmol

For cytochrome c the calculated and experimental numbers are as follows:

- Change in heat capacity: 1.3 and 1.6 kcal/°Kmol

- Change in enthalpy: 78 and 78 kcal/mol

- Change in entropy: 257 and 208 cal/°Kmol

For lysozyme the calculated and experimental numbers are as follows:

- Change in heat capacity: 1.7 and 1.6 kcal/°Kmol

- Change in enthalpy: 124 and 112 kcal/mol

- Change in entropy: 318 and 310 cal/°Kmol

Dendritic Ice Growth

When viewed on a microscopic scale, the moving solid boundary during freezing is not flat, but consists of dendritic, or fingerlike crystals protruding forward from a moving solid front (Kurz and Fisher 1989; Koerber 1988; Rubinsky and Eto 1990). Such an interface is difficult to describe and model (Egolf and Manz 1994). A frequently used modeling simplification is to treat the solid-liquid interface as a linear transition surface.

Dendrites are composed of pure ice, while the solutes are located in the interdendritic spaces with their solidified form reaching the eutectic composition or glassy state (Franks 1993). The moving solidification front with an array of extended dendrites can entrap solutes in the interdendritic spaces. There is a discrete distribution of the ice and solutes on a microscopic scale, but on a macroscopic level the solute distribution within the frozen mass may appear uniform. In the interdendritic space the concentration of solutes increases from the tip of the dendrite where it is close to the bulk solution concentration, to the maximum or eutectic concentration at the base of the dendrite. Such a concentration gradient would normally cause a diffusion of solute molecules toward the bulk liquid if the dendritic front becomes stationary. Refer to Table 2.1 for diffusion coefficients for proteins, small molecules, and ions.

In addition to the solute concentration distribution in the interdendritic spaces, there is also a temperature distribution along the dendrites and within the interdendritic space, with temperature declining from the tip of a dendrite toward the frozen mass.

Table 2.1. Diffusion Coefficients in Aqueous Solutions

Proteins	cm^2/sec (unit $\times$ 10^{-7})
Cytochrome c (M.W. 12,310)[a]	13.00
Chymotrypsinogen (M.W. 25,670)[a]	9.48
Hemoglobin (M.W. 64,610)[a]	6.02
BSA (M.W. 67,500)[b]	6.81
HSA (M.W. 72,300)[b]	5.93
Urease (M.W. 482,700)[b]	4.01
Small Molecules and Ions	**cm^2/sec (unit $\times$ 10^{-7})**
KCl[b]	187.00
NaCl[c]	140.00
Urea (M.W. 60.1)[b]	120.00
Sucrose (M.W. 342.3)[b]	46.00
Glycerol (M.W. 92.1)[b]	82.50

[a]Creighton, T. 1993. *Proteins.* New York: W. H. Freeman.

[b]Geankoplis, C. 1983. *Transport processes: Momentum, heat and mass.* Boston: Allyn and Bacon.

[c]Reid, P., J. Prausnitz, and T. Sherwood. 1977. *Properties of gases and liquids.* New York: McGraw-Hill.

Temperature gradients along dendrites may facilitate solidification at the eutectic or glassy state composition in the interdendritic spaces. Since the layer of solidified material grows during the freezing process, the conduction heat transfer resistance increases and the solidification rate decreases. To overcome the decrease in freezing rate due to heat transfer resistance and for better control of dendritic growth, the cooling medium temperature may be decreased as freezing progresses.

Rubinsky et al. (1993) investigated solidification phenomena of saline solutions. Experiments were performed using a thin layer of saline solution (0.154 M) on a cooled microscope stage with strict temperature control. Initially, a flat front of the solidified material developed instabilities in the form of waves with an amplitude of about 10 μm, which grew into dendrites. Due to the controlled directional heat flow, the dendrites formed a regular parallel pattern with dendrites spaced approximately 90 μm apart.

The moving dendritic ice front allows solutes to be entrapped in the interdendritic space, which promotes a uniform distribution of solutes in the frozen mass. If the moving solid-liquid interface were flat, solutes could be excluded from the frozen mass and become increasingly concentrated. One of the important conditions for controlling dendritic growth for freezing large volumes is to assure directional heat flow.

Convection in the liquid phase may affect the formation of dendrites and their shape. By changing the liquid phase viscosity, Chen (1992) showed detrimental effects of convection in the liquid phase on dendrite formation. Natural convection may also occur in the interdendritic spaces (Worster 1991).

Concentration Phenomenon

Intensive convection in the liquid phase of the solution during freezing may cause an exclusion of solute molecules from the solution's solidifying mass and gradual cryoconcentration of solutes in the liquid phase. This effect occurs due to the sweeping effect of the turbulent liquid motion at the solid surface and the suppression of dendritic ice growth. As a result, a flat interface forms. This phenomenon is utilized in the food industry to concentrate fruit juice by applying forced convection in the liquid phase, causing solidification of an almost pure ice with solutes remaining in the liquid phase (Davis 1990; Kyprianidou-Leonidou and Botsaris 1990, 364–372; Shimoyamada et al. 1994; Spicer 1974). In these processes ice crystals are separated from the solutes, which are recovered in the concentrated liquid form. The phenomenon of cryoconcentration is very undesirable during the freezing of pharmaceutical formulations; therefore, efforts must be taken to design the process in a way to minimize convection in the liquid phase during freezing.

The moving solid-liquid interface also causes solute concentration polarization (e.g., there is an increased concentration of solutes in the liquid phase adjacent to the interface [Koerber et al. 1983; Lombrana and Diaz 1987]). This phenomenon has been clearly observed on a small scale. Increasing the concentration of solutes in the liquid phase may have destabilizing (Muecke and Schmid 1994) or stabilizing (Ahmad and Bigelow 1986; Arakawa and Timasheff 1982a) effects on protein molecules. Therefore, the formulation should include components that ensure protein stability at increasing concentrations.

Interaction of Solutes with the Ice-Liquid Interface

In addition to the phenomena associated with phase changes during solidification and melting, one must consider product interactions with other formulation solutes and water at the molecular level and at the solid-liquid interface (Huyskens et al. 1991; Jeffrey and Saenger 1991; Tiller 1991).

There are two areas of concern at the molecular level near the solid-liquid interface during freezing: (1) the interaction of water and ice and (2) the interaction of solutes and ice. An accepted theory of the interaction of water and ice is that the ice surface has exposed hydroxide groups that can form hydrogen bonds with the surrounding liquid water or solute molecules (Franks 1982). Investigations of the freezing phenomena are closely associated with the ice structure. The crystalline ice structure when formed under atmospheric pressure assumes a hexagonal, hydrogen-bonded pattern (Fletcher 1970; Fukusako 1990).

Interaction Between Proteins and Ice

Studies on the phenomena at the ice-water interface may shed light on the possible interactions of ice and solutes. Intermolecular distances in the ice lattice are larger than those in liquid phase water clusters; for this reason the density of ice is lower than water.

Karim and Haymet (1988) reported on molecular dynamics studies of the ice-water interface. The density profile, molecular orientation, and diffusion constants were calculated as a function of the distance normal to the interface. The interface effects extend from the solid to liquid phase, with a transitional zone of structural changes measuring approximately 10–15 Å. This range may be sufficient for the protein surface residues to be affected in their interaction with the ice surface. The size of proteins are on the order of tens of angstroms. For example, hemoglobin (MW 64610) has the approximate dimensions $70 \times 55 \times 55$ Å, trypsin (MW 23200) is $50 \times 40 \times 40$ Å, and lysozyme (MW 14320) is $45 \times 30 \times 30$ Å (Creighton 1993).

In general, adsorption of proteins to solid surfaces is a complex phenomenon involving multiple effects on surfaces of the protein molecule and the solid (Johnson et al 1994). Adsorption of proteins to solid surfaces may depend on the protein molecule surface charges and on the exposed hydrophobic area. Proteins usually adsorb well to hydrophobic surfaces.

The interaction of proteins with ice has been studied in diverse fields such as biological cryoprotectants (Avanov 1990), polar fish (DeVries 1984) and lyophilization (Pikal 1990). Protein-ice adsorption may depend on the structural characteristics of amino acid or oligosaccharide structures of the protein molecules and the interaction with water molecules involved in protein hydration, which may affect matching lattices of ice crystals. Such lattice matching may involve the formation of hydrogen bonds. Hydrogen bonds play a major role in protein secondary structure and its stability (Bordo and Argos 1994; Jeffrey and Saenger 1991; Stickle et al. 1992).

In ice the regular spacing of surface oxygens that may form hydrogen bonds is 7.36 Å (DeVries 1984) and the spacing of alpha-helix turns in proteins is 5.4 Å (Branden and Tooze 1991). The average length of alpha-helices is approximately 15 Å; and therefore the regular helices may not match well with the ice structure. Some alanine-rich alpha-helical proteins are known to adsorb to ice (Holmberg et al. 1994).

Influence of Proteins on Ice Crystal Growth. Ice-protein interactions are well researched in the area of protein antifreeze activity. DeVries (1984) and Avanov (1990) support an opinion that antifreeze glycoproteins may form hydrogen bonds with ice crystals and compete with water molecules. Hydroxyl groups of antifreeze molecules play an important role in such hydrogen bond formation. Wen and Laursen (1992) proposed a model for binding antifreeze polypeptides to ice. Hew and Yang (1992) published a review on protein interaction with ice. Proteins can have both inhibiting and promoting influences upon the growth of ice crystals. Results were cited showing the exclusion of sodium chloride ions from ice crystals and the incorporation of antifreeze proteins into the ice structure. The antifreeze proteins adsorb with a preference to certain planes of ice crystals. Since they do not adsorb uniformly to all ice surfaces, they have a detrimental effect upon ice crystal growth. A result of such an effect is a lowering of the temperature of crystal formation (supercooling). It was suggested that ice nucleation-promoting proteins may have a highly repetitive structure and they may consist mostly of beta sheets. The tertiary structure of such ice nucleation proteins may also possess a surface structure that is lattice-matching with ice.

Chakrabartty et al. (1989) investigated the minimum number of ice-interaction residues and the helix length required for antifreeze activity (e.g., for adsorption to ice lattice). The ability of the peptides to develop antifreeze activity depended on the presence of appropriately positioned amino acid residue side chains that can form hydrogen bonds with ice. Polar amino acid residues were observed aligning along one face of the helix and were reported as probable ice-interaction sites.

Adsorption of glycopeptides and glycoproteins to ice during freezing may vary with molecular size. Larger molecules may adsorb more than smaller ones (DeVries 1984). For glycopeptides that exhibit antifreeze activity, the adsorption diminishes at molecular masses below 2000 Da. Carbohydrate moieties of glycoproteins may also play a role in protein-ice adsorption and incorporation into the ice structure (Mashimo et al. 1992; Mashimo and Miura 1993).

Adsorbing proteins may also affect the recrystallization of ice during warming of the frozen mass prior to thawing (Carpenter and Hansen 1992). Warren et al. (1993) attempted to engineer peptides to adsorb to ice. They concluded that it is reasonable to expect molecular adsorption effects to become stronger in longer molecules that may have more sites available for interaction with the substrate. The high hydrophobicity factor of these peptides may indicate that hydrogen bonding may not be predominant in their adsorption to ice, although they may reach a certain molecular orientation in the process of adsorption. The molecular weights were in the range of 2,145–5,733 with corresponding hydropathy indices in the range of 0.673–1.050. Considering that the size of the protein molecules are larger, there might be enough hydrogen bonding between the molecule and the ice to affect the adsorption phenomena.

At the molecular level the phenomenon of protein hydration further complicates the protein freezing process. The protein hydration water may not freeze together with the bulk water, but may freeze at temperatures below 0°C (Kuntz and Kauzmann 1974). Measurement of such nonfreezing water was proposed as a method to estimate protein hydration (Rupley and Careri 1991). Hydrated water in proteins may crystallize during slow cooling or can be vitrified at high rates of cooling. In hydrated proteins a fraction of water (usually below 0.3 g/g of protein) may remain unfrozen (mobile) even at low temperatures and does not crystallize even during long periods. Change in dynamics of hydrated proteins usually occurs near –70°C to –80°C (a glasslike transition) (Chang and Randall 1992; Sartor et al. 1994).

The data on adsorption of peptides and proteins to ice and antifreeze activity may provide an indication of the behavior of similar biomolecules. Since the adsorption of macromolecules to ice depends on molecular structure and conformation, individual studies for particular products are required.

Interaction of Small Molecules with Ice

Since protein formulations include a variety of components, ranging from simple ions to macromolecular complexes, interactions of these molecules with ice during freezing and thawing must be well understood. Recent research work with small molecules suggests that this may also be a preliminary step to better understanding protein-ice interactions. Small ions are usually rejected from ice due to the disturbed water structure in their hydration shells (Conway 1981; Floris et al. 1994). Recently, Schaff and Roberts (1994) announced results of work on the adsorption of acetone to amorphous and crystalline ice. The authors reported that while acetone adsorbs to amorphous ice via hydrogen bonds, its adsorption to crystalline ice is controlled via dispersive forces. They concluded that the presence of free hydroxyl (OH) groups on the crystalline ice surface is much lower than on the amorphous surface. These results may have relevance when considering the methodology of freezing and its effect on product-ice interactions. Silva and Devlin (1994) reported results of interactions of acetylene, ethylene, and benzene with ice surfaces. This work may lead to a better understanding of the interactions of biomolecules with ice, since the interaction between water/ice and benzene is similar to the interaction between water and amino groups with aromatic residues found in proteins. The interactions between water and acetylene or water and ethylene have similarity to hydrogen bond phenomena in peptide-to-peptide and water-to-peptide interactions. These organic molecules have been demonstrated to act as proton acceptors in their interaction with ice. The infrared spectroscopic studies showed that these molecules bonded tightly to the ice surface. Bonding to crystalline ice was about 25–30 percent lower compared to amorphous ice. Strong interactions with the hydroxyl groups on ice molecules with the formation of hydrogen bonds were noted in both cases.

The hydration shells of charged salt ions in aqueous solutions are disturbed areas of water structures (Floris et al. 1994), which may prevent incorporation of ions into the ice crystal structure. Since there is a solute concentration effect occurring in the interdendritic space, the protein product may be exposed to high ionic strength solutions. Interactions of proteins with salts in concentrated solutions were summarized by Arakawa and Timasheff (1982b). The presence of additional solute molecules can affect protein behavior at ambient and low temperatures (Conway 1981; Makhatadze and Privalov 1992; Pace and Tanford 1968). Mashimo et al. (1992) investigated the structures of mixtures of water with glucose, polysaccharides, and ascorbic acid. The authors demonstrated that the glucose molecule can be readily incorporated into the ice lattice (e.g., it can easily replace the hexagonal cluster in the lattice of ice). The ice lattice might be slightly distorted by the presence of the glucose molecule, but it is also stabilized by several hydrogen bonds between the glucose and the lattice. The glucose molecule is similar in size and shape to the water clusters and, therefore, can be incorporated into the ice lattice. Polysaccharides that are larger than the typical water clusters (larger than maltotriose) cannot be incorporated into the ice lattice in place of the clusters. Ascorbic acid, although similar in size to glucose can, in principle, replace the water cluster and enter the ice lattice, but the lattice is not stable since only two hydrogen bonds could form between the lattice and the molecule.

Later, Mashimo and Miura (1993) demonstrated that trehalose and maltose were also incorporated into the ice lattice due to the fact that their length was similar to the water cluster size. The authors also concluded that water forms two classes of structures: (1) the local structure consisting of 6 water molecules and (2) the high order structure consisting of 30 molecules, which is less ordered, but similar to the ordinary ice lattice. These works demonstrate the importance of similarity of molecular size and shape to water clusters and the ability to form multiple hydrogen bonds as a requirement for the sugar molecules to be incorporated into the ice lattice. Larger sugars, which are excluded from the ice lattice, are concentrated in the solution in the interdendritic space and may reach the glassy state there.

In summary, while ions, some small and most of the large molecules may be rejected from the ice structure and are entrapped as eutectics or in the form of a glassy state in the interdendritic space, some proteins may be incorporated into the ice structure. Protein adsorption has been observed in proteins and peptides that exhibit antifreeze activity. Since these molecules are only a particular subset of a large variety of biomolecules, one might anticipate that the protein of interest may not adsorb well to the ice surface; therefore, the protein will be excluded from ice and entrapped in the interdendritic space. Individual studies of protein distribution are required for each product, due to differences in molecular structure. Interactions among ice and solutes in freezing solutions are not well understood and additional research efforts in this area are needed.

THAWING

Frozen material requires thawing prior to subsequent processing steps, such as final purification, dilution, or filling. The thawing step should be approached with caution, since it requires delivery of energy to melt the frozen mass (Sartor et al. 1994). A strict temperature limit for the product during the thawing operation can be applied. The wall temperature of heat transfer surfaces and the heat transfer media must not exceed an allowable temperature limit established for the product. This product temperature maximum should be supported by product stability studies. Typically, biotechnology product stability studies are performed at 2–8°C, 25°C, and at higher temperatures for accelerated stability studies (Manning et al. 1989; Wang and Hanson 1988).

The general process of melting and dissolving was described by Woods (1992). An important factor during the thawing process is the use of convection in the liquid phase. The liquid phase first occurs next to the heat transfer surface. If there is no forced convection in the liquid phase, only natural convection and conduction participates in energy transfer through the liquid from the heat transfer surface towards the solid-liquid interface where the thawing takes place (Bareis and Beer 1984; Benard et al. 1985). Theoretical treatment of melting with convection is described by Bejan (1989). Energy requirements are mostly for the latent heat of phase change and also for the heating of the liquid and solid. Forced convection in the liquid phase provides increased heat transfer near the heat transfer surfaces and at the solid-liquid interfaces. Liquid streams moving along or against the melting surface may significantly increase the rate of phase change from solid to liquid in the areas affected by the moving liquid streams (Yen and Zehnder 1973; Yen 1975). The liquid streams can virtually "drill" through the block of frozen material under the condition that sufficient thermal energy is supplied to the liquid phase. Solid surface ablation phenomenon plays an important role in the solid phase removal process (Storti 1995; Swedish et al. 1979). Liquid stream velocities should be kept sufficiently low to prevent foaming and product degradation due to hydrodynamic shear.

FREEZE–THAW PROCESS DEVELOPMENT

Freeze-thaw studies may be performed with small (i.e., 20–50 mL) stainless steel or polymer containers. The use of glass vials should be avoided since glass tends to crack, especially when formulations contain multiple excipients that crystallize and expand at different temperatures. Multiple freeze-thaw cycles should be tested in the small containers, with the product sampled after each freeze-thaw cycle. Thawing should be conducted at the highest allowable temperature determined by stability studies.

A pilot-scale freeze-thaw vessel should be used to qualify products prior to performing freeze-thaw studies at production scale. Development studies using scaled-down vessels can provide conditions similar to the production process with the benefit of using a small quantity (i.e., a few liters) of product.

The distribution of solutes in a large frozen mass may be analyzed by cutting the frozen mass into sections, thawing the sections, and assaying the sections for distribution of proteins and salts. Figure 2.2 illustrates a cross section of a frozen mass for 20 liters of formulated Activase® solution (2.5 mg/mL recombinant-tissue-type plasminogen activator, 85 mg/mL L-arginine, 25 mg/mL phosphoric acid, 0.2 mg/mL polysorbate 80), which was frozen in a 12-inch (305 mm) diameter pilot-scale freeze-thaw vessel used for development. The frozen mass was removed from the vessel with four heat transfer fins embedded; five frozen sections were cut horizontally from the core (C) and outside the core (A). Samples were assayed for protein concentration and conductivity to examine the distribution of proteins and ionic solutes. Protein concentration and conductivity results are shown in Figure 2.3 and Figure 2.4. The pH of the original solution was 7.25. The pH measured for different frozen sections did not show

Figure 2.2. Illustration of frozen section analysis for protein concentration and conductivity to determine the cryoconcentration effects for Activase® frozen in a 20-liter pilot-scale freeze-thaw vessel.

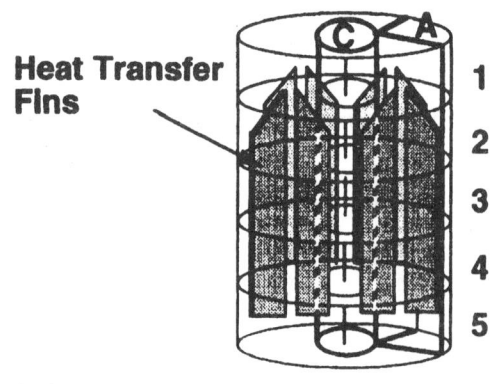

Figure 2.3. Protein concentrations were measured to determine the cryoconcentration effects for Activase® frozen in a 20-liter pilot-scale freeze-thaw vessel.

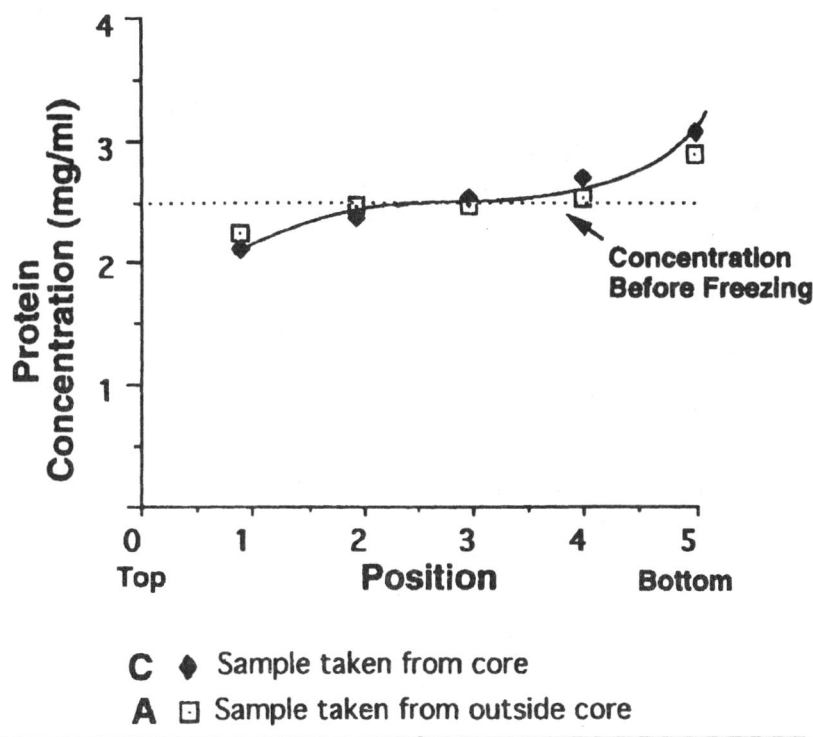

C ◆ Sample taken from core

A ☐ Sample taken from outside core

a significant trend with values ranging between pH 7.14 and 7.23. The data indicate a higher protein concentration at the bottom of the vessel and a lower concentration at the top. These differences may be attributed to density differences in the liquid phase and to the descending convectional currents during freezing. The rate of sedimentation of proteins depends on their molecular weight, density, shape in solution, and interactions with the aqueous medium. Sedimentation of proteins is countered by their diffusion. Calculated densities of proteins from partial specific volumes (Creighton 1993) are as follows: cytochrome c (MW 12,310) is 1.3986 g/mL, chymotrypsinogen (MW 25,670) is 1.38696 g/mL, and hemoglobin (MW 64,610) is 1.3333 g/mL. Higher concentrations of proteins and salts at the bottom of the vessel may also occur due to the decreased solubility of solutes with decreasing temperature and partial precipitation.

Figure 2.4. Conductivity was measured to determine the distribution of ionic solutes for Activase® frozen in a 20-liter pilot-scale freeze-thaw vessel.

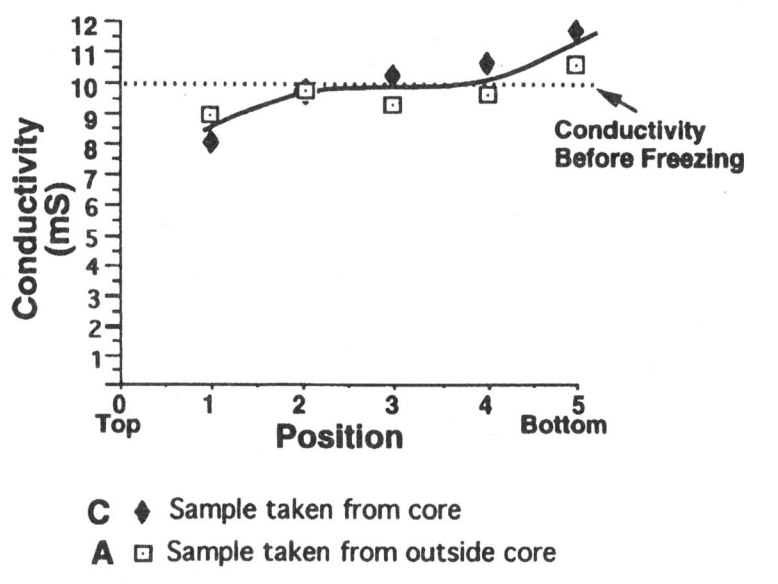

C ♦ Sample taken from core
A ▫ Sample taken from outside core

Knowledge of the range of concentrations of the proteins and salts in the large-scale production vessel is valuable for conducting laboratory-scale freeze-thaw stability experiments at various temperatures in small containers. Due to the larger size of the production-scale vessel, it may not be possible to remove the entire frozen mass from the vessel to examine solute distribution. However, frozen bulk at production scale may be analyzed by samples obtained by coring the frozen mass, or by taking scrapings from the top and bottom of the frozen mass if ports are provided at the top and bottom of the freeze-thaw vessel.

An important task is to identify the warmest point in the frozen mass using temperature surveys by placing arrays of thermocouples in the vessel. Since the top-center area of the frozen mass is designed to freeze last as a precaution against building up any excessive stresses, it should be the warmest point in the vessel. This warm spot location will allow temperature monitoring with an infrared thermometer mounted at the top center of the container to determine the completion of the freezing process. An infrared thermometer may be used while maintaining integrity of the container by using an infrared-transparent sightglass. An infrared thermometer that is offered by Mikron Instrument Co. (Wyckoff, NJ) was found to be suitable for temperatures down to –40°C.

Freezing and thawing experiments with various formulations may be performed using a microscope and a thermoelectric cooling/warming device. Dendritic ice crystal growth may be observed during freezing; the size of dendrites may be estimated using graded microscope oculars. A thermoelectric cooling/warming instrument provided by Physitemp, Inc. (Clifton, NJ), was used in this work. Figure 2.5 illustrates an experimental setup for observing dendritic ice crystals. A 120 mM saline solution was frozen at –40°C and surface dendrites were observed. Dendrites had a width of 50–90 μm with projecting needle lengths of 150–200 μm. Similar experiments were performed with protein formulations.

Figure 2.5. Experimental setup for observing dendritic ice growth.

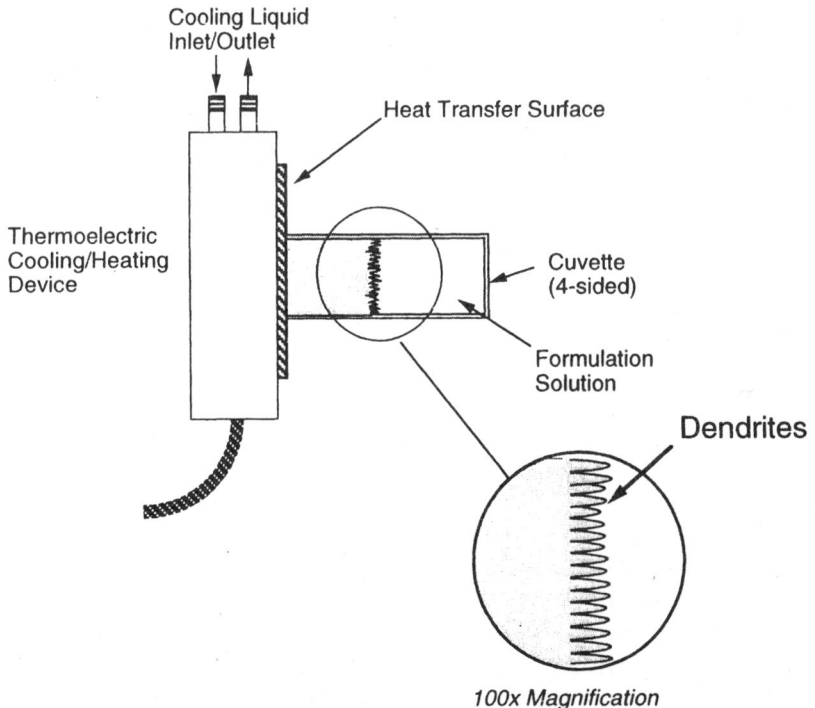

Cooling Liquid
Inlet/Outlet

Heat Transfer Surface

Thermoelectric
Cooling/Heating
Device

Cuvette
(4-sided)

Formulation
Solution

Dendrites

100x Magnification

As previously mentioned, maintaining dendritic growth is believed to be beneficial for freezing proteins. The dendrites encompass the proteins and small molecules and reduce convectional effects in the liquid phase. Maintaining conditions that facilitate dendritic growth may be influenced by the shape and configuration of the cooling surfaces, by controlling the cooling rate, and by minimizing convection in the liquid phase.

Freezing Rate

The effect of freezing rate on human growth hormone formulations was investigated by Eckhardt et al. (1991). Aggregation of human growth hormone (hGH) was studied with respect to cooling rate, excipients, and pH of the formulation. Insoluble aggregates in hGH formulations at pH 7.4 and 7.8 were measured by light scattering and results indicated that insoluble aggregates increased for the pH 7.4 formulations with increased freezing rate. The fastest freezing rate studied was 50°C/min, which produced the highest level of insoluble aggregates. The authors suggested that smaller ice crystals are formed during faster freezing, which may provide greater surface area for the denaturation of protein molecules.

Due to the size of the systems discussed here for bulk freezing processes, freezing rate is inherently slow. For example, a 120-liter freeze-thaw vessel that utilizes mechanical refrigeration for cooling provides cooling rates of approximately 0.5°C/min at the beginning of the freezing process.

LARGE–SCALE FREEZING AND THAWING OF BIOPHARMACEUTICALS

Large-Scale Freezing

There are numerous concerns in large-scale freezing that may not be apparent at smaller scales. The involved scales (volume, time, dimensions) and scale-associated phenomena require attention to details that may not be considered when performing freezing at the milliliter scale. These concerns include minimizing convection in the liquid phase, minimizing cryoconcentration effects, and controlling dendritic ice growth. Another consideration is to make the freezing and thawing processes rapid enough to prevent any potential product deterioration and to make the operating time reasonable from a manufacturing point of view.

There are several design considerations for the monitoring and control of the freezing process. Ideally, process control should be performed by a temperature sensor that measures the warmest point in the vessel to provide direct determination that freezing has been completed. If the freeze-thaw vessel is designed in such a way that the warmest area is at the top of the freezing bulk, then an infrared temperature sensor may be implemented. Since batch sizes vary, the infrared beam offers the advantage of being able to accommodate a range of liquid volumes in the vessel. If a temperature sensor cannot be located at the warmest point in the vessel, a welded, sidewall thermowell, used commonly in portable tanks, may be implemented for measuring the temperature of the bulk. The thermowell may have inserted into it a temperature sensor or thermocouple to monitor the temperature of the bulk during freezing and thawing for recording and control.

One process control approach for freezing completion is to use both, a setpoint temperature at the product thermowell and a time requirement below or at the temperature set point. For example, freezing may be considered complete after –36°C is achieved at the vessel thermowell and after 5 hours have elapsed. The temperature and time setpoint approach makes up for potential performance variations in the refrigeration system and its ability to reach low temperatures at the end of the freezing process. These variations may be caused by moisture in the system or variations in the refrigeration system performance.

Large-Scale Thawing

Forced convection has been utilized during the thawing step in the production-scale system. After initial warming using the heat transfer surfaces (i.e., the vessel jacket and internal heat exchanger), and sufficient liquid volume has formed between the heat transfer surfaces and the frozen mass, the bottom valve is opened and the liquid product is recirculated using a peristaltic pump through sterilized silicone tubing. The liquid is returned to the top of the container and directed against the frozen mass in a pattern, which allows local melting by a moving stream of liquid. This approach not only accelerates melting (as a result of the liquid stream contacting the frozen mass), but also significantly increases convection in the liquid phase and, therefore, improves heat transfer from the heat transfer surfaces to the melting solid-liquid interface.

The effectiveness of such an approach has been tested by thawing with and without liquid recirculation; liquid recirculation has proven to increase the thawing rate significantly. For example, the thawing time for 100 L of a frozen aqueous solution initially at −25°C was shortened from 22 hours without liquid recirculation to 8 hours with liquid recirculation in a specially designed vessel with heat transfer surfaces maintained at 25°C.

Experimental work and subsequent optimization of the thawing step has been done with consideration of the maximum temperature to which product can be exposed. The monitoring and control of temperature deviations from the set point for the heat transfer fluid was a critical factor of system performance.

The optimization of the thawing process included determination of the time when product recirculation can begin. Liquid phase recirculation can be initiated after the heat is applied to the heat transfer surfaces and when enough liquid forms to permit opening of the bottom valve and filling the recirculation system. Disappearance of frozen mass from thawed liquid at different initial volumes was also investigated.

A concept for controlling the flow of heat transfer agent into the vessel's jacket and heat exchanger depending on the temperature pattern measured in the thermowell was developed. Initially, the thermowell was embedded in a frozen mass and the measured temperatures were below 0°C. When the thermowell was submerged in the liquid phase and the remaining frozen mass was relatively large, liquid temperatures were steady and remained near 0°C. The presence of frozen mass maintains the liquid temperature at low levels (below the heat transfer agent temperature); early in the thawing process the energy delivered through the heat transfer surfaces is used for the latent heat of melting without significant heating of the liquid phase. An increase in liquid temperature and a subsequent temperature trend towards the level of heat transfer agent indicates diminishing and final disappearance of the frozen mass.

The thawing times were established for various product volumes. Recirculation at a slow rate during thawing also provided a gentle method for maintaining product homogeneity, prevented the product from becoming overconcentrated, and decreased the possibility of aggregation or precipitation. Experiments have shown that product thawed without recirculation is more concentrated at the bottom of the vessel.

FORMULATION ISSUES ASSOCIATED WITH LARGE–SCALE FREEZE–THAW

Freezing behavior of simple formulations using limited amounts of well-known compounds may be predicted using published phase diagrams (Cocks and Brower 1974). However, the formulations used for biopharmaceutical products may be complex, including a large variety of compounds. Needed physical data might not have been published for certain substances. Therefore, one may anticipate that experimental work will be required to determine the formulation behavior during the processes of freezing and thawing.

If bulk freezing is planned to be a part of the manufacturing process from the outset of formulation development, the formulation components should be appropriately selected. Operational parameters of the freezing and thawing processing steps depend not only on the characteristics of the product molecule, but also on the characteristics of the solute molecules that make up its formulation. Stabilizing additives such as sugars, certain salts, amino acids, or polyols, may be added to the formulation (Carpenter et al. 1991; Tamiya et al. 1985). Some enzymes (e.g., phosphofructokinase) may lose activity after a freezing and thawing cycle if performed without protective additives. A good review of solvent-protein interactions in pharmaceutical formulations, which also addresses the effects of freeze-thaw on proteins, was published by Arakawa et al. (1991).

There are three potential pitfalls of formulation behavior during the freezing and thawing steps:

1. The possibility of cryoconcentration of small molecules

2. The adverse effects of potentially high concentrations on the product molecules

3. Precipitation of the product or the formulation components

Therefore, a process development approach should be undertaken to reduce possible problems caused by the presence of formulation compounds at significantly varying concentrations. Freezing and thawing steps can be performed in small volumes with precise temperature monitoring to determine eutectic and transitional points. The next step may involve scale-up into a pilot-scale vessel similar in design to the production vessel. After freezing, the frozen bulk may be cut into sections and these sections analyzed to determine the distribution of solutes.

In general, development of formulations that provide stability of the product at higher temperatures is preferable (for example, -20°C is preferred rather than -70°C). Storage temperature of the frozen product may depend on whether the protein requires storage below or above the eutectic temperature or below the glass transition point of proteins at the temperature range between -65°C (More et al. 1995) and -80°C (Chang and Randall 1992). Below this transition temperature the molecular mobility of the protein almost ceases (Steinbach and Brooks 1994).

In the early stages of process development, it may be desirable to concentrate the protein as much as possible at the bulk storage step in an effort to minimize the freeze-thaw vessel capacity requirements. Product can be thawed, a portion can be removed for dilution, and the bulk can be refrozen. Holding product concentrated at this frozen storage step also lends flexibility in the product inventory if there is more than one dosage form, allowing the manufacture of different formulations or protein concentrations to be produced from the same bulk.

When considering frozen storage temperatures of bulk product on the large scale, it may not be necessary, or practical, to freeze the bulk product to temperatures below the eutectic temperature to achieve adequate product stability for the storage periods required for manufacturing. Biologicals are commonly stored at –70°C or lower in the laboratory during product development; however, these materials may be stable at –20°C. DiMagno et al. (1989) from the Mayo Clinic has examined the stability of various blood proteins at –20°C and –70°C over a 10-year period. It was reported that many proteins in blood demonstrate stability at –20°C.

There are several advantages in handling frozen bulk materials at the production scale at –20°C as opposed to –70°C. The storage of multiple vessels in large walk-in freezers is more desirable at –20°C than at –70°C for operational logistics. Also, if the product requires shipment to a second site for further processing, product shipment in air cargo containers is more easily managed at higher temperatures.

A typical approach in formulation development is to consider product stability in liquid or lyophilized forms, but not taking into account transitional steps involved in storage or handling. However, transitional steps may involve transporting product in liquid form in large containers with a possibility of foaming or product oxidation. The approach involving freezing and thawing of bulk material eliminates the foaming problem as well as minimizes product degradation by oxidation or proteases.

HEAT AND MASS TRANSFER

The freezing process is generally applied to biopharmaceutical formulations that are low concentration aqueous solutions. Governing principles applied to the freezing process are those of a general solidification problem (Huppert 1990; Kurz and Fisher 1989; Tiller 1991). The first step in the development process is to determine whether a phase diagram is available for the excipient formulation (e.g., without the protein) (Cocks and Brower 1974; Taylor 1987, 3–71). If phase diagrams are not available, it is advisable to conduct a series of experiments to determine the compositions and to estimate eutectic temperatures as well as formation of glassy states. Energy changes during freezing and thawing for the formulation of interest may be estimated by differential scanning calorimetry. Assuming that the product formulation is aqueous, preliminary heat transfer calculations based on water alone can be adequate since pure water has a relatively high latent heat capacity (334.8 J/g). This assumption will provide a good estimate for heat and mass transfer calculations.

After cooling the liquid to the temperature of solidification (near 0°C for aqueous solutions), solidification involves a phase change at the solid-liquid interface and a subsequent cooling of the solidified material. The heat to be removed is the heat of phase change:

$$H_m = m \times h_m$$

where H_m is total heat of phase change, m is solidifying mass, and h_m is latent heat. The heat of cooling of the frozen mass is

$$H = m \times C_p \times (T_m - T_1)$$

where H is heat of temperature change, C_p is specific heat of solid, T_m is temperature of solidification/melting, T_1 is final temperature to cool mass m $(T_1 < T_m)$.

Heat is removed through the cooling wall with a heat transfer agent, and the traditional equations for forced convection heat transfer should be applied. The heat transfer is complicated since the liquid-solid interface moves and the layer of heat conducting solid material increases. Therefore, the temperature profile of the solidified layer changes continuously. Classical approaches to unsteady heat transfer/heat conduction must be modified to include movement of the solid-liquid interface and to take into account the phase change latent heat occurring at the interface during solidification or melting.

In addition to the moving boundary and latent heat change at the surface, the liquid phase includes density difference-based natural convection effects, caused mostly by temperature, but also by composition differences. Contemporary investigations and modeling of solidification and melting involving convection and diffusion processes use the following assumptions:

- Parabolic heat transfer equation is used (Fourier law).

- Phase change of pure substances at the solid-liquid interface uses Stefan's conditions and models of the dendritic ice or mushy region are employed for multisolute liquids.

- Natural convection in the liquid phase is described by Navier-Stokes equations with Bussinesq laminar flow approach.

- Flows in the mushy or dendritic regions are modeled as flows in simplified porous media.

All of these problems are strongly nonlinear. The equations describing heat and mass transfer processes during the phase change are based on laws of conservation of momentum and mass and energy, and are written for solid and liquid phases (Fukusako and Seki 1987; Samarskii et al. 1993).

The volumetric solidification process itself could be approached in macroscopic terms using the Stefan approach (Carlslaw and Jaeger 1959; Grigull and Sandner 1984). The model is called a moving boundary problem (Crank 1984). This can be a first approximation, providing means for calculation of times of solidification for simple geometries. The quasi-steady state approximations can provide freezing times for aqueous or water-containing products with an error in the range of 4–8 percent (Grigull and Sandner 1984). In addition, there is difficulty with handling the solid-liquid boundary since there is a latent heat of phase change involved in addition to a boundary movement (Crank 1984). More accurate calculations involve numerical methods, such as finite difference (Crank 1984; Crowley 1978; Rostami et al. 1992) and finite elements analysis (Cleland et al. 1984; Johnson 1987; Sutanto et al. 1992). The most popular are the finite difference methods (Crank 1984, 1985; Smith 1985).

Actual solidification and melting phenomena are more complicated than described by these computational approaches, which assume that the moving solid-liquid boundary is flat. During actual freezing and thawing processes, convectional phenomena in the liquid phase occur due to liquid density differences, which result from temperature gradients (Nishimura et al. 1994). This temperature-induced liquid circulation deforms the solid-liquid interface, producing a curvilinear surface. Experimental work by many authors (Christenson and Incropera 1989, Viskanta 1985, 845–877; Zhang and Bejan 1990) showed that for vertical heat transfer surfaces, natural convection during freezing may cause thickening of the solidified layer at the bottom due to the descending stream of liquid along the solidified surface. As this liquid stream descends, it cools until it reaches a point of solidification.

During thawing, natural convection causes the liquid to rise along the heat transfer surface, therefore, the warmest liquid is at the top, resulting in thinning of the solid material there. As a result, in both freezing and thawing processes, one may expect a thicker layer of solid material at the bottom. Figures 2.6 and 2.7 illustrate the above phenomena during freezing and thawing.

Contemporary numerical approaches to the solidification and melting phenomena take into account the effects of natural convection in the liquid phase and the formation of the curvilinear solid-liquid interface (Bennon and Incropera 1988; Christenson et al. 1989).

A discussion of detailed convectional and heat transfer problems in the liquid phase during the simultaneous phase change phenomena is beyond the scope of this chapter and the reader should refer to works of Lacroix (1992); Nishimura et al. (1994); Samarskii et al. (1993); Zabaras and Nguyen (1995).

Figure 2.6. Freezing at a vertical heat transfer surface.

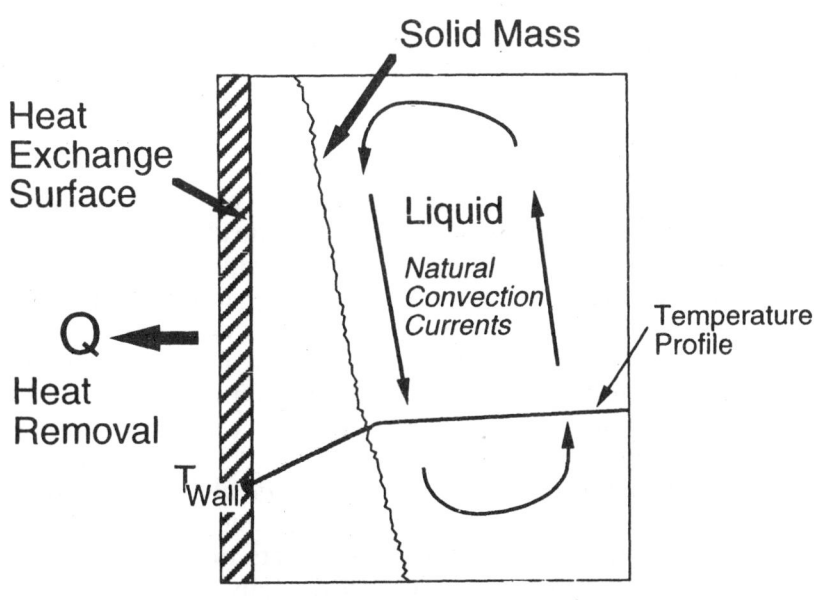

Figure 2.7. Thawing at a vertical heat transfer surface.

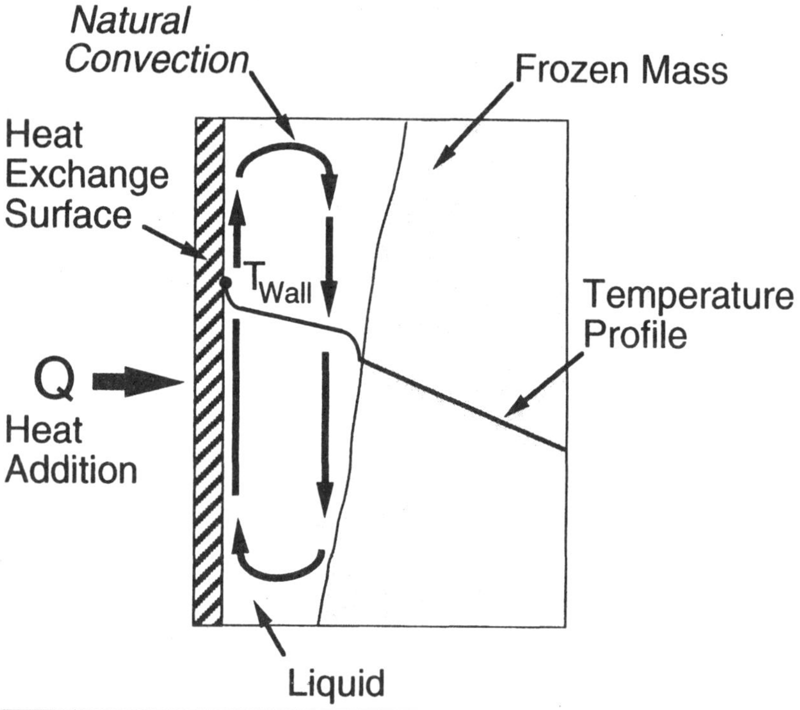

VESSEL DESIGN

The design of the container used to perform controlled freezing and thawing of protein solutions is the most critical part of the system design process. The container should provide adequate product containment during filling, freezing, handling, thawing, and product transfer procedures. The vessel design must also prevent product contamination by the heat transfer fluid. The freezing and thawing processes should occur under conditions that do not promote any physicochemical changes of the solutes, nor cause any loss of biological activity.

The requirements for the process are the ability to freeze large volumes of liquid formulation in a reproducible, rapid, and uniform fashion without causing detrimental effects on the product. The goal is to produce a frozen mass without any significant zones of increased concentration of product or formulation solutes that may be detrimental to the stability of the product. Such prerequisites impose stringent requirements on the process design approach.

Freezing in a rigid container requires that the freezing process occurs directionally from the bottom to the top of the liquid volume, so that there are no entrapped liquid volumes that may freeze and expand later, potentially resulting in damage to the vessel.

Freezing and thawing by recirculating heat exchange medium, through the jacket of a portable tank was investigated using a computer model. This method was rejected due to extended freezing and thawing times and the possibility of unwanted cryoconcentration effects. These results suggested adding heat transfer surfaces to the inside of the vessel. An internal heat exchanger with extended surfaces was designed. The internal heat exchanger design must be reliable and must take into account forces acting upon it during freezing (i.e., the heat exchanger must be designed to withstand structural stress during the freezing process). Due to the presence of the free liquid surface at the top of the vessel, the volumetric expansion of the freezing mass should be directed toward the head space (i.e., the vessel contents should be frozen from the bottom towards the top of the vessel). This can be accomplished by a jacketed vessel with a tapered design (Burton et al. 1995). However, the tapered design significantly increases the cost of the container and increases its size. A cylindrical-shaped vessel with an internal heat exchanger designed to promote the required freezing pattern from the bottom to the top may be the most economical and practical design. Such freezing patterns can be accomplished by providing larger heat transfer surface areas in the lower portion of the vessel. Freezing in the direction from the lower portion of the bulk to the top of the vessel also has the advantage of minimizing molecular stratification effects that result in settling and a high concentration of solutes at the bottom of the vessel, since the lower part solidifies faster.

The internal heat transfer surfaces should be configured to divide the vessel volume into compartments to decrease the freezing and thawing time and to reduce cryoconcentration effects. Compartmentation of the vessel is especially effective for maintaining liquid in a static state to minimize cryoconcentration. Configuring the heat transfer surfaces of the internal heat exchanger allows for control over the heat flow directions and, therefore, influences dendritic ice growth. A jacket that extends to the vessel bottom should be provided, and the vessel must be well insulated with chloride-free insulation. A freeze-thaw vessel design is illustrated in Figure 2.8. The

Figure 2.8. Freeze-thaw vessel shown in thawing mode.

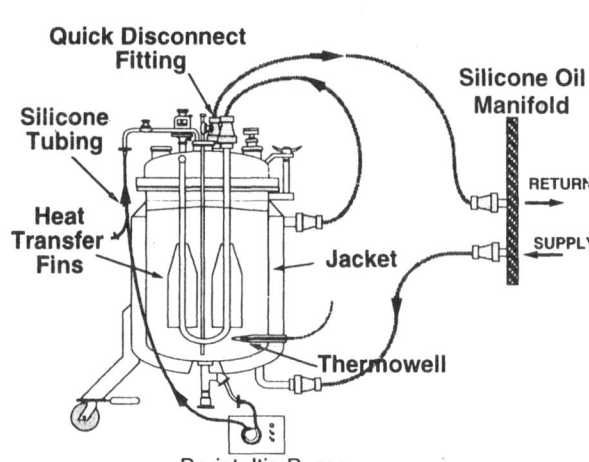

vessel is shown with a peristaltic pump that is used for recirculation of product during the thawing process only.

The internal heat exchanger may be fabricated from a seamless, thick-walled, stainless steel pipe (316L) to eliminate potential leakage from the heat transfer side to the product side. The heat exchanger should be constructed to minimize stress caused by the freezing process by allowing flexibility in its design. The stainless steel pipe may be equipped with multiple-finned, heat transfer surfaces. There are literature references on the behavior of finned heat transfer surfaces applied to phase change systems (Kalhori and Ramadhyani 1986). The finned heat transfer surfaces perform well under conditions where heat conduction is involved through the fin and through the solidified mass around the fin. The heat conduction coefficient through the fin material should be much higher than through the solidified mass. This principle can be applied to the freeze-thaw vessel design, since the thermal conductivity of stainless steel is higher than ice. The thermal conductivity of stainless steel is 15 W/m°K and the thermal conductivity of ice is 2.25 W/m°K. In comparison, copper has a thermal conductivity of 372 W/m°K (Grigull and Sandner 1984). The fin thickness may be optimized and change with distance, but for practical purposes, the fin can have a uniform thickness. Optimized thickness of the well-performing fin depends on the material used and the fin width.

The internal heat exchanger should be designed in a configuration that facilitates efficient CIP and SIP procedures. The design should have smooth vertical surfaces and no crevices, which facilitates sprayball coverage and cleaning. Multiple CIP spray devices may be required for the vessel to provide efficient cleaning of the internal heat exchange surfaces. To facilitate cleaning and inspection, the internal surfaces of the vessel including the internal heat exchanger surfaces may be polished to 240–320 grit (Ra = 0.4–0.25 μm) and electropolished to provide a mirror finish. The vessel must be pressure rated to withstand steam sterilization pressures and temperatures and must be rated for full vacuum.

The temperature sensor that monitors temperature during the freezing and thawing processes may be located in a thermowell located in a fixed position on the sidewall of the vessel. The thermowell position should be selected to provide representative temperature readings for varying liquid volumes in the vessel. The vessel thermowell length and wall thickness should be optimized when considering heat conduction. Ideally, the temperature sensor should be located at the warmest point in the vessel.

For those vessels that are to be shipped after freezing the product, an additional design constraint for the vessel is its ability to fit into a shipping container. The dimensions of the vessel may be restricted by available air cargo space. The shipping container should be well insulated thermally and capable of maintaining low temperature. Dry ice blocks are commonly used for maintaining the temperature of the frozen bulk in the shipping container. The vessel may be designed with eyebolts or special supports to fasten it to the shipping container.

FREEZE–THAW REFRIGERATION SYSTEM

Design

Systems designed for freezing and for thawing may be constructed as a single system, or separate units for freezing and thawing can be designed, depending on the application. The systems can be designed for freezing and thawing in single or multiple vessels, depending on production schedule requirements and batch sizes.

The major components of a freeze-thaw system include a heat exchange medium reservoir, a recirculation pump, a refrigeration system, heat exchangers, a heater, filters, and instrumentation. Components may be assembled on a structural frame with supply and return piping connected to a manifold, with quick disconnect fittings for attachment of the vessel(s).

Figure 2.9 shows a freeze-thaw system design capable of providing recirculated heat exchange medium at controlled temperatures to the vessel jackets and internal heat transfer surfaces of 1–4 vessels. A mechanical refrigeration system cools recirculated heat exchange medium to temperatures in the range of –40°C to –50°C during the freezing process. A heater, utilized in conjunction with the refrigeration system, allows recirculated heat exchange medium supplied to the vessels to be maintained at approximately 25°C during the thawing process.

Heat Exchange Media

In order to process the product in the freeze-thaw vessel, heat exchange fluid must be supplied to the vessel and recirculated. During the freezing and thawing processes, heat exchange fluid is provided at controlled temperatures to the vessel jacket and internal heat

Figure 2.9. A freeze-thaw system capable of freezing and thawing multiple vessels is illustrated in the thaw mode.

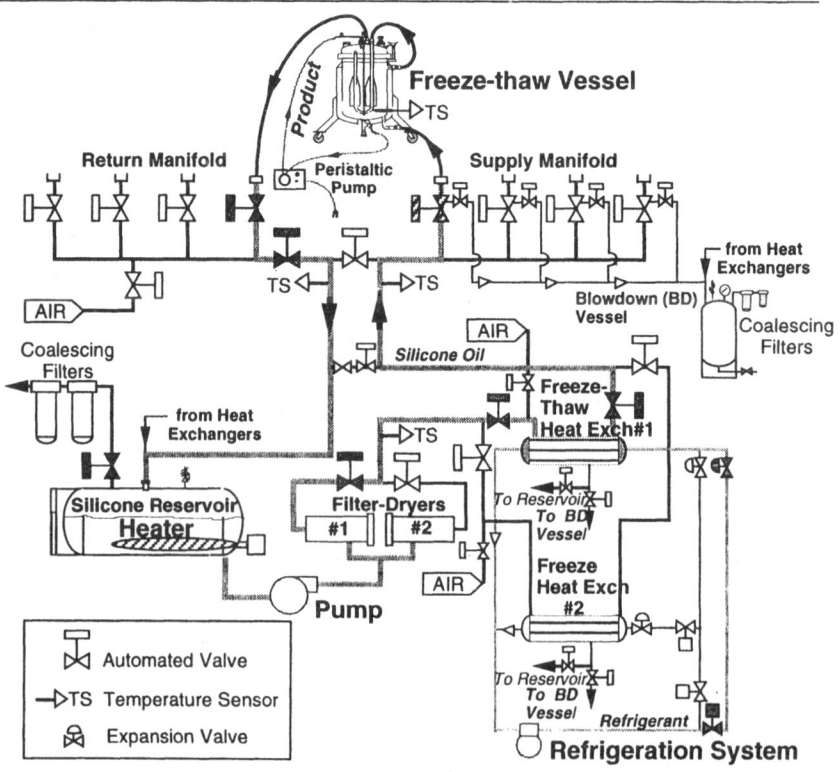

exchanger. The heat exchange fluid must have certain characteristics at low and elevated temperatures for the freezing and thawing operations. It should be nontoxic, have a very low freezing point, and low viscosity at low temperatures. The viscosity at the lowest required process temperatures should allow efficient pumping and fluid recirculation. Its thermal properties should assure sufficient heat transfer coefficients in the tank jacket, the internal heat exchanger, and the evaporator of the refrigeration system. During the thawing process the heat transfer medium is heated; therefore, it should not evaporate or degrade during heating. It should also be nonflammable, noncorrosive, and compatible with stainless steel (chloride-free).

A nonflammable, low viscosity, silicone fluid was determined to be suitable due to its thermal and physical characteristics and acceptability in the pharmaceutical manufacturing environment. For example, Dow 200 Fluid® with 5 cSt viscosity can achieve approximately -60°C, and its boiling point is still high enough for heating during thawing. The recommended upper operating temperature limit for 5 cSt Dow 200 Fluid® is 65°C due to its flammability temperature limit. Although lower viscosity silicone fluids are preferable for pumping, these fluids have lower flammability temperature limits.

Managing Moisture in the System

Protecting the system against entry of moisture and the formation of ice is a concern. The reservoir holding the fluid should be equipped with a vent that includes a cartridge with a dessicating agent.

Moisture in the heat transfer medium can create operational problems, including ice buildup on the evaporator tubes. A moisture trap should be installed in the system, such as dessicant-type filter-dryer cores. A multiple filter-dryer design is recommended to allow an undisturbed system performance in the event that filter dryers must be changed during the operation. There is also a possibility of ice crystal formation in the filter-dryer cores (Ozawa and Kinosita 1989) due to a laminar parallel flow in the pores. A dual filter-dryer system allows switching from one set of filters to the other when a certain pressure differential limit across the filters is achieved.

If water is present in the heat transfer fluid, it will freeze first at the lowest temperature area and where the heat exchange fluid velocity is the lowest. Such an area for ice buildup is the refrigerant evaporator, with the lowest temperature in the recirculation loop and where the heat transfer fluid velocity is low since it flows outside the heat exchanger tubes on the shell side. Any frozen water within the heat exchanger will lower its thermal performance due to the insulating effect of ice.

A solution to managing ice buildup on the heat exchanger tubes and to allow low temperatures to be achieved at the end of the freezing cycle is to provide two heat exchangers. The first heat exchanger may be run for a specified time period; if any water is present in the heat transfer agent, ice may build up on its tubes. The system then automatically switches to a second heat exchanger, which is free of ice, and completes the freezing process run. To remove ice from the heat exchanger tubes after freezing, the heat exchangers can be provided with a silicone oil blowdown by purging with dry compressed air to the reservoir.

Additional precautions should be undertaken to prevent water from entering the freeze-thaw vessel jacket and heat exchanger prior to the attachment to the heat transfer recirculation loop, including blowing down the freezing vessel jacket and internal heat exchanger with dry compressed air prior to beginning the freezing process. Standard operating procedures should not allow the use of steam or cooling water in the vessel jacket or internal heat exchanger during SIP procedures.

Mechanical Refrigeration Systems

The refrigeration requirements to freeze a bulk vessel are the highest at the beginning of the process when the heat loads are highest. The temperature of the heat transfer fluid gradually decreases as the thickness of the layer of the frozen material increases. As the freezing progresses, the load decreases; the heat exchange fluid temperature drops and stabilizes at the lowest achievable temperature of the selected refrigerant. During the freezing process the refrigeration system may run at its maximum capacity to achieve its lowest temperatures. For special applications (e.g., for validation purposes, to provide a worst-case freezing cycle) a higher than usual silicone oil temperature may be used for the freezing process by providing a special freezing validation cycle that controls the silicone temperature by utilizing the heater in conjunction with the refrigeration system.

After the heat loads and the lowest required temperature of the heat transfer agent are established, the subsequent step is a selection of an adequate refrigerant, and determination of heat exchange equipment and compressor size. Selection of the expansion valve for the refrigerant line is very important. The valve performance determines the overall performance of the heat exchanger-cooler for the recirculating heat transfer fluid. Due to changing loads, the operational range of the expansion valve should accommodate a wide range of refrigerant flow rates.

There are several points to consider in the design of the refrigeration system:

- Since the load on the refrigeration system varies significantly, and there is a prolonged period of operation at a very low load at the end of the freezing cycle, selection of the evaporator expansion valve is particularly important to avoid evaporator flooding at low loads.

- A synthetic lubricating oil for the compressor that performs well for prolonged work and at low temperature should be selected over hydrocarbon oils that may degrade. The lubricating oil must be compatible with the refrigerant, since there is mixing of lubricant and refrigerant in the compressor cylinder.

- The condenser should be cooled with refrigerated water or glycol to keep the temperature of the condensed refrigerant as low as possible. To aid in the fine-tuning of the refrigeration system, thermocouples may be attached to the refrigerant piping at critical points in the system to monitor the refrigeration system performance. These temperature readings can become a part of an overall system control and diagnostic scheme.

- The design of the refrigerant evaporator should ensure turbulent, high velocity flow of heat transfer medium around the bundle of evaporator tubes.

- The heater used to heat the heat transfer medium during the thawing process can be on a separate branch of the piping, or it can be installed in the heat transfer fluid reservoir. Attention should be paid to the specification of the surface temperature of the heater elements to prevent local overheating of the silicone fluid at the heater surfaces.

- To maintain temperature control of the heat transfer fluid during thawing, cooling is required to prevent overheating of the heat transfer fluid. The same refrigeration unit used for the freezing operation may be used for cooling during the thawing process by utilizing a second smaller expansion valve for the evaporator. Alternatively, a separate, smaller refrigeration system may be used to provide cooling or a chilled glycol system can be used.

- The heat transfer agent recirculating pump should have a seal-less design to prevent any fluid leaks. The pump design also should ensure that a minimum amount of heat from the pump is added to the fluid. Heat might be added by conduction from the motor through the pump body. It is also generated internally due to inherent characteristics of any centrifugal pump (since its operational efficiency is less than 100 percent). A pump with optimal characteristics should be chosen, considering the change in the heat transfer agent viscosity (Lobanoff and Ross 1986). A magnetically coupled pump is a better choice than a canned pump, since less heat will be added from the motor to the recirculating fluid.

Compressor-based refrigeration systems, when used in the freeze-thaw system design, generally offer high reliability and predictability. The earlier designs were based on R502, R13B, and R12 refrigerants. Current designs are based on more environmentally acceptable agents, such as Dupont Suva HP62®.

Mechanical refrigeration systems used to cool the heat transfer medium have limits regarding the lowest achievable temperatures, depending on the refrigerant used and the design principle. For instance, refrigerant R502 allows temperatures in the evaporator to reach a level as low as –53 to –55°C; the refrigerant R13B may achieve about –65 to –67°C with a two-stage compressor (Hamm 1986, 8.15–8.17). If very low temperature applications are required, a cascade refrigeration design may be considered, or the heat transfer fluid may be cooled using liquefied gases.

Further details on freeze-thaw system design can be found in the authors' earlier publication (Wisniewski and Wu 1992).

Instrumentation and Controls

There are two main functions of the freeze-thaw system instrumentation and controls:

1. To ensure temperature control of heat transfer fluid during the freezing and the thawing processes (including preprogrammed temperature profiles).

2. To monitor and control the freeze-thaw processes in individual vessels. The number of vessels and the loads of individual vessels may vary.

A traditional, process control approach can be taken that utilizes proportional, integral, and derivative control for maintaining heat exchange medium temperatures during thawing that utilizes a heater and a cooling system. Freezing may allow a refrigeration system to run at its maximum to permit maximal cooling of heat exchange medium. In addition to standard controls (for the heat transfer fluid loop and for the refrigeration system), multiple thermocouples may be located on the piping of both refrigeration and heat transfer loop systems, permitting monitoring, diagnosis, and optimization of the system performance. Critical points on the refrigerant loop to monitor temperatures are as follows: after the compressor, after the condenser, after the expansion valve, after the evaporator/heat exchanger, and on the inlet to the compressor. The heat transfer fluid temperatures are monitored at locations before and after the heat exchanger, after the recirculating pump, and in the reservoir. The presence of a flowmeter on the heat transfer fluid recirculating loop allows system performance monitoring and calculation of thermal and mass balances.

Monitoring and control of product temperature in the vessels poses a significant challenge to the design of the control system, if there is a need to accommodate freezing or thawing multiple vessels that may contain varying liquid volumes. Temperature sensors in each vessel can be used to make such control possible. During thawing the flow of heat transfer fluid to individual vessels can be controlled according to the temperature of each vessel. Freezing and thawing completion can be based on temperature and time set points established for the maximum liquid volume capacity of the vessel, since liquid volumes less than the maximum will be frozen or thawed within the time frame required for the maximum liquid volume (see also "Large-Scale Freezing and Thawing of Biopharmaceuticals").

The control system may be based on a combination of individual controllers/recorders and programmable logic controllers (PLCs), or can be fully computerized. Various process control approaches may be taken with satisfactory results since the process dynamics are relatively slow. The computerized process control offers the advantages of flexibility and ease of data recording and analysis. Process development results may readily be implemented into manufacturing processes. Computerized control also may be used for system performance diagnostics, by applying data analysis, and trend monitoring of system temperature profiles.

Liquefied Gas Refrigeration Systems

An alternative to mechanical refrigeration is a liquefied gas-based cooling system for the heat transfer agent recirculation loop. Liquid nitrogen is commonly used for biological freezing applications. Liquid nitrogen has a boiling point of 77.4 K (-195.6°C). Advantages of a liquefied gas system are its design simplicity, flexibility in temperature control, and its ability to achieve very low temperatures. An evaporative cryogenic heat exchanger with injection of liquid nitrogen controlled by a cryogenic metering valve can be coupled with a computer or PLC–based temperature control loop. This heat exchanger is placed in the heat transfer agent recirculating loop. A cryogenic shell-and-tube-type heat exchanger with tubes having internal fins is preferred due to its extensive heat transfer area. The heat transfer agent flows through the shell space, while the liquid nitrogen is injected into the tubes and evaporates on finned surfaces. The temperature of the heat transfer agent may be rapidly lowered to the desired low level, or a gradual temperature decrease may be programmed. The cold gas formed by evaporation of liquid nitrogen may be vented outside, passing on its way through heat recovery coils. The amount of liquid nitrogen used for cooling can be controlled so that it can follow the actual process load, which declines as freezing progresses.

A recirculating heat transfer agent system needs only a heat exchanger with controls and an electric heater with temperature control for thawing. A small metering valve for liquid nitrogen injection into the heat exchanger may be used as a device to control the heat transfer agent temperature during thawing to prevent overheating.

The system can operate using portable Dewar tanks or a permanent cryogenic tank to store the liquid nitrogen. The connecting piping lengths should be minimized when designing the system, to reduce heat gains. Adequate thermal insulation is needed to minimize heat gains, to provide frostbite protection, and to eliminate condensation of water and a possibility of formation of liquid oxygen on locally exposed surfaces (the boiling point of oxygen is 90.2 K). Such condensation of liquid oxygen may present an explosion or fire hazard. Insulation used in cryogenic systems can be categorized as rigid foam, vacuum jacketed, evacuated powder (perlite), and multilayer evacuated aluminized Mylar®.

Capital expenditures for a liquid nitrogen system can be kept low if cryogenic nitrogen transfer piping length is minimized by locating the bulk nitrogen source close to the system. A major operating expense is the cost of liquid nitrogen.

The decision on system selection should also include considerations of the safety aspects associated with handling liquefied gases. These precautions include the need for proper ventilation and the use of oxygen sensors to prevent suffocation in the mechanical area in the event of nitrogen gas leakage.

PRODUCT STORAGE AND SHIPPING

Handling product prior to freezing, in the frozen state, and after thawing requires special considerations. The product storage time prior to freezing should be as short as possible; cold storage is preferred during this period.

Adequate freezer space should be provided for the storage of frozen product for several months or years. Pallets may be designed for forklift handling of the vessels containing frozen bulk, or forklift supports may be incorporated into the design of the vessels.

Shipping of the frozen product requires the design of special containers that provide a low temperature environment for a sufficient time period. The shipping container requires a support structure to secure the vessel to the container floor, a ramp for rolling the vessel into the container and temperature recording devices. Insulated containers with a compartment to store adequate amounts of solid carbon dioxide blocks are available for shipping purposes. The containers are built on a pallet frame with forklift provisions and are designed to fit into air cargo storage areas and into trucks. Figure 2.10 shows a freeze-thaw vessel in an air cargo shipping container with dry ice blocks.

Cold room storage located near the formulations area should be designed to accommodate several vessels that will require storage after thawing and prior to aliquoting or pooling.

PRODUCT RELEASE AND SAMPLING

The product is sterile filtered into the freezing vessel prior to freezing and samples of the product are taken prior to the freezing step. A bioburden sample and a protein concentration sample may be taken after the filtration step. Other samples can be frozen and

Figure 2.10. Configuration of a freeze-thaw vessel in an air cargo shipping container with dry ice blocks.

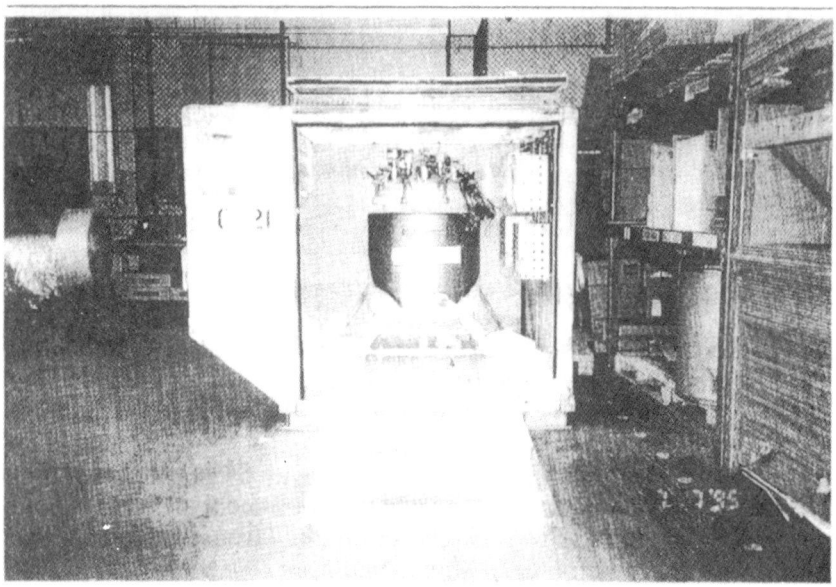

stored with the frozen bulk and can be used for product identity testing. After completing the thawing process, bioburden and protein samples should be taken to assure sterility has been maintained and to confirm that the thawed product is homogeneous.

STABILITY CONSIDERATIONS

The effect of the freeze-thaw process on the protein product and its effect on the stability of the protein after prolonged storage periods must be examined. It is often desirable to qualify the product for multiple freeze-thaw cycles so that the product may be thawed, aliquotted, and refrozen multiple times. During freeze-thaw development it is desirable to conduct multiple freeze-thaw cycles to exaggerate the effects of freeze-thaw on the product and to identify product attributes that may fail to meet specifications. Protein product subjected to multiple freeze-thaw cycles should be assayed after each freeze-thaw cycle for activity, pH, aggregation, deamidation, clarity/color and appearance, protein concentration, and oxidation.

The concept of the freeze-thaw processing steps should be included as early as possible in the production scheme development and the process should be incorporated into the final product stability testing program. Product that has been subjected to single and multiple freeze-thaw cycles can be compared to bulks that have not been frozen.

By conducting stability fills over a period of time, expiration dating of the frozen bulk product may be extended. For example, the bulk product may be frozen, held for many months, and then thawed. An aliquot may be taken from the thawed bulk, which is then diluted and filled. The filled product can then be placed on a stability program. The production-scale bulk can be frozen and thawed multiple times and sampled at intervals to extend the expiration dating of the bulk product. Hold times should also be established for liquid product storage at 2–8°C (e.g., for product stored prior to freezing and after thawing steps).

Small stainless steel containers (20–50 mL) filled with product may provide a more convenient sampling system for performing stability studies. However, the effect of container size and a possibility of cryoconcentration of solutes should be investigated. For example, if the production scale vessel has different compositions in different parts of the vessel, then the small-scale containers may be filled with product with the same compositions in an effort to simulate large-scale conditions.

VALIDATION OF THE FREEZING AND THAWING PROCESSES

Temperature monitoring surveys must be performed to test minimum and maximum thermal loads during the freezing and thawing processes. If the system is designed for freezing and thawing multiple vessels, then the system should be tested with the minimum and maximum number of vessels and with the minimum and maximum liquid volumes in the vessels. Reproducibility of the processes should be confirmed by multiple test runs.

Routine validation procedures are applicable to freeze-thaw systems including installation qualification, operational qualification, and performance qualification (Carleton and Agalloco 1986). The control systems may require particular attention, and validation should be conducted according to generally accepted guidelines (Akers et al. 1994a,b; McEntire 1994). Implementation of computerized systems involves validation of the computer system for both hardware and software (Grigonis and Wyrick 1994).

Freezing Validation

Freezing validation involves the verification that the bulk product achieves a desired setpoint temperature at its warmest point. Due to varying distances to heat transfer surfaces, the temperature at different points in the vessel may vary. For large-scale systems, such as those that have been described, temperature surveys indicate that the warmest point in the solution is at the top (center) of the frozen mass. The bottom of the vessel is the coldest area, since the solid-liquid freezing front moves from the bottom toward the top of the vessel.

A temperature set point may be established for the thermowell temperature based on a corresponding temperature with a thermocouple placed at the warmest point in the vessel (i.e., top center) during the validation run. The criteria of meeting both the thermowell temperature and the time for completing freezing may be validated by monitoring the warmest point in the vessel with a thermocouple (i.e., placed at the top center of the solution) with the requirement that the bulk be frozen, for example, to –20°C (at its warmest point), upon meeting the vessel thermowell temperature and time parameters.

Figure 2.11 illustrates temperature profiles for freezing 120 L of r-tPA formulation buffer to –20°C in a freeze vessel. The heat transfer medium temperature decreases rapidly in the beginning and decreases slowly as the bulk temperature decreases. At the vessel thermowell: (a) product is cooled to near 0°C, (b) the thermowell is exposed to liquid product as latent heat is removed, (c) the thermowell is exposed to solid product. Product temperature at the warmest point is at the top center of the bulk. Also shown is the performance of a two-stage refrigeration system using R502 refrigerant without a freezing load.

Thawing Validation

Validation of the thawing process should consider a maximum product temperature limit. Multiple thermocouples may be placed axially and radially in the vessel, at the vessel thermowell, and at the warmest point in the vessel. Visual verification of the absence of ice at the end of the thawing cycle is required, since temperature monitoring alone will not be suitable to detect small diminishing ice masses.

Figure 2.11. Temperature profiles for freezing 120 L of r-tPA formulation buffer to –22°C in a freeze vessel.

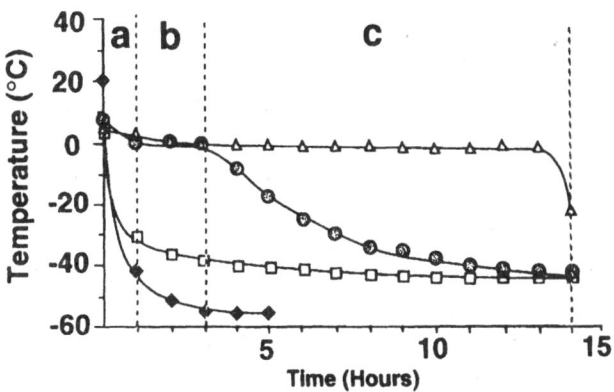

□ Heat transfer media supply temperature during freezing
◍ Product temperature at vessel thermowell during freezing
△ Product temperature at warmest point during freezing
◆ Heat transfer media supply temperature with no load (cooling)

If a control scheme is used that modulates the flow of heat transfer fluid to the vessel according to the bulk temperature, then this control scheme must be validated. Attention should be paid to the heat transfer fluid supply temperature and system thermal performance under varying loads.

Figure 2.12 illustrates temperature profiles for thawing 120 L of an arginine phosphate formulation buffer by recirculating 25°C silicone oil through the freeze-vessel jacket and internal heat transfer coil. At (a) the thermowell is embedded in the frozen mass, at (b) the thermowell is exposed to liquid product, and at (c) product is recirculated.

SUMMARY

Freezing and thawing bulk product can be an essential step in the manufacture of many biopharmaceuticals. It offers flexibility to the biopharmaceutical manufacturer and plays a key role in the management of multiproduct facilities. The ability to freeze and thaw large quantities of product provides an economical solution to the management of biopharmaceutical bulk production.

Figure 2.12. Temperature profiles for thawing 120 ℓ of arginine phosphate formulation buffer in a freeze vessel.

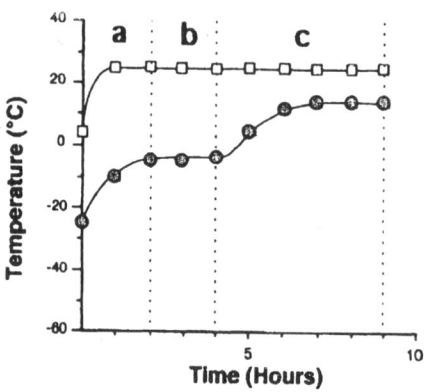

□ Heat transfer media supply temperature during thawing
⊚ Product temperature at tank thermowell during thawing

The use of a portable, jacketed, stainless steel vessel with internal heat transfer surfaces, as described in this chapter, is an approach that has been successful for protein products manufactured at Genentech. Its design is consistent with conventional pharmaceutical manufacturing and current good manufacturing practices.

Freezing and thawing biopharmaceutical product formulations in large volumes involves complex phenomena. Biopharmaceutical formulations contain a variety of solutes, including salt ions, sugars, amino acids, and the protein product. A significant development effort is involved in the design of properly functioning systems that perform without compromising product quality.

Important considerations for the large-scale freezing process includes minimizing freezing time, minimizing convection, promoting dendritic ice growth, minimizing cryoconcentration, avoiding mechanical stresses in the vessel, and providing a sanitary vessel design. A jacketed vessel with an internal heat exchanger design with heat transfer fins is effective for dividing the vessel into compartments, to provide rapid freezing, and to provide directional freezing. Attention should be paid to the methods for monitoring and validation.

Important considerations for the large-scale thawing process include avoiding overheating the product by maintaining tight control of the vessel wall temperature and maximizing convection in the liquid phase. Recirculation of product during thawing is an effective and gentle method that provides forced convection and surface ablation effects that increase the thawing rate and provide mixing.

Research and development requires investigation of a very broad range of problems, which include molecular and microscopic interactions related to formulation, heat and mass transfer, and solving unique issues of mechanical system design. There is only a limited amount of literature that may be directly applied to the problems associated with freezing and thawing protein solutions in large volumes. References, such as those on protein cold denaturation, protein antifreeze activity, and studies on the interaction of small molecules with ice, may provide an indication of the mechanisms that may be involved in the freezing phenomena. Developmental studies for molecular and macroscopic interactions are required for particular protein products and formulations.

ACKNOWLEDGEMENTS

The authors would like to acknowledge Bill Young and Paul Hohenschuh for their continuous support of the freeze-thaw project.

REFERENCES

Agarwal, S., and R. Sohal. 1994. Aging and proteolysis of oxidized proteins. *Arch. Biochem. Biophys.* 309:24–28.

Ahmad, F., and C. Bigelow. 1986. Thermodynamic stability of proteins in salt solutions: A comparison of the effectiveness of protein stabilizers. *J. Protein Chem.* 5:355–367.

Akers, J., J. McEntire, and G. Sofer. 1994a. Biotechnology product validation, part 1: Identifying the pitfalls. *BioPharm* 7 (1):40–44.

Akers, J., J. McEntire, and G. Sofer. 1994b. Biotechnology product validation, part 2: A logical plan. *BioPharm* 7 (2):54–56.

Arakawa, T., and S. Timasheff. 1982a. Stabilization of protein structure by sugars. *Biochemistry* 21:6536–6544.

Arakawa, T., and S. Timasheff. 1982b. Preferential interactions of proteins with salts in concentrated solutions. *Biochemistry* 21: 6545–6552.

Arakawa, T., Y. Kita, and J. Carpenter. 1991. Protein-solvent interactions in pharmaceutical formulations. *Pharm. Res.* 8:285–291.

Avanov, A. 1990. Biological antifreezes and the mechanism of their activity. *Mol. Biol.* 24:473–487.

Azuaga, A. et al. 1992. Heat and cold denaturation of beta-lactoglobulin B. *FEBS Lett.* 309:258–260.

Bareis, M. and H. Beer. 1984. Experimental investigation of melting heat transfer with regard to different geometric arrangements. *Int. Comm. Heat Mass Transfer* 11:323–333.

Bejan, A. 1989. Analysis of melting by natural convection in an enclosure. *Int. J. Heat and Fluid Flow* 10:245–252.

Benard, C., D. Gobin, and F. Martinez. 1985. Melting in rectangular enclosures: Experiments and numerical simulations. *J. Heat Transfer* 107:794–803.

Bennon, W., and F. Incropera. 1988. Numerical analysis of binary solid-liquid phase change using a continuum model. *Num. Heat Transfer* 13:277–296.

Biringer, R., and A. Fink. 1988. Intermediates in the refolding of ribonuclease at subzero temperatures. *Biochemistry* 27:301–311, 311–315, 315–325.

Bordo, D., and P. Argos. 1994. The role of side-chain hydrogen bonds in the formation and stabilization of secondary structure in soluble proteins. *J. Mol. Biol.* 243:504–519.

Branden, C., and J. Tooze. 1991. *Introduction to protein structure.* New York: Garland Publications.

Burton, R. et al. 1995. An experimental investigation of the solidification process in a V-shaped sump. *Int. J. Heat and Mass Transfer* 38:2383–2393.

Carleton, F., and J. Agalloco, eds. 1986. *Validation of aseptic pharmaceutical processes.* New York: Marcel Dekker, Inc.

Carpenter, J., and J. Crowe. 1988. The mechanisms of cryoprotection of proteins by solutes. *Cryobiology* 25:244–255.

Carpenter, J., and T. Hansen. 1992. Antifreeze protein modulates cell survival during cryopreservation: Mediation through influence on ice crystal growth. *Proc. Natl. Acad. Sci. USA* 89:8953–8957.

Carpenter, J., T. Arakawa, and J. Crowe. 1991. Interactions of stabilizing additives with proteins during freeze-thawing and freeze-drying. *Dev. Biol. Standard.* 74:225–239.

Carlslaw, H., and J. Jaeger. 1959. *Conduction of heat in solids.* Oxford: Oxford University Press.

Chakrabartty, A., D. Yang, and C. Hew. 1989. Structure-function relationship in a winter flounder antifreeze polypeptide. *J. Biol. Chem.* 264:11313–11316.

Chang, B., and C. Randall. 1992. Use of subambient thermal analysis to optimize protein lyophilization. *Cryobiology* 29:632–656.

Chen, C. 1992. Viscosity effects on the directional solidification of NH4Cl solution in a Hele-Shaw cell. *Phys. Fluids* 4:1879.

Christenson, M., and F. Incropera. 1989. Solidification of an aqueous ammonium chloride solution in a rectangular cavity I. *Int. J. Heat Mass Transfer* 32:47–68.

Christenson, M., W. Bennon, and F. Incropera. 1989. Solidification of an aqueous ammonium chloride solution in a rectangular cavity II. *Int. J. Heat Mass Transfer* 32:69–79.

Cleland, D. et al. 1984. Prediction of rates of freezing, thawing or cooling in solids of arbitrary shape using the finite element method. *Int. J. Refriger.* 7:6–13.

Cocks, F., and W. Brower. 1974. Phase diagram relationships in cryobiology. *Cryobiology* 11:340–358.

Conway, B. 1981. *Ionic hydration in chemistry and biophysics.* Amsterdam: Elsevier.

Crank, J. 1984. *Free and moving boundary problems.* Oxford: Clarendon Press.

Crank, J. 1985. *The mathematics of diffusion.* Oxford: Clarendon Press.

Creighton, T. 1993. *Proteins: Structures and molecular properties.* New York: W.H. Freeman.

Crowley, A. 1978. Numerical solution of Stefan problems. *Int. J. Heat Mass Transfer* 21:215–219.

Davis, S. 1990. Hydrodynamic interactions in directional solidification. *J. Fluid Mech.* 212:241–262.

DeVries, A. 1984. Role of glycopeptides and peptides in inhibition of crystallization of water in polar fishes. *Phil. Trans. R. Soc. Lond.* B304:575–588.

Dill, K. 1990. Dominant forces in protein folding. *Biochemistry* 29:7133–7155.

Diller, K. 1992. Modeling of bioheat transfer processes at high and low temperatures. *Adv. Heat Transfer* 22:157–357.

DiMagno, E. et al. 1989. Effect of long-term freezer storage, thawing and refreezing on selected constituents of serum. *Mayo Clin. Proc.* 64:1226–1234.

Douzou, P. 1980. Cryoenzymology in aqueous media. *Adv. Enzymol.* 51:1–73.

Eckhardt, B. M., J. Q. Oeswein, and T. A. Bewley. 1991. Effect of freezing on aggregation of human growth hormone. *Pharm. Res.* 8 (11):1360–1364.

Egolf, P., and H. Manz. 1994. Theory and modeling of phase change materials with and without mushy regions. *Int. J. Heat Mass Transfer* 37:2917–2924.

Fennema, O. 1982. Behavior of proteins at low temperatures. In *Food protein deterioration: Mechanisms and functionality*, edited by J. Cherry. Washington, DC: ACS Symposium Series 206:109–133.

Fink, A. 1986. Effect of cryoprotectants on enzyme structure. *Cryobiology* 23:28–37.

Fletcher, N. 1970. *The chemical physics of ice.* London: Cambridge University Press.

Floris, F. et al. 1994. Hydration shell structure of the calcium ion from simulations with ab initio effective pair potentials. *Chem. Phys. Lett.* 227:126–132.

Franks, F., ed. 1982. *Water–a comprehensive treatise,* vol. 7. New York: Plenum Press.

Franks, F. 1993. Solid aqueous solutions. *Pure & Appl. Chem.* 65:2527–2537.

Franks, F. et al. 1988. The thermodynamics of protein stability: Cold destabilization as a general phenomenon. *Biophys. Chem.* 31:307–315.

Fukusako, S. 1990. Thermophysical properties of ice, snow and sea ice. *Intl J. Thermophys.* 11:353–372.

Fukusako, S., and N. Seki. 1987. Fundamental aspects of analytical and numerical methods on freezing and melting heat-transfer problems. *Ann. Rev. Num. Fluid Mech. Heat Transfer* 1:351–402.

Grigonis, G., and M. Wyrick. 1994. Computer system validation: Auditing computer systems for quality. *BioPharm* 7 (7):22–31.

Grigull, U., and H. Sandner. 1984. *Heat conduction.* Washington, DC: Hemisphere Publishing Corporation.

Griko, Y. 1989. Heat and cold denaturation of phosphoglycerate kinase (interaction of domains). *FEBS Lett.* 244:276–278.

Griko, Y., and V. Kutyshenko. 1994. Differences in the processes of beta-lactoglobulin cold and heat denaturations. *Biophys. J.* 67:356–363.

Griko, Y., and P. Privalov. 1992. Calorimetric study of the heat and cold denaturation of beta-lactoglobulin. *Biochemistry* 31:8810–8815.

Hamm, F. A., ed. 1986. *ASHRAE handbook: Refrigeration systems and applications.* Atlanta: American Society of Heating, Refrigeration and Air Conditioning Engineers, Inc.

Hew, C., and D. Yang. 1992. Protein interaction with ice. *Eur. J. Biochem.* 203:33–42.

Holmberg, N., G. Lilius, and L. Bulow. 1994. Artificial antifreeze proteins can improve NaCl tolerance when expressed in *E. coli. FEBS Lett.* 349:354–358.

Huppert, H. 1990. The fluid mechanics of solidification. *J. Fluid Mech.* 212:209–240.

Huyskens, P., W. Luck, and T. Zeegers-Huyskens. 1991. *Intermolecular forces.* Berlin: Springer.

Jeffrey, G., and W. Saenger. 1991. *Hydrogen bonding in biological structures.* Berlin: Springer-Verlag.

Johnson, C. 1987. *Numerical solution of partial differential equations by the finite element method.* Cambridge: Cambridge University Press.

Johnson, C. A., P. Wu, and A. Lenhoff. 1994. Electrostatic and van der Waals contributions to protein adsorption. *Langmuir* 10:3705–3713.

Kalhori, B., and S. Ramadhyani. 1986. Studies on heat transfer from a vertical cylinder, with or without fins, embedded in a solid phase change medium. *J. Heat Transfer* 107:44–51.

Karim, Q., and A. Haymet. 1988. The ice/water interface: A molecular dynamics simulation study. *J. Chem. Phys.* 89:6889–6896.

Koerber, C. 1988. Phenomena at the advancing ice-liquid interface: Solutes, particles and biological cells. *Quart. Rev. Biophys.* 21:229–298.

Koerber, C. et al. 1983. Solute polarization during planar freezing of aqueous solutions. *Int. J. Heat Mass Transfer* 26:1241–1253.

Kuntz, I., and W. Kauzmann. 1974. Hydration of proteins and polypeptides. *Adv. Protein Chem.* 28:239–345.

Kurz, W., and D. Fisher. 1989. *Fundamentals of solidification.* Aedermannsdorf, Switzerland: Trans Tech Publications.

Kyprianidou-Leonidou, T., and G. Botsaris. 1990. Freeze concentration of aqueous solutions. In *Crystallization as separation process,* edited by A. Myerson, and K. Toyokura. Washington, DC: American Chemical Society.

Lacroix, M. 1992. Predictions of natural convection dominated phase change problems by the vorticity-velocity formulation of the Navier-Stokes equation. *Num. Heat Transfer* 22:79–93.

Lobanoff, V., and R. Ross. 1986. *Centrifugal pumps: Design and application.* Houston: Gulf Publications.

Lombrana, J., and J. Diaz. 1987. Solute redistribution during the freezing of aqueous solutions under unstability conditions. *Cryoletters* 8:244–259.

Makhatadze, G., and P. Privalov. 1992. Protein interactions with urea and guanidinum chloride. *J. Mol. Biol.* 226:491–505.

Manning, M. et al. 1989. Stability of protein pharmaceuticals. *Pharm. Res.* 6:903–918.

Mashimo, S., and N. Miura. 1993. High order and local structure of water determined by microwave dielectric study. *J. Chem. Phys.* 99:9874–9881.

Mashimo, S., N. Miura, and T. Umehara. 1992. The structure of water determined by microwave dielectric study on water mixtures with glucose, polysaccharides and L-ascorbic acid. *J. Chem. Phys.* 97:6759–6765.

McEntire, J. 1994. Biotechnology product validation, part 5: Selection and validation of analytical techniques. *BioPharm* 7 (5):68–80.

More, N., R. Caniel, and H. Petach. 1995. The effect of low temperatures on enzyme activity. *Biochem. J.* 305:17–20.

Muecke, M., and F. Schmid. 1994. A kinetic method to evaluate the two-state character of solvent-induced protein denaturation. *Biochemistry* 33:12930–12935.

Murphy, K., and E. Freire. 1992. Thermodynamics of structural stability and cooperative folding behavior in proteins. *Adv. Protein Chem.* 43:313–361.

Nishimura, T. et al. 1994. Occurrence and development of double-diffusive convection during solidification of a binary system. *Int. J. Heat Mass Transfer* 37:1455–1464.

Ozawa, H., and S. Kinosita. 1989. Segregated ice growth on a microporous filter. *J. Colloid Interface Sci.* 132:113–124.

Pace, N., and C. Tanford. 1968. Thermodynamics of the unfolding of beta-lactoglobulin A in aqueous urea solutions between 5 and 55 deg. *Biochemistry* 7:198–208.

Pikal, M. 1990. Freeze-drying of proteins, Part II: Formulation selection. *Biopharm* 9:26–30.

Privalov, P., 1989. Thermodynamic problems of protein structure. *Ann. Rev. Biophys. Chem.* 18:47–69.

Privalov, P. 1990. Cold denaturation of proteins. CRC Critical Review. *Biochem. Mol. Biol.* 25:281–305.

Rostami, A., R. Greif, and R. Russo. 1992. Modified enthalpy method applied to rapid melting and solidification. *Int. J. Heat Mass Transfer* 35:2161–2172.

Rubinsky, B., and T. Eto. 1990. Heat transfer during freezing of biological materials. *Ann. Rev. Heat Transfer* 3:1–38.

Rubinsky, B., C. Lee, and M. Chaw. 1993. Experimental observations and theoretical studies on solidification processes in saline solutions. *Experim. Thermal Fluid Sci.* 6:157–167.

Rupley, J., and G. Careri. 1991. Protein hydration and function. *Adv. Protein Chem.* 41:7–172.

Samarskii, A. et al. 1993. Numerical simulation of convection/diffusion phase change problems–a review. *Int. J. Heat Mass Transfer* 36:4095–4106.

Sartor, G. et al. 1994. Calorimetric studies of the kinetic unfreezing of molecular motions in hydrated lysozyme, hemoglobin and myoglobin. *Biophys. J.* 66:249–258.

Schaff, J., and J. Roberts. 1994. Structure sensitivity in the surface chemistry of ice: Acetone adsorption on amorphous and crystalline ice films. *J. Phys. Chem.* 98:6900–6902.

Shimoyamada, M. et al. 1994. Freezing and eutectic points of an aqueous amino acid solution containing ethanol and the effect of ethanol addition on the freeze concentration process. *Biosci. Biotech. Biochem.* 58:836–838.

Silva, S., and P. Devlin. 1994. Interaction of acetylene, ethylene and benzene with ice. *J. Phys. Chem.* 98:10847–10852.

Smith, G. 1985. *Numerical solution of partial differential equations: Finite difference methods.* Oxford: Clarendon Press.

Spicer, A., ed. 1974. *Advances in preconcentration and dehydration of foods.* London: Applied Science Publications.

Steinbach, P., and B. Brooks. 1994. Protein simulation below the glass-transition temperature: Dependence on cooling protocol. *Chem. Phys. Lett.* 226:447–452.

Stickle, D. et al. 1992. Hydrogen bonding in globular proteins. *J. Mol. Biol.* 226:1143–1159.

Storti, M. 1995. Numerical modeling of ablation phenomena as two-phase Stefan problems. *Int. J. Heat Mass Transfer* 38:2843–2854.

Sutanto, E., T. Davis, and L. Scriven. 1992. Adaptive finite element analysis of axisymmetric freezing. *Int. J. Heat Mass Transfer* 35:3301–3312.

Swedish, M. et al. 1979. Surface ablation in the impingement region of a liquid jet. *AIChE J.* 25:630–636.

Tamiya, T. et al. 1985. Freeze denaturation of enzymes and its prevention with additives. *Cryobiology* 22:446–456.

Taylor, M. 1987. Physico-chemical principles in low temperature biology. In: *The effects of low temperatures on biological systems,* edited by B. Grout, and G. Morris. London: Edward Arnold.

Tiller, W. 1991. *The science of crystallization. Microscopic interfacial phenomena.* Cambridge: Cambridge University Press.

Viskanta, R. 1985. Natural convection in melting and solidification. In *Natural convection fundamentals and applications,* edited by S. Kakac et al. Washington DC: Hemisphere Publishing Corporation.

Wang, Y., and M. Hanson. 1988. Parenteral formulations of proteins and peptides: Stability and stabilizers. *J. Parent. Sci. Technol.* 42 (Suppl.):S4–S26.

Warren, G. 1993. Properties of engineered antifreeze peptides. *FEBS J.* 321:116–120.

Wen, D., and R. Laursen. 1992. A model for binding of an antifreeze polypeptide to ice. *Biophys. J.* 63:1659–1662.

Wisniewski, R., and V. Wu. 1992. Large scale freezing and thawing of biopharmaceutical drug product. *Proceedings of the International Congress: Advanced Technologies for Manufacturing of Aseptic and Terminally Sterilized Pharmaceuticals and Biopharmaceuticals,* 17–19 February, in Basel, Switzerland.

Woods, A. 1992. Melting and dissolving. *J. Fluid Mech.* 239:429–448.

Worster, G. 1991. Natural convection in a mushy layer. *J. Fluid Mech.* 224:335–359.

Yen, Y., and C. Zehnder. 1973. Melting heat transfer with water jet. *Int. J. Heat Mass Transfer* 16:219–228.

Yen, Y. 1975. Heat-transfer characteristics of a bubble-induced water jet impinging on an ice surface. *Int. J. Heat Mass Transfer* 18:917–928.

Zabaras, N., and T. H. Nguyen. 1995. Control of the freezing interface morphology in solidification processes in the presence of natural convection. *Intl. J. Numer. Meth. Eng.* 38:1555–1578.

Zhang, Z., and A. Bejan. 1990. Solidification in the presence of high Rayleigh number convection in an enclosure cooled from the side. *Int. J. Heat Mass Transfer* 33:661–671.

3

PROCESS DESIGN CONSIDERATIONS FOR LARGE–SCALE CHROMATOGRAPHY OF BIOMOLECULES

Richard Wisniewski

NASA Ames Research Center

Egisto Boschetti

BioSepra, Inc.

Alois Jungbauer

University of Agriculture, Forestry, and Biotechnology (Vienna)

This chapter reviews process development, process design, and design and operation concepts of large-scale chromatography systems used in biopharmaceutical manufacturing. Liquid chromatography is an essential purification step in achieving the high product purities required for biopharmaceuticals. Chromatographic media, system components, and system integration and performance are described. Process development, scale-up, and optimization stages are also discussed.

The principal requirement in the large-scale biopharmaceutical production of therapeutic proteins is very high product purity. In

61

the manufacturing process liquid chromatography is an essential technique, which allows the achievement of such high purity levels. The majority of publications on the purification of biomolecules using chromatography techniques pertains to analytical applications. Industrial chromatography has a different purpose from analytical- and laboratory-scale preparative techniques; thus, different criteria are applied. In addition to product purity, productivity and cost minimization are of primary interest (Sadana and Beelaram 1994).

While analytical-scale separations operate in the linear range of adsorption isotherms, production-scale processes operate primarily in the nonlinear range (Goldshan-Shirazi and Guiochon 1992; Gu et al. 1993; Katti and Guiochon 1992).

Although there are many good reviews and publications on the subject of large-scale industrial chromatography of biomolecules (Bonnerjea and Terras 1994, 160–185; Janson and Ryden 1989; Sofer and Nystrom 1989), the authors believe that certain topics may need more attention among field practitioners. The information presented herein addresses aspects of industrial chromatography that may aid users in process development, scale-up, and final design of manufacturing operations.

In general, the task of process development is to ensure consistent product purity and yield, and at the same time maintain sufficient process reliability, robustness, and economics. It is important that development efforts of downstream processing (purifications) be combined with the process development of upstream processing (fermentation, cell culture, product release from cells). An "ideal" desired situation in the industrial chromatography purification step would be a process based on a simple adsorption/desorption principle, where either all contaminants flow through the column and the product is bound to a resin, or the product flows through and the contaminants bind. In either case the binding step is followed by an elution step. In practice, in most processes the product binds to a resin and an attempt is made to allow the contaminants to flow through by selection of an environment, which can favorably affect the molecular interactions associated with the binding of desired molecules (ionic strength, pH, buffer composition, and stationary phase surface chemistry). Binding of the product permits concentration during elution and also allows the strict control of buffer composition for product handling.

The typical steps of chromatography separations are as follows:

- Column equilibration (stationary and mobile phases reach binding conditions)

- Sample loading (application of controlled amount of protein mixture; binding)
- Column washing–single or multiple step (removal of unbound and some bound contaminants)
- Elution [desorption of molecule(s) of interest by changing the parameters of the mobile phase]
- Column regeneration (removal of strongly bound contaminants by applying extreme composition of mobile phase)
- Column cleaning (application of a specially composed mobile phase to remove accumulated contaminants and restore column performance)

The key component of a chromatography system, which determines purification success, is the chromatographic stationary phase. Molecular interactions among the stationary phase and solutes in the buffer environment must be well understood during the development of the purification process (Ceulemans 1991). Molecular interactions involving product, contaminants, buffer solutes, and active sites of the stationary chromatographic medium are relatively straightforward in ion-exchange chromatography (Gerstner et al. 1994; Yamamoto et al. 1988), more complicated in hydrophobic interaction (Kato 1987) or reversed-phase (Cretier and Rocca 1994; Gooding and Regnier 1990; Mant and Hodges 1991), and are very complex in affinity chromatography techniques (Chase 1986; Labrou and Clonis 1994; Liapis 1989; Mohr and Pommerening 1985, 19–115, 209–214). Understanding the molecular interactions may not always be an easy task due to the complexity of biological macromolecules. All of these techniques require knowledge of ligand-molecule interactions, not only during binding but also during elution. Binding and elution conditions should be optimized in order to achieve high productivity, and also from the point of view of preventing or minimizing detrimental effects to the product (such as unfolding, precipitation, oxidation, deamidation, or multimer formation).

Several modern stationary phases have been introduced in the past few years (Arshady 1991; Boschetti 1994; Horvath et al. 1994; Liapis and McCoy 1994; Rippel et al. 1994). Due to the proprietary technologies involved in manufacturing chromatographic media, a user is advised to consult media manufacturers in individual cases. Media manufacturers can provide extensive documentation on safety, reliability, and performance of particular media; however, typically, users must develop their own purification procedures for individual products. Process conditions should also be selected to ensure compatibility, consistent performance, and long life of the chromatographic resin (the leaching of components, permanent binding of contaminants or product, or particle cracking are not allowed).

The selection of chromatography stationary phases may follow manufacturers' data and recommendations; however, it is up to the user to test media applicability for a particular separation. For example, the average load capacities for typical proteins as given by media manufacturers may prove to be completely different from the real product capacity; in addition, the capacity may depend on liquid phase velocity and the mixture of biomolecules. More information on chromatographic media is given in "Chromatographic Media and Their Use."

Equipment material selection is dictated by process conditions. In most cases stainless steel (316L grade), glass (borosilicate), and certain polymers and elastomers (such as EPDM or Kalrez®) are used to ensure good material compatibility and stability. However, buffers containing chloride ions may not be compatible with stainless steels (Fontana and Greene 1978). Metallic components that are in contact with buffers containing high levels of chloride ions may be made of Hastelloy C or titanium. The elution of product and contaminants may be accomplished using step/isocratic elutions, gradient elution, or a combination of both techniques. The gradient elution requirement poses a design challenge to large-scale systems. Gradient formation may be accomplished by low or high pressure mixing (Truei et al. 1992). Low pressure mixing involves rapid operation delivery valves and mixing chamber(s) in front of or after the pump. High pressure mixing requires two individually controlled pumps, each delivering a separate gradient component.

The most often applied principle of scale-up from the bench developmental level to the industrial scale is to keep the bed height approximately constant and increase the column diameter. At similar liquid phase velocity, the flow rates can be estimated for various column cross sections (Groundwater 1985). This approach may work only up to certain column diameters; above these diameters the liquid distribution effects (nonuniformity) might adversely affect the quality of separation. The quality of column packing may also change with an increase in column diameter.

In addition to solving scale-up problems, industrial-scale chromatography also involves process optimization. Process optimization may be approached at many levels of sophistication. For example, one may consider the following factors: maximize productivity, minimize costs, minimize the number of purification steps, reduce risks of system failure, simplify buffer composition, minimize buffer usage, extend the operational life of resins, and remove specific contaminants. These factors should be considered at an early stage in purification process development. However, they may be interconnected in such a complex way that thorough investigation of their interdependence may be impractical; some of them should be given a priority during process development, depending on individual user situations.

Several interrelated factors are involved in process development work that can affect the outcome of the purification step:

- Packing characteristics, including surface chemistry, particle size, and internal porosity

- Composition of eluting agents and the method of elution (step, gradient, or combined)

- Ionic strength and pH

- Column (bed) height

- Sample load (including concentration)

- Flow rate (to a different degree, depending on the type of packing)

- Cleaning and regeneration

Development work is frequently done using a readily available workstation/pilot system (for example, BioPilot® by Pharmacia, BioCad® by Perseptive Biosystems, ProSys® by BioSepra). These systems provide high precision equipment combined with sophisticated development software. This software can aid in chromatogram analysis (peak area calculation, peak height, resolution, number of theoretical separation plates, shape of gradient elution, fractions cutoff, normalization of baselines, etc.). Depending on the applied type of detector, such analysis may also be performed at multiple wavelengths. The capability to compare (overlay) multiple chromatograms is a typical feature of such software packages. The software can also analyze the reproducibility of the purification. Development strategies can be evaluated by manipulating many variables (pH, ionic strength, flow rate, gradient slope, etc.). In the case of ion-exchange chromatography, pH maps can be prepared to find the optimum separation conditions. Software packages may also provide simulation algorithms. These can predict purification results under new conditions from previous experiments. Scale-up and validation tools may also be included in workstation software packages. Validation software contains documentation routines that may include tools for testing run repeatability, resin deterioration and lifetime, product characterization, and system diagnostics capability. The scale-up part may also include routines for flow, porosity, particle size effects, and column geometry. In special cases such systems can also be applied for the manufacture of products to be used in clinical trials. Users may consider applying some of the software capabilities of these systems in production chromatography. Aspects of scale-up and process optimization are discussed further in "Process Development and Scale-Up."

MAJOR CHROMATOGRAPHY TECHNIQUES USED IN LARGE–SCALE PROCESSES

Industrial chromatography introduces specific features and requirements when compared to an analytical environment. Separation resolution may not be as important in industrial chromatography as it is in analytical chromatography. Column loads are much higher and the loss of resolution due to overload may approach the limits of acceptable separation quality. The buffers used should be of low cost, easy to prepare and store, compatible with materials of construction, nontoxic, and easy to dispose. Widely used techniques are ion-exchange (Horvath et al. 1994; Yamamoto et al. 1988), hydrophobic interaction (Kato 1987; Szepesy and Rippel 1994) and size exclusion (Kato 1989, 87–123) chromatography. Reversed-phase chromatography (Kroeff et al. 1989) is seldom used in large-scale protein purification, because it involves the use of solvents and more expensive equipment and facilities. It has been used in the purification of synthetic peptides (Mant and Hodges 1991). Product-specific techniques (such as affinity chromatography) are individually tailored to particular separation processes (Jack et al. 1987; Labrou and Clonis 1994; Mohr and Pommerening 1985; Narayanan 1994; Wainer and Noctor 1993).

Many industrial processes opt for the reliability and low cost of ion-exchange chromatography as a basic purification step. The ion-exchange step can be accompanied by hydrophobic interaction and size exclusion (gel filtration) chromatographic steps. In many cases this approach to purification may provide satisfactory results, although product-specific binding and affinity techniques are also needed.

Affinity chromatography can capture even very dilute product from a vast number of contaminants. Product concentration can be accomplished in the same step. In certain cases affinity chromatography may be used as a single-step technique, selectively removing desired product molecules from the stream, while all contaminants flow through.

While analytical chromatography separations may utilize complex profiles of the mobile phase elution gradients (Jandera and Churacek 1985), industrial chromatography usually employs linear or step gradients, or a combination of both. The number of separation steps may vary, but a larger number of purification steps usually means higher product losses and lower overall product yield. Therefore, an attempt should be made to minimize the number of steps (see also "Chromatographic Media and Their Use"). One of the early approaches to reducing the number of separation steps was the use of product-specific purification techniques, such as affinity chromatography, although it has often been an additional benefit on the quest for product purity.

Since the purification process also involves membrane separation steps (such as ultrafiltration), additional efforts might be undertaken to reduce, if possible, the number of membrane separations to a minimum. Since the ultrafiltrations are typically used between chromatography steps for buffer exchange and product concentration, there is a possibility of eliminating at least some of them. Product concentration can be accomplished as an additional effect on chromatographic columns during the purification steps. Purification development work may consider media and buffer selection for individual chromatography steps, which at a proper sequence may allow the avoidance of some membrane separations (e.g., the high salt concentration elution buffer for ion-exchange chromatography might become a base for an initial buffer for hydrophobic interaction chromatography). Further steps in the direction of limiting the number of steps in downstream processing could be an application of an expanded bed adsorption column, which can combine product specificity and tolerance to the presence of cells, cell debris, and other contaminants (Chase and Draeger 1992). This single step could eliminate cell separation steps (microfiltration or centrifugation) and product concentration/buffer exchange steps (ultrafiltration) by providing the capability of capturing the product directly from the bioreactor broth (Yang and Goto 1993).

Principles of Chromatographic Separations

Table 3.1 lists the principles of separations for the major chromatographic techniques.

Table 3.1. Types of Chromatography Distinguished According to the Nature of the Retention Forces and the Principle of Separation

(Only chromatography types with a major impact in industrial chromatography are listed. Modified from Jungbauer [1993].)

Name	Action Principle	Separation According To
Adsorption chromatography	Surface binding	Molecular structure
Ion-exchange chromatography	Ion binding	Surface charge
Molecular sieve chromatography (gel filtration)	Steric exclusion	Molecular size and shape
Affinity chromatography	Biospecific adsorption/desorption	Molecular structure
Hydrophobic (interaction) chromatography	Hydrophobic complex formation	Hydrophobicity and hydrophobic patches
(Metal) chelate chromatography	Coordination complex formation	Complex formation with transition metals
Reversed-phase chromatography	Hydrophobic complex formation	Hydrophobicity

Major Techniques

Ion-Exchange Chromatography

Ion-exchange chromatography (IEX) is the most widely used method in industrial chromatography. An ion exchanger consists of an insoluble matrix, to which charged groups have been covalently bound. The charged groups are associated with mobile counterions. These counterions can be reversibly exchanged with other ions of the same charge. An amphoteric macromolecule may also displace a counterion. Various charged groups can be immobilized to the matrix. Resins for different applications, in different particle sizes, different ligand densities, and pore sizes are easily available (see "Media for Ion Exchange").

Separation in ion-exchange chromatography is obtained by reversible adsorption. The protein can be bound at low salt concentration; after washing out the unbound material, the protein can be displaced by a high salt concentration. Elution can also be performed by a change in buffer pH. Both types of elution can be accomplished by step gradients or linear gradients. A fundamental description of the ion-exchange process is provided, for example, by Yamamoto et al. (1988). The most prominent advantages of IEX are its high dynamic capacity (up to 150 mg protein per mL sorbent), the use of simple buffers, and the overall low cost of this technique compared to other types of chromatography.

Hydrophobic Interaction Chromatography

Hydrophobic interaction chromatography (HIC) has gained increasing attention, because it is an effective step that can be linked directly to IEX, affinity chromatography, and gel filtration or nonchromatographic steps. Since HIC uses high salt concentrations in the loading buffer, the effluent from an ion exchanger or clarified culture broth can be added with salt and applied on an HIC column. If many proteins precipitate due to the high salt concentration, a clarification step prior to loading may be required. The effect of salt concentration on HIC at sufficient high ionic strength (m) can be described as follows:

$$\log \frac{k'}{k_0'} = \lambda \times m$$

where λ is an empirical parameter that is related to the retention strength and is similar to the salting-out constant (Melander et al. 1984). k' and k_0' are the capacity factors of a protein (relative retention time) at a particular salt concentration and at zero salt concentration. Attention must be paid to the conformational change of proteins at high salt concentrations (Pahlman et al. 1977; Wu et al. 1986). In addition, HIC is very sensitive to the temperature of the loading step and to the residence time in the column. By modifying the ligand, the selectivity of the salt-promoted interaction, as reported by Porath (1986), can be increased.

Thiophilic adsorption demonstrates how the selectivity of HIC can be improved. For example, by introducing sulfur atoms into the hydrophobic ligand, a specificity for IgG can be created. Antibodies can be specifically bound in the presence of albumin and other serum protein contaminants. Sulk et al. (1992) described monoclonal antibody purification from hybridoma culture supernatant by thiophilic adsorption.

Affinity Chromatography

Affinity chromatography, first described by Cuatrecasas et al. (1968), utilizes biospecific interaction with a natural or synthetic ligand. Support material and activation principles for covalent linkage of a ligand were comprehensively reviewed by Clonis (1990), Narayanan and Crane (1990) and Carlson et al. (1989). The method becomes essential if the three-step concept of capture, purification, and polishing should be realized.

There are many examples of applications that use affinity chromatography techniques: immobilized monoclonal antibodies are used in industrial scale for Factor VIII, Factor IX, and interferon purification. In fusion protein technology a protein fragment possessing a specific affinity to a ligand is fused to a parent protein. The fusion protein can be affinity purified, after purification the affinity tag is cleaved off (Moks et al. 1987). In another application, biological and synthetic peptide libraries (Kramer et al. 1993) are a rapid way for developing a small ligand. The small ligand may be more stable compared to a macromolecule, and ligand leakage may be small or not pronounced.

Metal (Chelate) Chromatography

Metal (chelate) chromatography has become a subject of great interest in the biotechnology industry. The method can be very efficient. The use of affinity tail interaction with complexed heavy metals may lead to a simplification of the purification flowsheet. An affinity tag is a small peptide that has affinity to metal ions. The principle of this system is illustrated in Figure 3.1. Metal chelate chromatography is also potent in endotoxin removal. However, the principle is not well understood. Especially at higher pH values, this method can be very efficient.

Reversed-Phase Chromatography

During the early 1980s protein purification of large proteins (MW > 50,000) by reversed-phase chromatography (RPC) was first mentioned (Lewis et al. 1980). The separation principle of RPC is based on a very hydrophobic stationary phase. The hydrophobic patches

Figure 3.1. Schematic structure of the nitrilotriacetic acids sorbent charged with nickel ions. The sorbent is an aquadridentate chelate former, which occupies four positions in the metal coordination sphere. The remaining two ligand positions in the octahedral coordination sphere are free for interaction with the adjacent histidines. Only proteins with a dihistitydl tag will bind to the sorbent (Hochuli 1990).

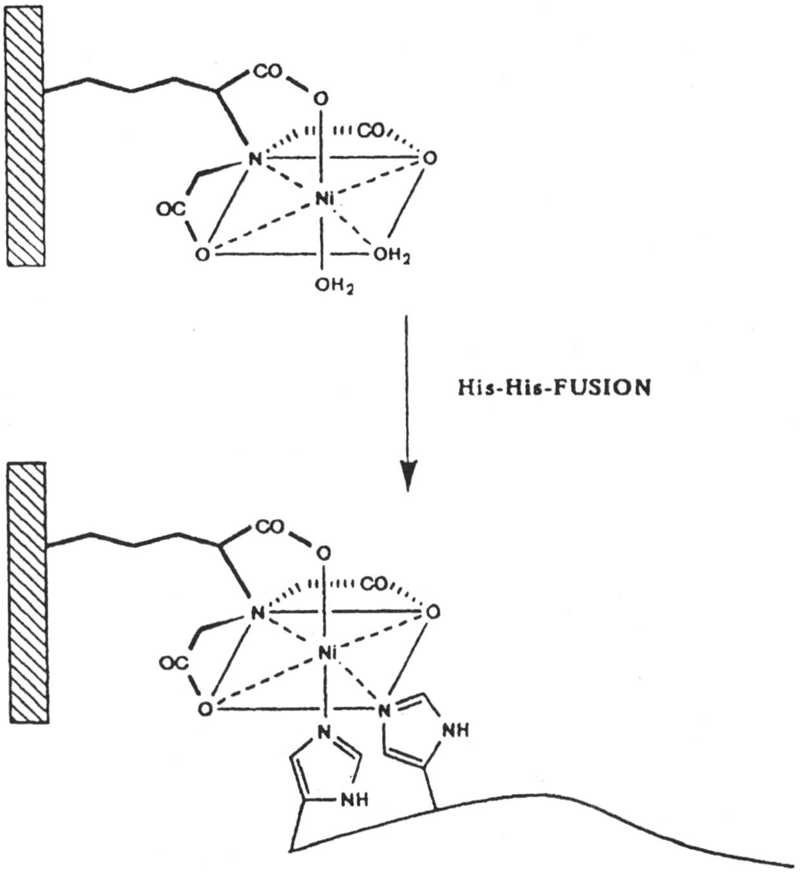

of a protein interact with this apolar phase. The mobile phase contains a water/buffer and an organic component, such as acetonitrile, methanol, or isopropanol (Corran 1989, 1527–1556), which is responsible for desorption from the stationary phase. Due to the

composition of the mobile phase, proteins can be optimally dissolved; however, denaturing conditions for proteins are often generated. The protein may be unfolded following the proposed kinetic
model (Sadana 1992), assuming first order deactivation kinetics for
a zero incubation time.

$$P = P_0 \times e^{-kt_e}$$

The incubation time is the time from the injection of the sample to the time when the gradient is started. P_0 is the amount of protein injected into the column and t_e is the time from injection until
elution of the native peak. The aforementioned equation demonstrates that the protein can be rapidly inactivated since k coefficient
values are in the range of 10^{-4} sec^{-1}.

The RPC method tends to disappear from the stage of large-
scale protein purification due to low recovery and the organic
phases that require certain precautions to be taken (solvent handling, explosion-proof design) in a production plant. In some cases
RPC may be the only technique able to deliver a final separation for
variants of the product molecule. Reversed-phase chromatography
is a valuable method for process control or for the separation of peptides from tryptic maps. It is carried out in an HPLC mode.

Size Exclusion (Gel Filtration) Chromatography

Size exclusion chromatography, also called gel filtration, is an essential method for desalting and the separation of aggregates or degradation products. The simple relationship between the distribution
coefficient and the elution volume can be expressed as follows:

$$\frac{V_e}{V_0} = 1 + K_{av}\varepsilon^{-1}$$

where V_e is the elution volume, V_0 is the void volume, K_{av} is the
available distribution coefficient, and ε is the fraction of the void
volume of the total column volume (Laurent and Killander 1964).
Furthermore, K_{av} is related to the molecular mass (M_R) of a macromolecule by a logistic equation:

$$K_{av} = \frac{1}{1 + \left(\dfrac{M_R}{c}\right)^b}$$

where b and c are constants depending on the particular separation
conditions (Rodbard 1976, 145–179). The above equations show

that the proteins are eluted in order of their molecular mass or Stokes radii, if other interactions than penetrating into the pores can be excluded.

The advantages of gel filtration are as follows:

- The product is collected in the required buffer.

- Low molecular contaminants are removed.

The disadvantages are as follows:

- Low sample volume (in general < 10 percent of total column volume)

- Very sensitive to viscosity and salt content in the protein solution (e.g., with a high protein concentration or salt concentration of the sample, "fingering" occurs, causing reduced resolution.)

- Dilution of the final product by a factor of 1.5 to 10

Size exclusion chromatography can be carried out in two different modes: the desalting mode and the resolution mode. In the desalting mode, the K_{av} value is close to zero, and the protein does not enter the pores of the gel chromatography medium. The protein is eluted with the void volume and the contaminants or salts, which are substantially smaller than the product, are retained. In that case the dilution of the product is less than fourfold.

In the resolution mode the K_{av} value is different from zero, the protein is able to enter the pores and is retained. High molecular mass contaminants can be removed by this technique. They elute earlier than the product. In that case the product is diluted between a factor of 5 and 10.

In general, a gel chromatography step requires long running times and large columns due to the small injected sample sizes and limits in resolution. It is preferred as the final step in a protein purification sequence, when the product purity is high and liquid volume is low. Recently, Kurnik et al. (1995) proposed an original method for the solution of a general chromatography equation with application to size exclusion chromatography using Green's function. "Chromatographic Media and Their Use" provides more details on chromatographic media and techniques.

PROCESS DEVELOPMENT AND SCALE–UP

Process development involves laboratory experiments at the bench, expansion to pilot scale, and a final scale-up to the industrial application. The elementary scale-up procedures involve maintaining the bed height and increasing the column diameter, with a corresponding increase in the flow rate if there is no change in chromatographic medium characteristics. Changes in particle diameter and column height introduce new factors that must be considered in scale-up. Early development work frequently employs gradient elution techniques, while the preferred way of operation for industrial scale may be isocratic or step gradient elution. Process development efforts may include such conditions in the early stages, or the linear gradient elution results may serve as a basis for planning the pilot experiments using isocratic, or stepwise, elution.

While many practical separations in the past have been conducted at low temperature (cold rooms were required), an attempt should be made to avoid low temperature separation conditions when developing a new process to facilitate operations and reduce investment expense. New chromatographic media may facilitate this task due to more defined binding capabilities and to much shorter purification times made possible by utilizing high liquid velocities. Users should test the high liquid velocity media for their dynamic binding capacity (this is often reduced with a liquid phase velocity increase, or with a large number of adsorbing contaminants). High velocity media are further described in "Chromatographic Media and Their Use."

Bench-scale and pilot-scale systems can be matched with software aids, which may significantly reduce man-hour requirements needed for process development. While in the bench scale for analytical and development of chromatography systems, and in some pilot-scale installations, such software may reach a high level of sophistication; in an industrial scale the manufacturing systems usually possess rather limited capabilities. In addition to monitoring, elementary calculations (such as flow totalizing), recording, and displaying, certain software capabilities can be very beneficial for industrial-scale operations. This includes peak area calculation, drift compensation, signal noise reduction, multiple chromatogram overlay with comparison (deviation detection), slope analysis, and derivative calculation/display. The software may also have features aiding in calibration procedures. If implemented, these features can clearly show the advantages of an integrated computer-based system over the systems based on individual controllers or programmable logic controllers (PLCs) and recorders.

Equipment and methodology used in bench-scale tests are frequently different from the subsequent pilot and industrial development steps. Anticipation of industrial-scale conditions and limitations is, therefore, very important during the early stages of process development. For example, column overload conditions may significantly affect the purification outcome when compared to separation using the injection of small samples.

Chromatography expert systems may have limited use in production chromatography, if they originally were developed with focus on analytical techniques (Bryant et al. 1994). Some approaches to process optimization consider the cost of separation as a factor to be minimized. For example, Wilhelm and Riba (1989) proposed a complex approach to scale-up and optimization of production liquid chromatography considering cost as the main criterion.

Phases in Process Development

There are five phases in process development that are strongly interrelated and that hypothetically should be done simultaneously:

1. De novo purification

2. Resin screening

3. Optimization of running conditions

4. Flow sheeting

5. Productivity optimization

First of all, it is necessary to clarify how much material is needed and what purity requirements will be expected. Although drug development is a process that has clearly defined rules, the regulatory authorities still decide on a case-by-case basis. This means that the exact purity and stability requirements probably will evolve during the course of preclinical and clinical testing.

De Novo Purification

De novo purification is mainly carried out in the biochemistry laboratory. Frequently, it is the purification of a protein that has an unknown structure and physicochemical properties, and which has only a biological effect known. Frequently, this phase predetermines the process scale. In the early phase (i.e., for development of a pharmaceutical), the goal is focused on the production of sufficient material, and the exploration whether or not the substance has the expected in vivo properties and potency. For pragmatic reasons, the refining of methods is not carried out at this stage. When the question of in vivo properties is solved, the product will often be moved directly to clinical trials, without "wasting" too much time for developing a good process.

Finally, when the clinical trials are successful, everything is fixed and the protein may be produced with a suboptimal process. Computer programs and strategies for rational process design may be helpful to determine in early stages if it is feasible to invest time and manpower in process development. Although everyone is aware that the development of pharmaceuticals is a race, the accelerating effect of optimal process development is underestimated in many cases. Those competitors who are using the knowledge of rational process design may gain an effective advantage in this race from the start.

Resin Screening

In order to start a purification process, a resin must be selected. The heuristic rules that can be applied for resin screening are not very advanced. The pragmatic question is: Under what conditions can a particular protein be bound? There also are very pragmatic points to follow, such as long-term availability or whether a drug master file (DMF) is available. At this stage some consideration on productivity should be made. The pragmatic considerations are valid for all types of chromatography. A complete description of all the rules would exceed the scope of this chapter. As an example, a few guidelines for IEX, HIC, affinity chromatography, and hydroxyapatite are discussed.

- *IEX:* The isoelectric point (Yang and Langer 1985) of the protein, the salt, the pH of the eluent buffers (Gooding and Schmuck 1983; Kopaciewicz and Regnier 1983), and the protein or peptide molecular weight and stability will determine the resin. The ligand density and porosity of the bead influence the retention time (Wu and Walters 1992) and the loading capacity (Rounds et al. 1986).

- *HIC:* The major concern is protein stability and solubility at high salt concentrations. Ligand density considerations may determine at which concentration of the eluent salt the protein is eluted.

- *Affinity chromatography:* One should identify if a generic resin is actually available (Protein A, Protein G, T-gel) for antibody purification. For successful metal chelating separation, histidine residues at the surface of the protein should be accessible. The biological nature of the protein should allow it to bind to a certain generic ligand. DNA–binding proteins may bind to dye-affinity resins (Dean and Watson 1979).

- *Hydroxyapatite:* Since the binding mechanisms for hydroxyapatite are not well understood, it is very difficult to make a priori considerations about binding. Only literature data, in which a protein from another source has been successfully purified, may be used as an indication of whether to consider this technique. It is necessary to make experiments show whether the protein binds or not (Jungbauer et al. 1989a).

Optimization of Running Conditions

Once the resin is selected, one can start to optimize the eluent buffers, and the velocity and shape of the elution gradient. Software is available for IEX to simulate different running conditions. A reliable map of the distribution coefficient K versus the protein concentration and the mobile phase modifier concentration (in IEX, generally, salt concentration) must be evaluated (Whitley et al. 1989; Kaltenbrunner and Jungbauer in press).

Several methods are available for this purpose. Batch determination must be avoided, since it requires too much material and the results are not precise. One can infer these data from chromatographic experiments, such as linear gradient experiments, pulse experiments, and breakthrough curves (frontal analysis). A software package called Prosym® (BioSepra Inc., Marlborough, MA) together with hardware known as Prosys® (BioSepra Inc.) has been recently introduced, which can carry out an optimization automatically. Once a dependence of the distribution coefficient (K) on the protein concentration and the salt concentration is evaluated, overloaded conditions can be simulated.

Pulse Experiments. Two functions can be used for the derivation of the distribution coefficient K. The most simple approach is as follows:

$$V_e = V_0 + K(V_t - V_0)$$

where the K value is directly related to the elution volume V_e or retention time (t_R)

$$t_R = \frac{V_e}{F}$$

where F is flow rate.

Over a limited range of salt concentrations, the relationship between $\log k'$ and $\log 1/C$ is often approximated to a linear dependency, given as

$$\log k' = \log K + Z \log\left(\frac{1}{C}\right)$$

where k' is the capacity factor, also known as the relative retention time

$$k' = \frac{t_R - t_0}{t_0},$$

the Z coefficient reflects the apparent number of ionic charges associated with the adsorption-desorption process at the sorbent surface, and C is protein concentration (Rounds and Regnier 1984; Hearn et al. 1988).

Linear Gradients. It is well understood that the peak position of an eluted protein varies with the steepness of a linear gradient. The peak position is defined as the molarity of displacer where the peak maximum elutes. This phenomenon can be used for the determination of the distribution coefficient.

Several runs with different gradient slopes and protein concentrations must be carried out. The relative peak position, Θ_R, is defined by the following equation:

$$\Theta_R = \frac{V_e}{V_0}$$

It varies with the steepness of the linear gradient (G), where V_0 is column void volume and V_e is elution volume (Figure 3.2).

The empirical relationship between the dependence of the distribution coefficient, $K(I)$, on the salt (Yamamoto et al. 1983) is as follows:

$$K(I) = A \times I^B + K'$$

where A and B are empirical parameters, K' is the distribution coefficient of the salt, I is ionic strength, and the change of the peak position $d(G\Phi)/dI$ allows the deduction of the K value from linear gradient experiments (Yamamoto et al. 1990).

$$\frac{d(G\Phi)}{dI} = \frac{1}{K(I) - K'}$$

Figure 3.2. Variation of the relative peak position Θ_R with the steepness of the linear gradient in IEX. Three gradients of different slope are compared.

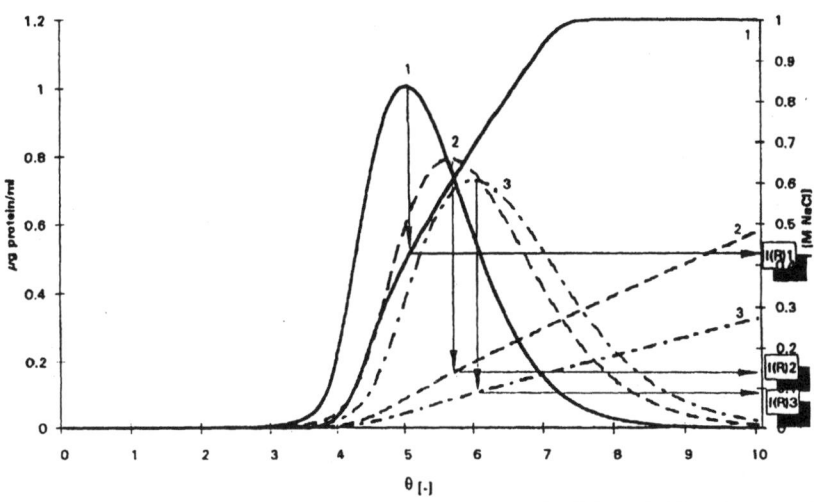

where G is the steepness of the linear gradient normalized in respect to V_0 and Φ is the stationary phase ratio (Φ = volume of liquid in sorbent pores/void volume).

Some authors assume that the distribution coefficient for salt is constant (Yamamoto et al. 1983), but a slight dependence of K' on I has been observed (Jungbauer 1993). Linear gradient experiments can only match a narrow range of salt concentrations–the range where the protein is eluted. After K is measured by a series of chromatographic runs at different slopes and different salt concentrations, a function must be found that allows for extrapolation of the high and low values.

Frontal Analysis. The breakthrough curve is used for the determination of the distribution coefficient. The simple relationship

$$K = \frac{\dfrac{q}{(1-\varepsilon) \cdot V_t}}{C_0}$$

can be used to map K versus the protein concentration and ionic strength, q is the maximum capacity, ε is the void volume, V_t is the total column volume, and C_0 is the protein concentration in equilibrium (Figure 3.3). As seen from the aforementioned equations, the separation parameter acquisition methods are based on chromatography results. They can now be automated easily, for interpretation computer programs are available. An example of a complex computational approach is described by Whitley et al. (1991). When the optimal running condition is found by simulation, this condition is verified by an experiment and one can move on to the next process step or scale up the operation.

Flow Sheeting

The process for the purification of a protein consists of several steps. Usually, there is a link between the performance of each step and the performances of the previous step and the subsequent steps. There are certain heuristic rules for flow sheeting: remove the solvent (water) first, which implies that concentration steps should be at the beginning. Then the main impurities must be removed. Finally, aggregates and minor impurities must be removed in parallel with transferring the protein in the required buffer. Wheelwright

Figure 3.3. Dependence of the distribution coefficient on protein concentration and ionic strength (BSA binding to Q-HyperD resin). The dots represent the experimental data obtained from chromatographic experiments.

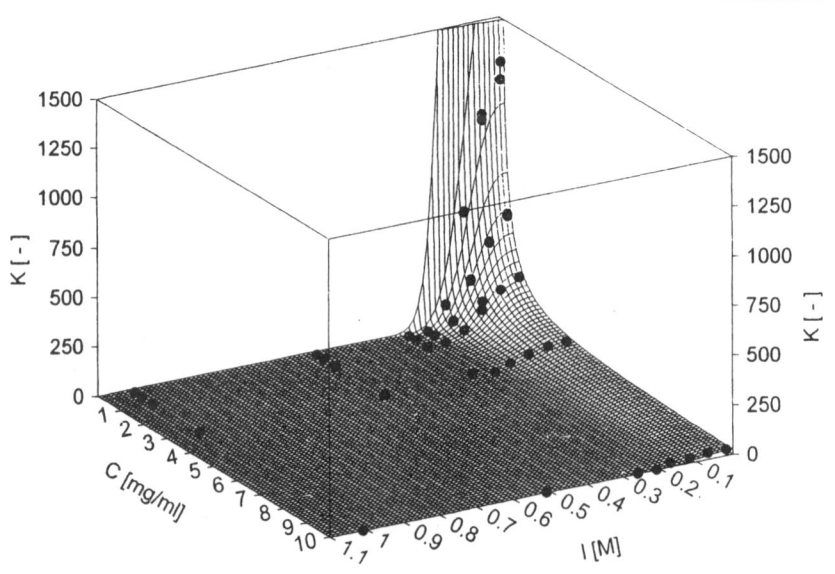

(1991) adapted the list of heuristics for multicomponent mixtures published by Nadgir and Liu (1983) to the separation of proteins and biomolecules (Table 3.2).

Recently, Watanabe et al. (1994) described the heuristics approach based on physical, chemical, and biochemical properties. Their proposed list of rules was as follows:

- Choose separation process based on different physical, chemical, or biochemical properties.

- Separate the most plentiful impurities first.

- Choose those processes that will exploit the differences in the physicochemical properties of the product and impurities in the most efficient manner.

- Use a high-resolution step as soon as possible.

- Do the most arduous step last.

Hypothetically, an optimal flow sheet consists of three steps: capture, purification, and polishing. More steps are required in practice, if process optimization is not carried out properly.

Table 3.2. Classification of Heuristics According to Wheelwright (1991) and Nadgir and Liu (1983)

Type	Application	Example
Method heuristics	Specify choice between different unit operations.	Describe conditions for preference of microfiltration over centrifugation.
Design heuristics	Specify order or sequence of process steps.	Perform low resolution step prior to high resolution step. Use large particles at the beginning of a purification sequence.
Species heuristics	Specify based on the properties of the components.	Choose separation method based on the greatest difference in properties of product and impurities. This rule tells us to always use affinity chromatography. There are certain other limitations.
Composition heuristics	Specify feed composition based on separation costs.	This rule tells us that affinity chromatography may be too expensive.

Productivity Optimization

Productivity can be considered as the highest throughput at a defined purification ratio (resolution) and column life time. Several mathematical functions are available for predicting the highest productivity. The performance of different processing steps should be compared on the basis of solute productivity. Yamamoto et al. (1990) defined productivity as follows:

$$\text{Productivity} = \frac{\dfrac{\text{recovery ratio} \times \text{sample feed volume}}{\text{column volume}}}{\text{cycle time}}$$

There are cases where productivity has an optimum range (Figure 3.4). This means that at very high flow rates the productivity again decreases (case II). This is due to lower resolution at higher flow rates. In the case where an optimum is not achieved, the resolution is not significantly influenced by the flow rate. The recovery ratio, better known as yield or recovery, is influenced by operating conditions, the stability of the protein, the source of the protein, and the presence of degrading enzymes. A general rule is: The faster the sequence of purification steps is performed, the higher may be the yield, because all degrading and precipitation processes during storage are minimized.

Janson and Hedman (1982, 43–99) found that the productivity of an ion-exchange column depends on

$$\left[\frac{\left(\dfrac{Z_I}{u} \right)}{\left(\dfrac{Z_{II}}{u} \right)} \right] = \left(\frac{N_{II}}{N_I} \right)^{\frac{2}{3}}$$

where u is fluid velocity, N_I and N_{II} are plate numbers, and Z_I and Z_{II} are column lengths. However, the situation is more complex than first assumed. Productivity is a very complicated function of various parameters:

$$\text{Productivity} = f(d_c, d_p, Z, C_0, u, Q_P, Q_R, \text{etc.})$$

where d_c is column diameter, d_p is particle diameter, Z is column length, C_0 is initial protein concentration applied to the column, u is liquid velocity, Q_P is the purity ratio, and Q_R is the recovery ratio (yield). In nonisocratic elution the feed is applied until the product appears in the breakthrough[1] (Figure 3.5).

---

[1]In practice, loading is finished earlier.

Figure 3.4. Productivity versus linear velocity. In case II an optimum in productivity is obtained. In some cases (I) the optimum may be far beyond the practically applicable linear velocity.

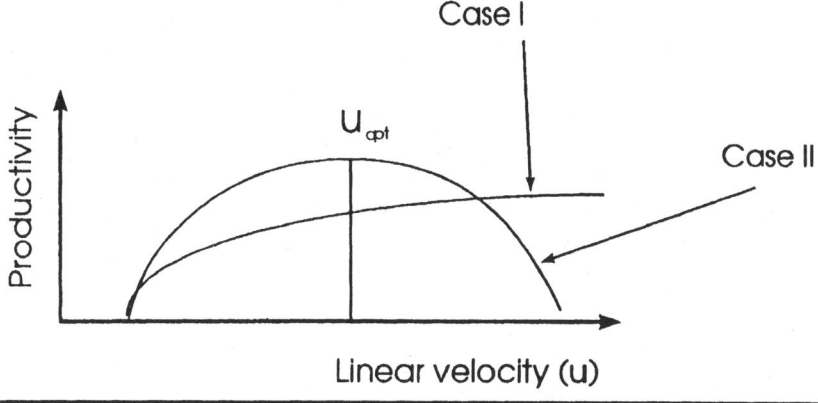

Figure 3.5. Breakthrough curve: *C* and *C*₀ are the actual and the initial feed concentrations.

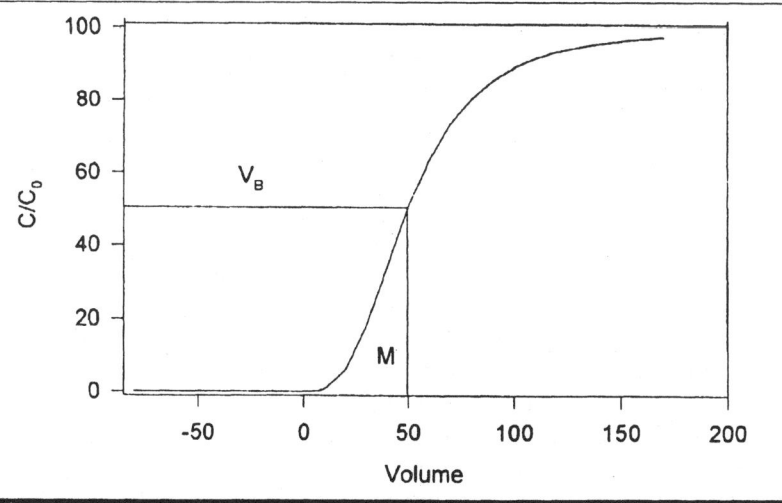

Productivity is, therefore, determined by the breakthrough time (V_B/F) and the amount of feed discarded before the breakthrough time, where V_B is the breakthrough volume and F is the flow rate.

$$P_r = Q_R \frac{(C_0 V_B - M)}{t_C \times V_t}$$

where M is volume remaining after breakthrough, V_t is total column volume, and t_C is the total operation time.

Very often, productivity is limited by nonchromatographic issues, such as the availability of system components, or that a certain infrastructure is available and the investment must be utilized. Therefore, a process may be a design, which is not optimal according to the mathematical functions. Determining the optimal productivity is a complex and time-consuming venture. If economic pressure is not too high, it is recommended to operate beyond the optimal/highest productivity limit. Frequently, purification processes are more stable beyond the optimal productivity. The purity ratio is the most important concern; deviations from the process conditions do not imply a change in purity ratio.

Scale-Up Philosophy

Several modes of scale-up are available. Once a process is fixed, it must be ensured that the resolution is maintained at the required level during scale-up. The most important modes of scale-up are as follows: constant height/change in column diameter, constant height-to-diameter ratio (H/D), and changing particle size ($H_2 > H_1$, where H_1 and H_2 are heights of the small and large column).

Constant Height/Change in Column Diameter; Particle Size Is Kept Constant

The conventional way to scale up preparative chromatography is to increase the column diameter using the adsorption/desorption mode, if the bead size is not changed from laboratory scale to preparative scale. The construction of the column inlet is an important feature, if this mode of scale-up is feasible. An even distribution can be achieved by nets and grids placed on the inlet adapter or by small, radially arranged baffles of frit profiles.

Since the packed bed has a higher flow resistance than the column space adjacent to the top of the bed, the liquid first tends to spread over this space with lower flow resistance (see also "System Design for Large-Scale Chromatography"). Nonhomogeneous packings, craters, and clogged frits are the major occurrences that may destroy resolution. Ion-exchange chromatography and affinity chromatography operated with stepwise elution are not very sensitive to changes in column geometry. The finding that the shape of the column has no influence on either the shape of the breakthrough curve (Chase 1986; Johnston et al. 1991), or the peak shape and volume, favors the use of short, wide columns to minimize the pressure drop and process time (Yamamoto et al. 1988; Jungbauer 1993). Linear gradients should be investigated more carefully prior to a change in column geometry. Very often, the column geometry must be changed because the exact size is not commercially available. Custom-made chromatography columns with the exact required volume and column diameter are rare in the biotechnology industry. The following relationships should be obeyed when column geometry is changed.

Linear Gradients. When only the diameter of the column is increased, the volumetric flow rate is increased and the slope of the gradient *(G)* must be decreased to give the same resolution *(R_s)* and retention time *(t_R)*. It is assumed that the large column is stable and that the same packing density and distribution of the liquid over the cross-sectional area of the packed bed can be achieved.

$$\frac{F_{II}}{F_I} = \frac{G_I}{G_{II}} = \frac{A_{II}}{A_I}$$

where *F* is the flow rate, *G* is the gradient steepness, and *A* is the column cross section. The parameter and the variables of the large and small columns are denoted by the subscripts *II* and *I*, respectively. The slope of the linear gradient can be calculated as follows:

$$G = \frac{(I_f - I_0)}{V_G}$$

where I_f is the final ionic strength, I_0 is the initial ionic strength, and V_G is the volume of the gradient.

Stepwise Elution. The only case to be considered is where the operational variables, such as the distribution coefficient of the protein of interest *(K)*, HETP (height equivalent to a theoretical plate), and the ionic strength where the protein is eluted *(I_{elu})* are known. For the method of determining *K*, refer to "Optimization of Running Conditions." If the distribution coefficient of the protein is close to that of the salt, *K'*—not to be confused with the peak capacity *k'*, which is defined as

$$k' = \frac{t_R - t_0}{t_0}$$

then the protein is eluted together with the salt wave (salt front). This type of elution is also called type one or fronting. When *K* is larger than K', the protein is eluted after the salt wave and a type two elution curve is observed.

Especially for the initial purification stages, a type one elution behavior should be selected, if possible. In some cases the nature of the protein solution is composed such that the contaminating material has K values very similar to the protein of interest in the given separation system. In type one elution the protein will be concentrated and it will be eluted after having passed approximately one void volume elution buffer through the column. A rule of thumb for estimating the elution volume is given by the following equation:

$$V_e = F \times t_R = V_0 + K'(V_t - V_0)$$

However, collection of the column effluent must start earlier, because the aforementioned equation describes the elution volume of the peak maximum. The elution volume V_{eII} is only dependent on the change of the cross-sectional area of the column:

$$\frac{V_{eI}}{V_{eII}} = \frac{F_I}{F_{II}} = \frac{A_I}{A_{II}}$$

If the retention time (t_R) remains constant, the overall process time remains constant, since the application of the regeneration solution or equilibration buffers should not consume more time at larger scale.

Type one elution is only suitable when the properties of the protein of interest and the contaminants are sufficiently different. If an appropriate ionic strength for elution is not found, type two elution or a linear gradient should be used. In the case of type two elution, the approximate retention time can be calculated by

$$t_R = \left(\frac{Z}{u}\right) \times \left(1 + H \cdot K_{elu}\right)$$

where Z is the column length, H is the stationary phase ratio

$$\left(H = \frac{1-\varepsilon}{\varepsilon}; \ \varepsilon\text{-void fraction}\right)$$

and K_{elu} is the distribution coefficient at elution. There is no indication that the overall process time should change when the scale of the column is increased only by increasing the column diameter.

Constant Ratio of Column Height and Diameter

Distribution of loaded protein onto the surface of the column may change with scale and, consequently, propagation of peak broadening will occur. Normally, the distribution is affected by the distribution plate, a net, or a grid at the top of the column.

In small-scale RPC, single point injection is commonly employed. In this case, the column size must be increased by a constant height-to-diameter ratio *(H/D)*. In single point injection a certain height of valuable packing is sacrificed for an even distribution of the sample over the cross-sectional area.

In some instances, scale-up processing by just increasing the column diameter is not successful. The loss of resolution may be caused by irregularities in the bed, an unequal distribution of the feed or eluent buffers over the cross-sectional area of the column, or propagation of disturbances in the gel. Vorauer et al. (1992) reported the purification of recombinant superoxide dismutase (SOD) as a model for the scale-up of HIC with constant *H/D*. The cycle time (t_1, t_2) increases with increasing size of the column according to

$$\frac{t_1}{t_2} = \frac{H_1}{H_2}$$

where H_1 and H_2 are the heights of the small and large column, respectively. The volumes of the columns, V_1 and V_2 also change:

$$\frac{V_1}{V_2} = \left(\frac{H_1}{H_2}\right)^3$$

This mode of scale-up should be avoided, if at all possible, since both the relative buffer consumption and the process time are not constant; the bigger the scale, the longer the process time.

Changing the Particle Size

Although sometimes the simple approach *dp/H* = constant was used to scale up with a change in particle diameter, a more versatile solution was needed. When the particle size is changed during scale-up, the column must be changed according to the change of the HETP values of the particle with diameters dp_1 and dp_2. An equation published by Ladish et al. (1991) can be used for rapid calculations:

$$H_1 = H_2 \times \left(\frac{N_1}{N_2}\right) \times \left(\frac{u_1}{u_2}\right) \times \left(\frac{dp_1}{dp_2}\right)^2$$

where N is the number of separation stages, u is the liquid velocity, dp is the particle size, and H is the bed height. Firouztale et al. (1992) show a good agreement between Amberlite XAD-7® and Amberchrom CG71® using the above equation.

Resin Mechanical Stability

Recent developments in chromatography resins have substantially improved their mechanical stability (refer to "Chromatographic Media and Their Use"). In low pressure chromatography the back pressure of a column with 20–30 cm height packed with a 30 μm bead may not exceed 3 bar when the column is operated at a velocity of 500 cm/h. This is an improvement of nearly two orders of magnitude compared to soft gels based on agarose, dextran, trisacryl, or polyacrylamide. The scale-up is no longer limited by the pressure drop of the packed bed when it is operated at high velocities. Moreover, scale-up is limited by practical concerns, such as the cost-effective delivery of a high capacity fluid stream.

An Extra Column Effect

Packed bed reactors (a chromatography column is one of them) are frequently described in terms of ergotic space. Chemical reactors considered as ergotic spaces will have ideal internal flow characteristics. An ergotic space is a system that gives the same residence time distribution (RTD) independent of the measuring method—a step input or a pulse input. A typical chromatography system is not an ergotic space. The system behavior might especially affect the dynamic capacity because different dilutions at the end of loading are observed at different scales. The band broadening of a chromatography system can be measured by a pulse experiment (also known as an injection of a small amount of tracer, usually a salt or a UV-absorbing compound) or by a step input, which is called a frontal analysis or breakthrough curve. Since the pulse input and the step input are related, they can be used for checking the chromatography system when it is scaled up.

The underlying theoretical model says that a rectangular pulse input (Dirac functionlike injection) into a reactor where plug flow occurs will yield a Gaussian distribution curve. This curve is also denoted as C curve. The step input will produce the related distribution function or probability function (sum-curve), which is known as an F curve (Figure 3.6a–b) (Noar and Shinnar 1963).

Figure 3.6 a–b. Residence time of a fluid in a vessel with step input (a) and pulse input (b).

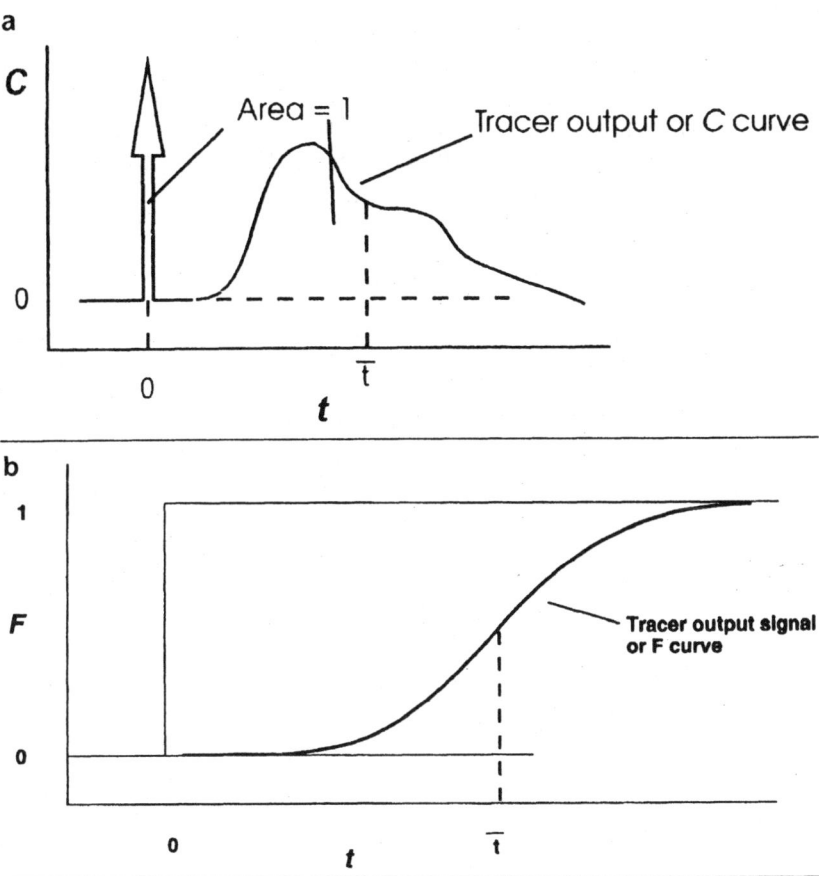

In an ergotic space the derived parameters of the functions should be identical. The first derivation of the F curve gives the C curve:

$$C(t) = \frac{d\left[F(t)\right]}{dt}$$

In an ergotic space the curve should be independent of the tracer concentration and velocity. But that, in fact, never happens.

Knowledge about the boundaries where the chromatography system behaves according to an ergotic space allows changes to the system without being confronted with a change of the peak profile due to external effects.

Once the different scales of a chromatography system are characterized in that manner, the scale-up calculation procedure can also include these changes. This will protect the user from unexpected shifts in peak position, change in dynamic capacity, and change in resolution during scale-up. Mathematical treatment of these theories is not far advanced, due to the fact that the rectangular input curve must be transformed either by a Laplace transformation or by another type of transformation in order to work with a continuous function. Furthermore, for many functions obtained by pulse input and step input, no analytical solution of the Laplace transformation is available (Sternberg 1966).

The theory of RTD and the rate theory are contradictory in their basic assumptions. This contradiction prohibits simple mathematical treatment or even a combination of both theories in order to facilitate the mathematical treatment of scale-up. The rate theory assumes that all peak broadening effects are additive, meaning that the variances of the different processes including extra column effects are also additive.

In the RTD theory the different band broadening mechanisms are multiplying each other. The outcoming C curve theoretically evolves by multiplication of the individual C curves when the system is virtually broken up into different zones where the band broadening occurs (Levenspiel 1962).

$$C_{\text{out}} = C_{\text{in } 1} \times C_{\text{in } 2} \times \dots C_{\text{in } n}$$

One should keep these inconsistencies in mind when a chromatographic system is characterized by a distribution function. When chromatography equipment is bought from a vendor, the customer might check if the chromatography system has certain minimum characteristics concerning the above-mentioned features. For example, the checklist may include the following:

- Minimum number of connections
- Knowledge of extra column volume
- Minimum restrictions in the tubing cross sections
- Low dead volume in the column (heads, piston)

- Knowledge of mixer characteristics
- Knowledge of behavior of an inert sample passing through the system

"System Design for Large-Scale Chromatography" provides more information on equipment design.

Large Bed Volumes

It may be more economical to operate two large columns in parallel than to operate an "extra-large" column. The weight and size of the extra-large type column might make it difficult to move and pack. The extra-large control and monitoring devices may not be available or the specification of flow rates may be out of range. Special design and extra validation may be necessary. Design and maintenance could become very expensive. Spare parts are not easily available and must be custom manufactured in some cases.

SYSTEM DESIGN FOR LARGE–SCALE CHROMATOGRAPHY

General Requirements

The large-scale manufacturing system usually does not have the versatility and flexibility of the process development workstation/ pilot unit. Such features are not needed since the process(es) to be conducted using the particular system is typically in the final stage of implementation (e.g., is developed to a point, where no serious changes may be anticipated). Therefore, the industrial system typically is developed from a successful scale-up of an already known process. This also includes satisfactory mechanical performance, which allows implementation of the purification concept. The software performance requirement is to make the mechanical part of the system function properly and in a repeatable fashion. The software must also fulfill a requirement of handling the manufacturing documentation; to a certain degree, it should also have a capability of data analysis.

System performance depends on system hydrodynamic design parameters combined with the molecular interactions between solutes and the stationary phase. An important factor in system performance is the resulting dispersion of solute bands. A recent review on dispersion of solutes in chromatographs and reactors was published by Balakotaiah and Chang (1995). Recent references and those most relevant among the earlier are listed. A paper by Wisniewski (1992) can serve as a supplementary reading on system design and provides an extensive list of references on the subject of large-scale high performance liquid chromatography (HPLC).

System Components

The major system components are the packed chromatographic column, the pumping system, the buffer delivery system, the elution/gradient forming system, detectors, fraction collection, and instrumentation/controls. Other subsystems, which may or may not be separate entities, are sample loading, the mixing chamber(s), the pulsation damper(s), and the bubble removal trap (Figure 3.7).

System components must have material compatibility with the product and all the process buffers and cleaning agents used. The design of individual components should comply with GMP requirements. Sanitary aspects of the mechanical design must be emphasized. This includes the proper selection of materials and surface finishes, the lack of crevices and dead pockets, and the use of proper radii to ensure flow patterns for adequate velocity and the penetration of cleaning agents (Timperley et al. 1992, 379–393). The finishes of metallic surfaces should be polished to at least "finish 4" (polished with 150–180 grit abrasive) or better (frequently 220 grit or better abrasive is used). The surface finish may be expressed in a more objective way (e.g., by use of profiling instru-

Figure 3.7. Block schematics showing system components.

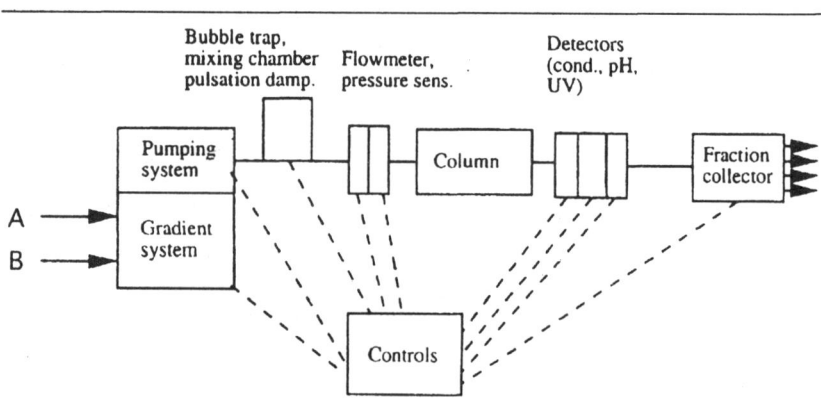

ments) and giving the readings in an arithmetic average (Ra) or root-mean-square (RMS) scale, with the RMS scale giving about 11 percent higher readings. Mechanical polishing using 180 grit abrasive gives a surface with Ra = 0.5–0.8 μm. High quality, sanitary finishes may have Ra values of about 0.1 to 0.25 μm. Electropolishing produces a smooth, mirrorlike surface; it is frequently applied as a final finishing step. While mechanical polishing removes metal particles leaving burrs and smears on the surface, electropolishing removes these tiny burrs and smears as well as smooths sharp microedges and micropeaks on the surface. Attention should also be paid to the surface state of nonmetallic components (no cavities, crevices, surface defects, or rough areas are allowed). Particular attention should be paid to the gaskets and static and dynamic seal design. Traditional industrial approaches (Brink et al. 1993) may not assure needed sanitary features, and special designs of sanitary seals should be employed (Wisniewski 1988, 11–21). If O-rings are used, they should have special grooves, located very close to the edge

Users should pay attention not only to the components to be purchased to build an in-house–designed system, but also to the components offered by a system vendor. Users may ask a vendor to fulfill a certain concept of the chromatographic system, and may require that certain components be used in system design. Insistence on particular components may increase the system cost, but might be beneficial in the long run if the components are compatible with those used in the user's manufacturing company. Frequently, users may have a preference regarding components from particular vendors based on past experience of performance and service. Current state of the art for commercial systems provides users with quality design and only process-related modifications may be required.

Column Design

Columns for Stationary Beds

A chromatography column contains a chromatographic medium (stationary phase), the key element of the separation process. Industrial-scale chromatography columns differ from analytical and preparative columns in many ways. The design of liquid distribution heads is very important due to large column diameters (up to 2 m). Since the packing step is usually performed in the field, a special arrangement of ports is needed; a moving head is very beneficial in accomplishing uniform internal bed configuration. Axial columns with an axially moving head are used most often in industry, although axial columns with fixed heads or columns with radial flow (Rice and Heft 1991) are also used.

In large diameter columns liquid flow distribution and the uniformity of the packed bed are two major factors affecting the quality of separation. The designs of fluid distributors may include several entry points into the column head. The performance of short-packed columns and columns consisting of membranes (Coffman et al. 1994) may be particularly sensitive to flow distribution quality. Production chromatography resins come with a certain range of particle size distribution. Since fines may be present, users should perform a fines separation step (such separation can be done by sedimentation).

The packing procedure, which may involve resins of a wide range of particle size, should ensure thorough mixing and homogeneity of the slurry prior to packing. Magnetic bar mixers are not recommended since they may damage resin beads and create fines due to the mechanical contact between the vessel bottom and the rotating bar; they may occasionally decouple from the drive and stall, causing mixing to cease and particle settling. At uniform particle size sedimentation packing may provide high packing densities (Wang et al. 1990; Porsch 1994). In the case of nonuniform particle size, pumping or pouring the slurry of resin beads into the column should be performed in uniform fashion to ensure bed homogeneity. Rapidly settling, uniform particles produce a good quality bed with no significant size segregation. A theoretical sedimentation rate of solid spherical particles can be determined from the Stokes equation. This equation is, however, valid for the infinite or close to infinite dilution (Batchelor 1972). Sedimentation of porous particles, at high slurry density and certain size distribution, cannot be described by the original Stokes equation. Batchelor (1982) and Batchelor and Wen (1982) used a rigorous analytical approach to sedimentation of dilute interacting polydisperse spheres. A review of sedimentation problems involving monodisperse and polydisperse particles was given by Davis and Acrivos (1985). One of the recently proposed equations (Vissers et al. 1995) applicable to chromatographic packing is as follows:

$$v = \frac{(1-\Phi)^{-K_2} \times dp^2 \times (\rho_s - \rho_v) \times (1-\varepsilon) \times g}{18 \times \eta}$$

where v is the sedimentation rate, Φ is the volume fraction of the particles, K_2 is the particle/solvent-dependent constant, ρ_s and ρ_v are the solid and liquid densities, η is the liquid viscosity, ϵ is the particle porosity

$$\varepsilon = \left(\frac{V_{pore}}{V_{pore} + \dfrac{1}{\rho_s}} \right),$$

with V_{pore} being the total pore volume per particle unit mass), and g is the gravitational constant. One must note that the particle diameter is squared (e.g., uniform sedimentation may be ensured at narrow particle size distribution, while at wide range of particle size, segregation may occur due to the faster settling of larger particles). One must ensure conditions of uniform sedimentation without hydrodynamic disturbances when pouring the slurry into the column.

A large range of particle size distribution may cause partial loss of capacity (an earlier bed breakthrough) and peak broadening during the separation due to diffusional effects the solutes undergo in intraparticular pores prior to binding and after elution. Therefore, one should select the stationary phase with regular spherical particles with as narrow as possible range of particle size distribution.

The flow path of the liquid phase depends on the initial flow distribution and to a certain degree on the outlet collector design; however, the most important factor determining the flow path is the packed bed itself. Initial uniform flow distribution may be accomplished by dividing the stream and delivering its parts to certain areas, uniformly located across the bed surface, or by employing a uniform grid/screen with a resistance to flow, which is large enough to cause the uniform flow of liquid regardless of inlet conditions. Usually, a carefully designed flow distributor is used, but a combination of both principles can also be applied. If a single liquid entry port is used, the jet deflecting device is placed prior to the screen. If the pressure drop across the screen is significantly lower than the pressure drop across the packed bed, then the bed itself becomes a flow distributor. Polymer screens/meshes, as well as sintered metal plates, have been used in industrial columns for bed support and flow distribution. A test of the quality of flow distribution by the column head alone could involve the pumping of the liquid through a very shallow packed bed, or with no bed at all. Such tests could also indicate to what degree the bed itself (at its working height) plays a role in flow distribution.

Since in typical large columns the major resistance to the fluid flow (pressure drop) occurs in the bed of the chromatographic medium, uniform packing is of utmost importance to ensure quality of separation. Any nonuniformities within the bed (such as densely and loosely packed volumes, or voids) may significantly affect the flow pattern and adversely affect the chromatographic peak shape (e.g., the quality of separation). The issues of fluid flow and dispersion phenomena in packed beds are well described in the literature. More recent publications are works by Koch and Brady (1985), Magnico and Martin (1990), and Salles et al. (1993). Lee and Ogawa (1994) proposed a new correlation for the pressure drop in packed beds and compared it to the widely used Ergun equation. The new equation was more accurate than the Ergun equation in predicting the pressure drop at higher Reynolds numbers, while at lower Reynolds numbers its accuracy was comparable.

The traditional approach to packed bed porosity distribution accounts for the wall effect, in which the bed voidage is affected by the wall up to five particle diameters, and beyond this zone the bed voidage becomes uniform (Benenati and Brosilow 1962). There are conflicting reports on bed uniformity in chromatographic columns (Knox and Parcher 1969; Knox et al. 1976; Baur et al. 1988; Farkas et al. 1994), but the packing wall effect per se may not affect large-scale separations due to the very large column/bead diameter ratio. Recently, Yun and Guiochon (1994) proposed a model for radial heterogeneity in chromatography columns. In chromatography columns the packing voidage distribution caused by the wall may reach beyond the five particle diameter zone due to conditions employed during packing procedures. Most probably, the bed uniformity variations are caused by the method by which the column is being packed. As a result, radial and axial bed nonuniformities may occur.

In axially compressed columns there are two factors to be considered during bed formation: (1) friction between the wall and the bed particles and (2) an internal friction among the particles within the bed. The granular material parameters are the angle of repose and the angle of internal friction. Characteristics of granular material in the column include the material/column wall friction coefficient and the angle of friction of the material and the wall (Harr 1977). Such information will be useful for the analysis of compressed columns; however, it is not easily available for chromatographic packings. Readily available data are for soils and typical granular materials. For example, for round quartz particles the angle of repose is about 36–38°, the angle of internal friction is 42–45°, and the particle/steel angle of friction is about 25°. Wet packing of axially compressed columns may use a multiple press and relieve packing pattern. This might yield a bed of better uniformity than a single press stroke. Sarkar and Guiochon (1995) reviewed packing behavior in axially compressed columns of 50 mm internal diameter. Column performance was long lasting, with no significant degradation. Bed height was declining due to bed consolidation (e.g., decrease in bed porosity). The phenomena of such bed settling, combined with wall support effects and interparticle friction within the bed, may be analyzed using an approach of mechanics of granular materials, particularly during the early stages of compression when piston travel is most pronounced.

The influence of wall friction effects decreases with an increase in column diameter. Large-scale HPLC columns, which employ a permanent axial pressure on the moving head, may experience a bed of rigid particles settling by several millimeters after a few runs. Radial compression is another way to provide better bed uniformity (Eon 1978). Sarker and Guiochon (1994) reported on the high stability of radially compressed columns and on the ability of this technology to restore the performance of columns suffering from channeling. Annular expansion columns are another form of the radial compression technology with additional axial compression effects. A tapered central rod is axially pressed through the packed bed, combining the radial and axial compression effects.

Low pressure columns are typically packed by sedimentation, with a subsequent lowering of the upper head. Packing quality may also be affected by the shape of particles (regular or irregular, uniform size, or with certain size distribution). Particle shape effects are further discussed in "Chromatographic Media and Their Use." The quality of packing may be tested by the use of a nonadsorbing tracer in the form of a short spike (Dirac functionlike) introduced on the column inlet side and monitored by the system or external detector (Lameloise and Viard 1994). Acetone may be used as a tracer. The shape of the outlet peak may indicate flow pattern deviations. Diffusional effects for porous beads must be taken under consideration during the interpretation of results. Recently, Baumeister et al. (1995) described a method to determine the radial and axial dispersion coefficients in chromatographic columns using pulsed field gradient nuclear magnetic resonance. The approach to packing testing and validation is further described in "Validation."

The most common design for a flow distribution device is a column head central inlet with deflector and radially cut grooves (Figure 3.8). The volume occupied by a liquid within the grooves should

Figure 3.8. Flow distribution device of an UpScale® column (BioSepra S.A., France).

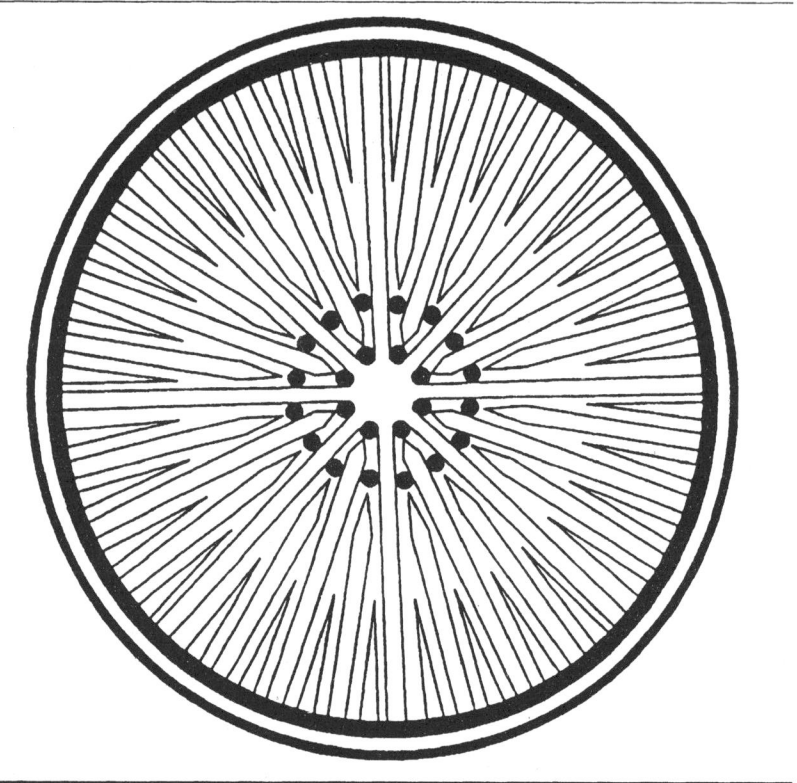

be minimized and may be optimized along the column radius (e.g., depth of grooves decreasing along the radius). The upper, axially moving head construction must provide room for the circumferential seal and the mounting ring for screen support. Column manufacturers design the upper head to ensure a pluglike flow through the whole column cross section. Typical designs have a narrow mounting ring on the head circumference next to the gasket. The result of this ring presence may be a small circumferential no-flow volume at the top of the packed bed. An influence of this ring depends on the column diameter in the standardized design and is more pronounced for smaller diameter columns (the percentage of the column cross section occupied by this ring is higher at smaller diameters). Negative effects can be seen at low bed heights. At higher beds this effect diminishes. Column manufacturers try to design the columns with this unswept edge area as small as possible, or eliminate it completely. One of the designs (BioSepra S.A., France) features a flow around the head edge, with an elastic sealing gasket far removed from the liquid distribution plate.

The distribution of liquid through multiple points may be an advisable solution for large diameter columns. The locations of the points should be symmetrical and offset from radius to radius. The areas of fittings or plate holes (their numbers or size) should increase proportionally to the radii. In the columns with an axially moving head, the seal design is of importance, since it should not only seal but also not allow beads to penetrate into the seal and cause damage during head movements. Column mechanical design with the upper moving head becomes complicated at large diameters due to the required head/column dimensional tolerances; head movement uniform guidance is needed to assure upper plate correct position against both the column walls and bottom plate. One design (BioSepra S.A.) facilitates head movements by the application of an inflatable seal. In such a design the dimensional tolerances between the moving head and the column internal diameter are not critical and can be large (thus making machining easier), since the seal adjusts itself to the proper geometry.

Since the major flow resistance occurs within the packed bed, the outlet collector cannot be used to correct flow deviations, and its flow pattern would reflect the pattern on the bed outlet. The stationary outlet head can be designed differently from the moving inlet head (e.g., without an inner seal and screen mounting ring protruding into the column). The gasket and ring may have an inner diameter equal to the internal column diameter (i.e., there is no unswept area and liquid can flow through the whole column cross section). Uniform flow in the collector is required and no mixing should occur in the liquid volume contained in the collecting head. While certain liquid mixing volumes may be acceptable on the inlet to the column, they should be avoided on the outlet side where they may negatively affect the quality of separation.

Current large-scale columns with transparent walls (glass or acrylic) are rated for higher operating pressures than past designs (pressures as high as 60–120 psi or 4–8 bars can be used in the process). Higher pressure ratings can be achieved by the use of metal column designs. High pressure rating facilitates the use of more efficient packing materials (e.g., of smaller diameter and of high flow type). Use of higher pressures may reduce the choice of the pumping unit to the diaphragm pump (see also "Pumping System").

Column setting requires knowledge of the stationary phase physical stability (whether it has any compressibility, or what the cracking pressure limit is for hard particles) and swelling properties. This information is available from stationary phase manufacturers. Columns are packed using preswollen beads. If the bed of particles demonstrates varying swelling during the process, additional internal pressure might develop inside the column if the heads are fixed and no void is left to compensate for bed volume changes. Fortunately, many modern stationary phases swell little if at all. Properties of chromatographic stationary phases are described in detail in "Chromatographic Media and Their Use."

Short, large diameter columns with fixed heads are difficult to pack in situ, due to problems with uniform resin delivery in the column cross section. Simple pumping of the resin slurry into such columns using a single port may not provide sufficient filling of the column with resin. Multiple ports may be needed, which might also be combined with reversed liquid flow pulses applied during the packing procedure. Due to these difficulties, typical packing procedures call for the removal of the column head. A design of large diameter (1.4 m), fixed head columns applied for gel filtration chromatography have been used in a stacked configuration of three beds (Pharmacia 1995). In this design liquid is introduced into the top head at four points. High strength, multilayered metal nets with uniform porosity were used for bed support and liquid distribution. Minimum dead zone sanitary gaskets were especially designed for this type of column. Packing was performed by a suction method followed by removal of the packing device and installation of the column head. This concept of a fixed head column with a three column-in-series configuration has been tested by checking the peak symmetry and determination of HETP. Peak symmetry was high, and for three columns in series the asymmetry was about 1.18. While the numbers of theoretical separation plates per 1 m of bed length for individual columns were 5782, 4368, and 4193, the number for three columns in series was 3336. This result points out the importance of system design and flow patterns in the interconnecting piping system (see "Piping and Valves" and "Hardware"). Decline in performance was possibly caused by the design of diaphragm valves used and the configuration of the flow path between the columns.

The columns with head positions fixed after packing may develop voids in the bed in the vicinity of the inlet distributor. Such voids may decrease column performance if they act as liquid mixing·

zones. This effect may be more pronounced for columns using fast flow resins (e.g., at high linear liquid velocities). The distributor design should permit uniform liquid distribution without local velocity differences that may cause internal liquid mixing in the voids. Columns with dynamic compression reduce the potential of developing such problems. The voids may be compensated by the head movement; the flow distributor design may play a less critical role if its screen remains in touch with the compressed bed, since the bed itself would act as an efficient flow distributor.

Large size, radial flow columns made of stainless steel have been recently introduced. Radial columns frequently operate at lower bed thickness than axial designs, although the liquid flow rates can be very high. High flow rates, combined with relatively thin beds, may demand more frequent cycling of the column. Straetkvern et al. (1991) compared performance of axial and radial columns and described the methodology of scale-up.

An emerging technique of chromatography separations are adsorptive membranes (Roper and Lightfoot 1995). However, some of the current designs experience flow nonuniformity, dead spaces, and extra-column dispersion. Single flat, spiral, or hollow fiber flow-through membranes represent small loading capacities and are sensitive to the nonuniformity of flow. Stacked, flat membranes packed in columns provide better separation and have higher total capacity.

Columns for Expanded Beds

Special attention should be focused on columns designed for expanded beds. The expanded bed column concept imposes a different set of design and performance requirements. The stationary phase should be of high density, monodisperse, and within a certain size range (further details are given in "Chromatographic Media and Their Use"). Since the bed works in an expanded state, the role of the flow distributor/supporting plate, which is located at the column bottom, is even more important than in the case of packed beds (Asif et al. 1991). The flow distribution must be uniform enough to avoid any expanded bed disturbances. Air bubbles must be removed prior to the column. Flow pulsations must be avoided, to prevent disturbances and internal mixing within the expanded bed. The column has an axially movable upper head, since the elution is typically performed in a compressed packed bed. If an elution is carried downward, then the flow distributor design adds a requirement of minimizing liquid volume in the space below the bed. Elution from the expanded bed column has usually been carried downward (opposite to loading), but it could also be performed in the same direction as loading. Then the top head becomes a flow collector and should be designed to minimize liquid volume contained in the head. Such solution may permit more flexibility in designing the bottom flow distributor (the volume of liquid within the distributor and the flow pattern there would not be as critical to elution peak quality as in the collector). However, if only a simple product adsorption/desorption is involved (as, for example, in affinity chromatography), then the liquid volume in the collector head is not as critical as in the case of gradient elution, since the eluted product is visible as a separate wide band and not as a peak–in other chromatographic techniques such a peak usually comes with the adjacent impurities on both sides. Additional mixing volume in the flow collector would only slightly affect the sides of such bands (making them less sharp).

The liquid distributor must have a capability of passing cells and cell debris without clogging (i.e., characteristics of its open area and porosity must be carefully evaluated [Draeger and Chase 1991]). The requirement of sufficiently large openings may need to be combined with a requirement for a certain pressure drop for even liquid distribution. Changes in the distributor pressure drop can be accomplished by applying distributors with different open areas at the same size of pores or holes. Bed-distributor interactions under working conditions, and the testing of such interactions at varying liquid velocities and bed depths, may be conducted in addition to testing for the uniformity of flow distribution without the bed present. Uniform flow under such conditions may assure uniform bed expansion, minimum disturbances of the expanded bed and liquid flow through the bed approaching the plug flow pattern. This check may be supplemented with a test, using only a thin layer of expanding/ fluidizing beads. Dyes could be injected upstream of the flow distributor and flow pattern observed in the liquid-only–filled column. Such tests may visually indicate any local flow nonuniformities. Rigorous testing of liquid velocity distribution may involve a hot film sensor or laser Doppler anemometry. Recently, Kuperman et al. (1995) proposed a new technique for the examination of phenomena occurring within the moving granular beds by using magnetic resonance imaging.

The stability of an expanded/fluidized bed depends not only on flow distributor design and performance but also on the operating conditions. Factors such as liquid viscosity and density, liquid velocity, and particle size and density all may affect the stability of the fluidized bed. Even at very uniform flow distribution, the bed may possess inherent instabilities. Foscolo and Gibilaro (1984) proposed a simple correlation for fluidized bed instability based on the particle Reynolds number. Batchelor (1988) proposed a theoretical approach to fluidized bed instability and related it to the Froude number. He concluded that the bed may become unstable above a certain Froude number. The Froude number is defined as follows:

$$Fr = \frac{8\rho_p}{3 \times \rho_f \times \gamma \times C_d}$$

where ρ_p is the particle density, ρ_f is the fluid density, C_d is the drag coefficient, and

$$\gamma = \frac{V}{F_h} \times \frac{\delta F_h}{\delta V} = \text{constant}$$

where V is the mean particle velocity and F_h is the mean force acting on a particle.

Later Foscolo et al. (1989) linked the stability criterion to the expanded bed voidage (bed expansion) in addition to liquid velocity, particle size, and media densities. For 2.5 mm glass beads fluidized in water, the stability limit was reached at voidage of about 0.65–0.68.

Johansson and Wnukowski (1992) investigated the hydrodynamic stability of liquid fluidized beds composed of small particles at Reynolds numbers < 1. The column diameter was 50 mm and bed voidage range was 0.6–0.85. The authors concluded that the Peclet number remains constant within the investigated range of parameters. The Peclet number is defined as follows:

$$Pe = \frac{u \cdot L}{D_z}$$

where u is the fluid velocity, L is the dimension (particle size), and D_z is a dispersion coefficient. Small Peclet numbers (close to zero) suggest an almost perfect mixing, while very large Peclet numbers (approaching infinity) indicate a plug flow.

Monitoring bed expansion and location of its upper level can be important when the liquid phase characteristics (such as viscosity or density) change. A level monitoring sensor can be installed at the bed top and become a part of a control concept (e.g., the pumping flow rate may be controlled by bed expansion). The flow is adjusted to maintain a steady bed top level.

De Luca et al. (1994) described a design of the flow distributors for expanded bed columns. The authors also investigated process dynamics and stability at changing characteristics of the liquid (viscosity change may significantly affect process stability). Yang and Goto (1993) described a process of affinity purification of fluidized beds in a tapered column. The authors claimed advantages of the tapered bed over the fluidized bed (e.g., breakthrough curves for the tapered bed were closer to those of the fixed bed than in the case of a fluidized bed). Elution curves approached those for the fixed bed. Pressure drop across the tapered fluidized bed was significantly lower than for the fixed bed. DiFelice et al. (1991) reported on the expansion characteristics of tapered fluidized beds. For the diverging taper they observed an increase in axial mixing due to the instabilities associated with the increase in bed density toward the top of the column. Use of tapered, expanded beds might provide a stability margin for the process if liquid properties suddenly change (such as a change in density or viscosity). The cost of tapered columns will be, however, higher than the cylindrical ones.

Fluidizing beds may also be stabilized by the use of magnetic fields. Recent work by Goto et al. (1995) reports that axial dispersion in magnetically stabilized expanded beds is comparable to the packed bed and smaller than for the fluidizing bed (for example, for Re = 0.5, the value of 1/Peclet is about 2 versus 10, respectively). Magnetic bed stabilization may become a technical problem for larger column diameters (size and weight of the coils, heat generation, etc.). Goto and colleagues used 20 mm ID column and the coil ID was 68 mm.

Usually, the expanded bed columns have been operated in configurations using large bed height-to-diameter ratio. However, the bed height may be limited if there is an elution step conducted in the compressed packed bed, and pressure is of concern (the pumping system and the column for expanded beds do not need high pressure ratings). This may not be a concern for the large particles with a solid core, since they give low pressure drop in the packed bed and have advantageous diffusional properties (controlled thickness of a porous layer); therefore, a fast flow gradient elution may be performed successfully. Expanded bed column design becomes a challenge for large diameter columns. The difficult requirement is to ensure steady and uniform flow of liquid and avoid any significant internal mixing within the bed. A combination of flow distribution means can be applied (e.g., the radial flow distributor and the screen plate with a certain pressure drop may ensure adequate pluglike liquid flow uniformity). The bed presence may also affect the uniformity of liquid flow when compared to the empty column due to bed-distributor hydrodynamic interactions.

Pumping System Before and After the Column

Pumping System

The performance of the pumping system is critical to the performance of the chromatography plant. The flow rate should follow a preprogrammed pattern regardless of changes in operational conditions, such as liquid viscosity and density change, or changing flow resistance.

There are several possible design solutions for the pumping system. The first step should be a determination of pump type. The selection of pump type depends on the flow rate, the required pressure, the required accuracy, the types of liquids to be pumped, sanitary/aseptic needs, and the applied control concept. The last factor may not be obvious at this stage of design, but an adequately designed control system should ensure desired flow patterns even if the pump alone behaves in a fashion strongly dependent on liquid properties and system back pressure. The selection of the pumping system may also depend on the applied concept of elution (e.g., gradient elution, step elution, or a combination of both).

Due to the low flow rates and relatively high system back pressures, the type of pump used in large-scale liquid chromatography systems is based on the positive displacement principle. The most common types of pumps used in modern, large-scale chromatography systems are the diaphragm pump and the lobe pump. Peristaltic pumps (Jaffrin and Shapiro 1971) cannot handle elevated pressures, and the limit of system back pressure may not exceed 25–30 psi (1.7–2.0 bar), although a small-scale peristaltic pump may pump against higher back pressures. Liquid delivery rates may drift from an original set point due to changes in flexible tubing characteristics occurring during operation. Peristaltic pumps might work with expanded bed columns due to the low pressures usually needed for these applications; however, the flow pulsations they generate may not be acceptable or may require dampening. Gear pumps may not be used because of their nonsanitary features and cleaning difficulties as well as the dependency of their performance on system back pressure. When considering any special or novel pump design, users should check the overall reliability, sanitary design aspects, practical cleanability, contamination potential, performance sensitivity to back pressure, liquid properties, range of flow rate, maximum available pressure, and level of flow pulsation. Examples of pump design concepts with potential in the chromatography field are the pump with sinusoidal rotor shape (its seal-less version) and the screw pump (in a rotor-stator configuration, or with independently driven, noncontact screw-type rotors). These pumps may provide approximately pulseless flow. However, the sinusoidal rotor pump may not be able to handle high back pressures. The performance of the pumping system should have little dependency on liquid characteristics and system back pressure (e.g., it should deliver required amounts of liquid in a predictable and repeatable fashion).

There are two approaches to ensure well-controlled fluid flow: (1) rely on the pump performance and its calibration or (2) rely on the pump-flowmeter-controller system. The first concept was derived from high precision laboratory instrumentation. Only high precision positive displacement diaphragm metering pumps may be used, since flow control is based on the open control loop concept (no feedback is received about flow rate). Maintaining high precision of liquid delivery using preset pumping systems in large scale without a flow control loop might make the system expensive due to the need for a very high quality pump. Further, frequent system adjustments and calibrations may be needed to maintain repeatable pump performance. Operational systems will lack the capability of complete run documentation since the flow rate in time history would not be recorded and only operator entries might provide data on average approximate flows (by measuring volumes processed in time) and on calibration data.

The second concept (the closed loop using flowmeter signal as a feedback) poses lesser demands on the pump itself, but requires more sophisticated controls. Additional requirements imposed on a chromatography system using the metering pump are the need for continuous flow and minimized pulsations. The continuous flow requirement eliminates the whole array of low cost, solenoid-driven metering pumps. The motor-driven pump remains a choice. Multiple pump heads and/or pulsation dampers must be applied to ensure pulseless performance of the pumping system. There are two possible ways to reduce pulsations: (1) increase the number of pump heads or (2) apply a pulsation damper after the pump (and sometimes on the pump inlet side, depending on piping configuration). A pump with a single head has a separate suction and discharge stroke; even with the use of a pulsation damper, the flow pattern may still be unsatisfactory. The double head (duplex) pump combined with the pulsation damper may provide satisfactory performance. The triple head pump (triplex) pump may give a satisfactory performance with a pulsation damper of limited capacity or even without a pulsation damper since its peak flow is $\pi/3$ (1.0472) times the average flow, and the flow variations are between 86.6 percent at minimum pulse flow rate to 100 percent at full maximum pulse flow rate (Figure 3.9).

Positive displacement pumps with rapid suction and slow discharge, although used in liquid chromatography laboratory instruments, have not yet found a place in industrial systems. Check valves in diaphragm pumps not only require periodic maintenance, but they also may cause problems such as worn seats or broken springs (in the spring-loaded valves). An additional negative aspect is the possibility of check valve wear material entering the process stream. Users should inspect the available check valve designs offered by a pump manufacturer and select the valves with the best sanitary features.

The pump diaphragm can be driven directly by mechanical linkage or indirectly by hydraulic fluid that is driven by a separate plunger. The mechanically driven diaphragms may be used for lower pressures (below 300 psi, or 20 bar) since they can deform under one side acting liquid pressure, causing pump accuracy to deteriorate. Hydraulically driven diaphragms can operate at very high pressures with pump accuracy unaffected since there is a force equilibrium condition on the diaphragm (Vetter et al. 1993). Diaphragm pumps can operate at high pressures, but there are limitations on the maximum flow rate. For higher flow rates (arbitrarily estimated at above 1.5–2.0 L/min), pump heads must be large (large diaphragm diameter), or multiple heads must be used; as a result, the overall pump cost increases. The diaphragm pump may incorporate a double diaphragm design (a sandwich type) with the diaphragm rupture sensing system. Considering the high value of proteinaceous products, such protection is highly recommended since it protects the product from being contaminated by hydraulic fluid and provides an instant indication of diaphragm failure.

The pump flow rate control concept must be considered together with the pump design selection. Rotation of the pump motor cannot be lower than a certain percentage of nominal speed, which is usually in the range of 10–20 percent. Recent reviews by Slemon (1994) and by Baliga (1994) describe types of motors used with variable frequency drives and semiconductor-based variable frequency drives. Slower motor speeds may be obtained using designs other

Figure 3.9. Flow pulsations vs. number of heads.

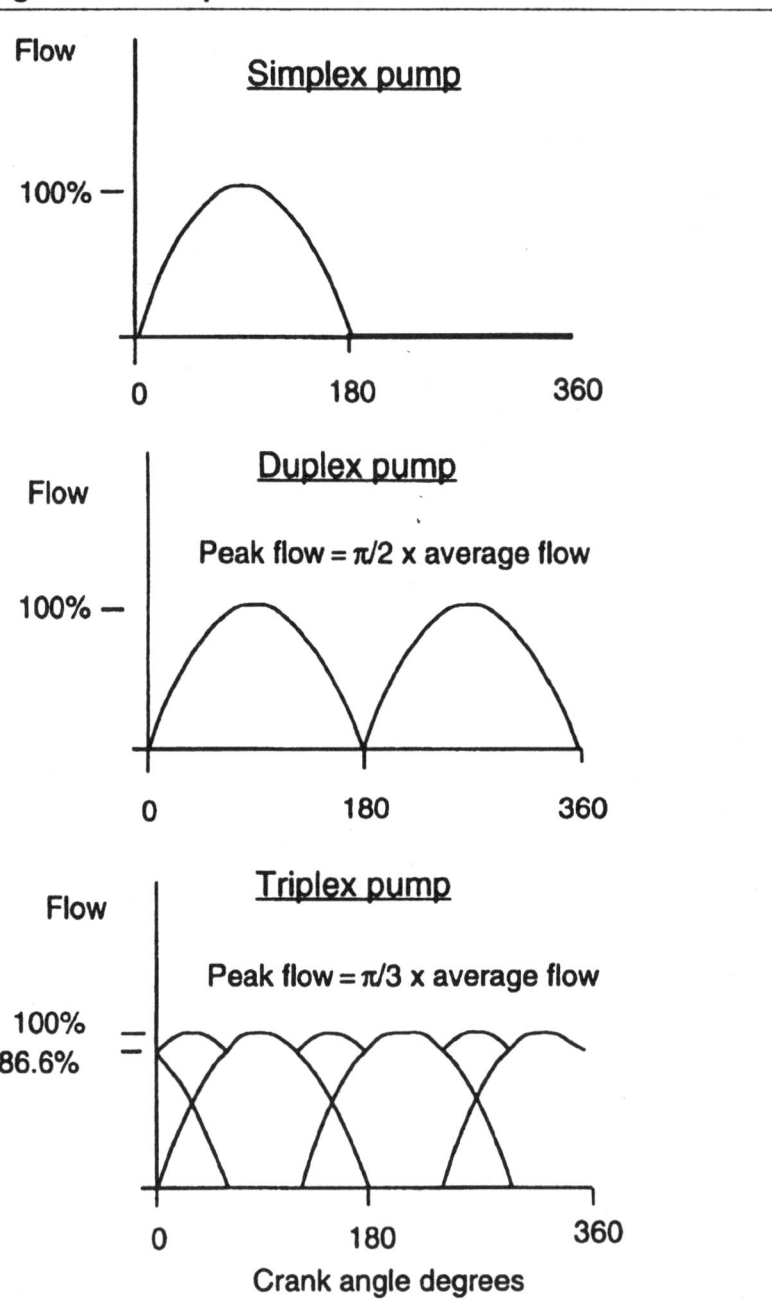

than standard AC motors (i.e., DC motors or stepping motors). Stepping motors can be operated at very low rotational speeds. Stepping motor technology has reached its maturity; economic, very accurate drive designs may provide good performance for lower flow rate systems. Since exact information on motor rotation and the rotor position in time is available, a properly calibrated pump may provide a lasting, high precision performance.

Stepping motor technology is also recommended for the automatic setting of actuators for the stroke control of metering pumps (it can provide higher precision than the typical electromechanical or pneumatic actuator designs). Linear stepping actuators of high accuracy are readily available. A traditional diaphragm pump with check valves cannot be operated in a well-controlled fashion below a certain level of shaft rotational speed and below a certain minimum stroke length (Wisniewski 1992). This is due to the performance characteristics of the diaphragm and check valves. The pump's mechanical characteristics (structural rigidity, dimensional tolerances) may also affect its accuracy. A pump with a diaphragm driven by an internal hydraulic circuit has its accuracy at low flow rates adversely affected by the presence of this circuit, fluid compressibility, the performance of internal valves, and so on. Diaphragm pumps may have unacceptable accuracy and repeatability at very low flow rates if the controlled flow depends on pump frequency (motor rotation) and an externally preset stroke length (manually, or using an electric or pneumatic actuator). Therefore, the introduction of a flowmeter controller may be necessary. The control system may vary the pump flow rate by changing the motor speed and the stroke length. The common approach to flow control has been to maintain the fixed stroke length and change the motor speed. Accuracy of the flowmeter controller system must be investigated since it may worsen at low flow rates. A combination of both poor accuracy of the flowmeter controller and inaccuracy of the pump at low flow rates may not provide an overall satisfactory solution (see also "Monitoring and Controls"). An accurate record of flow rates in time and preprogrammed flow patterns may be maintained in a properly designed system regardless of changing operational parameters, such as liquid characteristics or system back pressure.

Reciprocating pumps may have various maximum displacements per stroke depending on diaphragm design. To minimize pulsations, a shorter stroke and a smaller displacement volume can be selected. For a given volumetric flow the pump would then operate at shorter stroke and higher frequency. Long stroke diaphragm bellows or plunger pumps may generate pulses that may not be easily reduced by a small-volume pulsation damper. However, the combined design of a bubble trap, a gradient mixing chamber, and a pulsation damper may have volumes large enough to compensate for pulsations caused by longer pump strokes. Since flowmeter performance may be adversely affected by pulsations, the flowmeter should be positioned after the pulsation dampening chamber. The level of pulsation should be determined during system testing using a high frequency response pressure sensor. Shoikhet and Engelhardt (1994) proposed a photometric method to characterize pulsations in HPLC pumps.

The second approach to pump selection for industrial chromatography systems working at moderate pressures is to apply a double rotor, lobe type pump. Since there is no contact between the rotors or the rotors and the walls, this pump design may eliminate worn structural particulate material from entering the product stream. The pump does not have check valves, and this factor eliminates one of the possible trouble spots. Pulsation can be minimized by rotor design; therefore, no multiple pump heads or additional pulsation dampers are needed. Lobe pumps may have double, triple, or quintuple lobe rotors, with better flow uniformity reached at higher numbers of lobes.

A lobe-type rotary pump should be used in combination with a flowmeter. The pump alone is not recommended since flow rates would vary if the back pressure changes. The characteristics of lobe pumps are strongly dependent on liquid viscosity and back pressure due to minute leaks that occur through the gaps between the rotors and the pump walls. At high back pressures, this so-called slip backflow may reach a large proportion of the total flow. In such cases, the pump, even at high revolutions, can move much less liquid than its theoretical displacement indicates. Indeed, under such conditions the pump may act as an efficient mixing device. A pump working under certain back pressures may, therefore, perform as an additional mixer in a design with low pressure, gradient-mixing systems. However, the pump volume and the slip backflow should be carefully evaluated to provide sufficient volumetric mixing. Performance of buffer-switching valves in front of the pump may significantly affect such an approach to system design. The task may be difficult in the first place since pump mixing characteristics would change with a change in system back pressure; therefore, installing a mixing chamber is advisable. The mixing chamber may be installed in front of or after the pump.

Lobe pumps can be obtained with various dimensional toler-ances (gap sizes between rotors and walls). The largest tolerances are used in the sterilize-in-place (SIP) (up to 125°C) pumps. Since chromatography systems are not steam sterilized and operate at am-bient temperatures, standard or small tolerance rotors are usually selected. Lobe pumps can be equipped with a pressure relief cover, which provides an internal fluid recirculation if flow passage after the pump is blocked. Due to small dimensional tolerances and the existence of a slip backflow, lobe pumps should be protected from any fine particulate material that might enter the liquid stream.

Lobe pumps use rotary seals to seal the shafts and separate the pump interior from the environment. Sanitary and aseptic opera-tions should use mechanical seals in double configuration (Wis-niewski 1988, 11–21; Brink et al. 1993). Material selection for mechanical seals is important and depends on the process condi-tions (e.g., the material should not leach, corrode, crack, or chip off, and should not produce particulate wear material). The seals should be of sanitary design (e.g., with a proper selection of materials, with no crevices and deep pockets of stagnant liquid, and the ability to withstand the clean-in-place (CIP) and sanitization procedures). The barrier fluid is typically a sterile condensate for the aseptic operation of pumps. In a sanitary application a purified water or sterile con-densate may be used, with the last preferable, to minimize the pos-sibility of microbial contamination. The barrier fluid in double mechanical seals isolates the process stream from the environment and provides lubrication to the seal faces. A user should pay atten-tion to the design of mechanical seals proposed by the vendor. Dou-ble seal design, with the rings pressed by multiple spiral springs, single spiral springs, or wave springs, may be selected. Bellows springs are not acceptable since they create a deep pocket, which is practically impossible to clean. No elastomer rings should be used as a spring substitute. In the case of unavoidable pockets, they should be shallow and wide enough to be thoroughly cleaned dur-ing a CIP cycle. A user should request detailed information on the mechanical seals used in the pump for the chromatography system. Single mechanical seals have also been used for reason of simplicity and lower cost; however, this is not a recommended practice in the biopharmaceutical environment.

The pump configuration must ensure complete drainage (e.g., a vertical flow path should be selected). A lobe pump with a flowmeter may provide adequate solution for certain applications where the system back pressure is moderate. Depending on the pump size and the required range of flow rate control, the back pressure range may extend from 50 to 300 psi (3.3–20 bar). The flow rate range cannot be too wide since only the motor speed control can be used for flow control. Low flow rates may be obtained by combining the flowmeter with a bypass or throttling valve to recirculate liquid externally or internally (due to slip backflow) within the pump. Such solutions make the system complex and more costly, complicate the cleaning cycle and may cause the pump to run less efficiently (this factor may also add extra energy to the fluid, causing a temperature increase). In practice, backslip flow in the lobe pump is much more pronounced in small pumps than in larger ones. At higher back pressures, small pumps may produce very little actual flow. Due to backslip flow, the controllable flow range rapidly decreases with an increase in back pressure. In such cases, the diaphragm pump is a better choice, since it performs well at higher back pressures.

In cases when system back pressures are very high (as is common in HPLC systems [Wisniewski 1992]), positive displacement reciprocating diaphragm pumps are the choice, since they can handle elevated pressures very well and at the same time deliver repeatable flows.

Gradient-Forming Systems for Elution

Gradient elution requires system design that can formulate gradients precisely in a repeatable fashion. The major gradient-mixing systems used in preparative and industrial chromatography are of three types:

1. Two connected vessels discharge into the pump with agitation of solution in the vessel located closer to the pump (Figure 3.10a).

2. Two independently controlled pumps deliver gradient components to the mixing chamber. Such a system is also called high pressure gradient mixing (Figure 3.10b).

3. Switching valve(s) are located in front of the single pump and deliver liquid from two vessels by changing the valve opening times. A mixing chamber with static or dynamic mixing is required in this system. The system is called low pressure gradient mixing (Figure 3.10c).

The first system is the simplest, but offers limited flexibility. In practice it has been replaced by the low pressure and high pressure gradient-mixing systems. Information on other gradient-forming systems can be found in the work by Jandera and Churacek (1985).

Figure 3.10. Gradient-forming systems: (a) two vessel system, (b) high pressure, multipump system, and (c) low pressure, single-pump system.

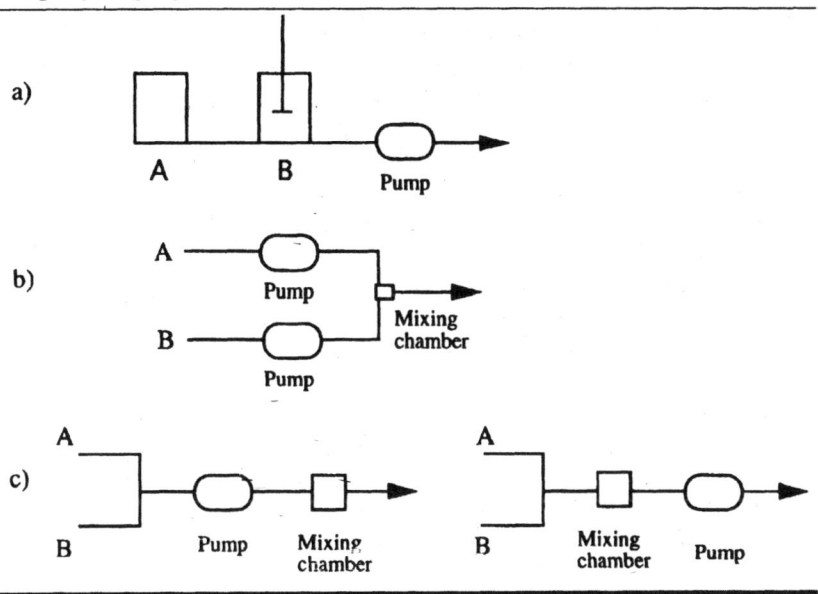

The typical high pressure gradient system requires two pumps (for a binary gradient) and a means of controlling the flow rates of the individual pumps. This can be accomplished by using a computerized control system and individual sets of a pump and a flowmeter for each gradient component. Such a system provides not only a feedback-based control of each component delivery, but also a recording capability for each stream. A secondary feedback from measurement of the final gradient parameter (e.g., electrical conductivity or pH) can be used by a computerized system for fine-tuning gradient formation. A disadvantage of such a gradient-forming system may be its high cost due to the need for two pumps and two flowmeters. The system may operate with one flowmeter only for total flow, and the computer may adjust the pumps according to a signal from the conductivity or pH sensor. However, a lack of information about individual pump performance may prove to be a significant shortcoming.

The low pressure, gradient-mixing system uses one pump and its performance depends mainly on the performance of the buffer delivery metering valve(s) and the mixing chamber(s). Since performance monitoring of metering valves is difficult, the control concept of gradient formation can be based on conductivity or pH sensing. The pump may be combined with a flowmeter to permit overall flow control, recording, and totalizing.

Performance of the gradient-mixing system depends mostly on the combined performance of the buffer metering valves and the mixing chamber(s). One or two mixing chambers may be employed –for preliminary mixing in front of the pump and for final mixing/pulse dampening/gas trapping after the pump. Usually, a single chamber located after the pump is used. Due to the requirement of sanitary design and flow characteristics, available designs of metering valves may not be able to operate at high speeds; as a result, the two components of an eluting buffer would arrive as "slugs," pass the pump (some preliminary mixing may occur there), and enter the mixing chamber. The mixing chamber design (in particular, its active volume) depends on performance of the metering valves (e.g., on volumes of the "slugs" these valves produce).

A computerized system can control the valve opening times, depending on the desired setpoint change in time for gradient formation, with fine-tuning depending on the measured conductivity or pH. In practice, such a system may not be able to produce good gradients at the ends (i.e., when one of the components should be delivered at a very low rate). Due to the limits of valve operational speed, there is a certain minimal achievable slug volume. Therefore, purification should be designed to elute product in the middle of the gradient. Then the ends of the gradient can be converted easily into step/isocratic elutions to elute large peaks of mixed contaminants. Valve selection for gradient mixing is an important decision. Conventional sanitary diaphragm valves with pneumatic or electric actuators move slowly, have limited diaphragm life, and poor flow control characteristics. Pure design PTFE diaphragm valves can operate faster and have longer life. Valves with specially compounded PTFE bellows have long life and may have finely tuned flow control characteristics (e.g., by selecting the orifice size). Whichever valve type is selected, the vendor should demonstrate the system's ability for gradient formation under worst-case scenarios (e.g., testing the gradient ends, checking the accuracy of flat or nonlinear gradients, etc.). Valving system cleanability must also be demonstrated.

The response speed of pneumatic actuators may be a limiting factor. Electrical actuators may provide better conditions for rapid valve action and can be directly operated by a computerized control system. The presence of a mixing chamber would dampen sharp step changes in composition of elution buffer, providing a sig-moidal-shape curve of concentration change. The shape of this curve can be altered by changing the liquid level (volume) in the mixing chamber, the flow rate, or both. The design of a mixing chamber is discussed in "Mixing Chambers, Pulsation Dampers, and Bubble Traps."

The high pressure gradient system may provide better operational flexibility since the well-controlled central gradient range may be wider than for the typical low pressure mixing system as a result of the different performance characteristics of pumps versus mixing valves. Due to the complexity of the gradient elution system design, operation, and maintenance, large-scale chromatographic separations, if possible, should be performed using stepwise/isocratic elutions. Despite these apparent difficulties (even for standardized gradient elution designs), system performance can be customized successfully to a particular large-scale separation as a result of collaboration between the user and vendor, if a sufficient lead time is available.

Sample Loading

The sample size loaded on the column has a strong influence on the shape of an eluted peak; column overload may reduce separation quality. Therefore, the purification process, to be fully repeatable, requires, as a first condition, a repeatable and precise sample loading. Selection of the loading method of product-containing solution on the column depends on the size of the system and on actual sample volume. The multiport valve and a sample loop concept used in small-scale chromatography cannot be applied due to the large sample size, although a similar concept with a small metering tank/reservoir instead of sample loop might work. A straightforward remedy is to use a system pump or a dedicated pump to load sample onto the column from the product tank. To monitor an exact volume loaded, a metering tank or a system flowmeter can be used. As an alternative, the number of fixed length pump strokes may be used for the volume estimate. At certain process conditions (small systems or small sample loads) the sample load dedicated pump may be driven by a stepping motor with no flowmeter needed (see also "Pumping System"). In each case, the computerized system would show its advantage since liquid volumes can be measured using the stepping motor rotation count or the flowmeter reading with corrections for time lags and liquid volume contained in the tubing. Information on sample load becomes a part of the production record and may serve as one of the variables in run repeatability and column performance calculations. Since the protein solution, buffers, and cleaning agents pass the sample loading pump, the pump design should comply with strict requirements regarding sanitary features and cleanability, analogous to those in the main pumping system described earlier.

Liquid Path Prior to and after the Column

Piping and Valves. The general principle to be used in piping design is to minimize the piping length and employ a turbulent flow pattern (flat velocity profile), at least after the column. The piping configuration should ensure complete drainability. Since the multi-port rotary valves used in analytical and preparative chromatography are considered a nonsanitary design, a valving system using single or multiple port sanitary diaphragm valves is typically applied. However, such a multivalve configuration may require a complicated sequence of the CIP pattern. The valves (manual and actuated) must be accessible for easy operation, maintenance, and visual inspection during the operation (e.g., to check the valve position when there are no feedback limit switches). The sanitary valves (diaphragm, bellows) can be installed on manifolds, or multiple port sanitary diaphragm valves may be clustered. Dead legs in manifolds may be eliminated by the use of zero-static diaphragm valves. Valve design must ensure a flow pattern similar to the pattern in the adjacent piping (e.g., valve internal volume and liquid mixing within the valve should be minimized). Most of the sanitary valve designs traditionally applied in industrial liquid chromatography affect negatively the quality of a final separation due to the presence of such internal mixing. The valves could be of pinch type, which at full opening perform like an empty tube.

Ball valves give the same flow pattern, but they cannot be considered a sanitary design (despite vendors' claims). If the diaphragm valves are used between such multiple columns as described in "Columns for Stationary Beds" or after the column, then the valve design should be selected to minimize internal liquid recirculation. For example, the 10 mm Gemu diaphragm valve has the valve chamber at full diaphragm opening only about 10 percent larger than the 10 mm ID tube of the same length (2.513 mL and 2.787 mL as, respectively, measured), it may be assumed to be equal to the tube volume, with no extra mixing volume involved. There is, however, a stream expansion (a diffusor effect) of approximately 36.5°; such configuration indicates stream separation from the walls in the expanding section (converging flow section is less critical [Schlichting 1979]). For comparison, the approximate parameters for ITT valves are as follows:

- The internal tube diameter for both Pure-Flo® and Biotech® valves is 9 mm.

- The valve chamber volume for the Pure-Flo® valve is about 7.51 ml and for Biotech valve is about 3.15 mL.

- The corresponding volumes of the tube equivalent to chamber lengths are respectively 3.43 and 2.42 mL, and this is approximately 119 percent and 30 percent more than the volumes of equivalent tubes.

- The angles of equivalent diffusors are, respectively, 52° and 45°.

This comparison demonstrates differences in the internal geometry of valves, and indicates anticipated behavior of the valves as mixing chambers. From the viewpoint of interest to the chromatographer, the best is the Gemu valve and the worst is the Pure-Flo® valve. The Pure-Flo® valve may act as an effective mixing chamber since it has both large volume and the diffusor angle (recirculating internal zones occur). Improper valve selection and/or use of a large number of valves after the column may degrade the quality of separation in a significant way (see also "Column Design"). A similar approach may be applied for the evaluation of flow-through chambers of instruments and sensors used in the system. Evaluations of the effects of mixing zones with different flow patterns are given in Levenspiel (1979).

The selection of metering valves for gradient-forming, single pump systems is of utmost importance. The valves should be of rapid action, have adequate flow characteristics, long life, and be of sanitary design. The piping system should have an air detector installed prior to the pump. It can indicate the end of the product batch and serve as an emergency device in case of liquid loss.

Mixing Chambers, Pulsation Dampers, and Bubble Traps. Gradient elution systems may require a well-designed mixing chamber (Jordan and Pardue 1992) if a low pressure, gradient-mixing concept is applied. The mixing chamber may be located in front of or after the pump. Location after the pump has several advantages. The mixing chamber design may also incorporate a bubble trap and a pulsation damper into a single design. The total volume of such a

chamber should include a sufficient liquid volume for mixing and a
volume for gas cushion above. The gas volume above the liquid surface performs a pulsation dampening role. A level control may be
used to maintain a desired level of liquid and to relieve gas bubbles
separating from the liquid. The liquid volume inside the chamber
and the flow pattern should be selected to permit the complete separation of gas bubbles and adequate liquid mixing. Although there
are mixing chambers employing an internal, magnetically driven ag-
itator, a design using purely hydrodynamic mixing is recommended
due to its simplicity. The two buffers composing the elution gradient may come in the form of liquid slugs of a size and frequency depending on the performance of the buffer's delivery system. Liquid
volume enclosed in the mixing chamber should accommodate several slugs of each buffer; the flow pattern inside the chamber should
mix the slugs thoroughly before the chamber outlet. This liquid
volume may be optimized considering mixing, gas separation, and
chamber dynamic response to changes in liquid composition. If a
positive displacement, lobe-type pump is used, then, due to its inherent slip backflow, such a pump also acts as a preliminary gradient mixer in front of the mixing chamber. The flow pattern inside
the chamber should ensure enough turbulence not only for the
process mixing, but also for the cleaning step, when the chamber
may become completely filled with cleaning solution. Flow rates for
process and cleaning may vary.

System configuration with an adequately designed mixing
chamber may ease the requirements imposed on the metering valving system located in front of the pump. If the mixing chamber is located before the pump, one must ensure sufficiently stable liquid
delivery conditions on the pump inlet side (no significant static
head changes). Low pressure mixing may be affected negatively by
changing liquid levels in the feed tanks (e.g., delivered liquid volume may vary at the same valve opening times depending on the
static head of liquid in front of the valve). Tanks under controlled
pressure may be used to stabilize liquid delivery, but such a system
design is more costly since special enclosed tanks must be used. At
long delivery pipelines, small constant liquid level transition tanks
may be used to unify the static liquid heads in front of the mixing
chamber and the metering valves. Properly designed control loops
for flow rate (flowmeter and pump) and gradient formation (metering valves–conductivity/pH) should be able to compensate for these
effects. These problems diminish if the mixing chamber is located
after the pump. Therefore, this location is preferred. The performance of metering valves should be synchronized, to ensure that at

least one valve is open when the pump is running. Valve operation in the low pressure mixing system would almost always give stepwise liquid composition changes after the pump; therefore, the design of a mixing/bubble trap chamber is of critical importance. A properly performing chamber would smooth the oscillations in concentration and might approximate a linear change in buffer composition. High pressure gradient mixing will circumvent all these difficulties, if a combination of two pumps and two flowmeters is used. The bubble trap/pulsation damper chamber can be smaller since no significant liquid mixing volume is needed.

A much simpler design of the large-scale chromatography system is required if only stepwise/isocratic elution is used in the process. In this case there is no need for a large mixing chamber and only a small bubble trap/pulsation damper may be used. Since operation of the expanded bed column requires a complete absence of pulsations and gas bubbles in order to avoid any significant internal mixing within the bed, particular attention should be paid to the design, testing, and operation of the bubble trap/pulsation damping chamber.

Detection and Fraction Collection

Literature on chromatography detectors pertains mostly to analytical chromatography (Scott 1986; Yeung 1986). The most universal detector for large-scale chromatography of biomolecules has been the flow-through UV absorbance detector set at a wavelength of 280 nm or 254 nm. The aromatic rings of tryptophan, tyrosine, and phenylalanine residues are responsible for most of the UV absorbance and fluorescence emission properties of proteins (Creighton 1993; Permyakov 1993). Tryptophan has two absorption bands: at 218 nm and at 280 nm. The 280 nm peak has a smaller side peak at 288 nm and a shoulder at 271 nm. Tyrosine has two absorption bands: at 222 nm and 275 nm. The 275 nm band has shoulders at 267 nm and 282 nm. The spectrum of phenylalanine has peaks at 187.5 nm, 205 nm, 242 nm, 252 nm, 257 nm, 263 nm, and 267 nm. The major peak is at 257 nm.

Typically, this type of detector is used together with electrical conductivity and pH detectors for monitoring and recording purposes. The conductivity detector allows monitoring of concentrations of eluting buffers in frequently used IEX and HIC processes, and its signal can be used as a feedback for gradient formation. The monitoring of pH is very important in all processes involving protein molecules (Creighton 1993; Matthew et al. 1985). In affinity chromatography and IEX, or chromatofocusing, pH values are an important parameter of the elution step. While in analytical instruments the detector cell must have a minimum volume for high peak resolution and a sufficiently long UV beam path for high sensitivity, these factors are not as important in industrial chromatography. Due to high product concentrations, the UV beam path length is not critical for detection sensitivity; due to broad peaks, the cell volume is not critical for resolution. The response time of an industrial detector may be slower than that of an analytical one due to broader peaks.

Microprocessor-controlled analytical systems frequently use high resolution (20–24 bits) analog to digital converters; however, such resolution may not be required for computerized production systems due to applied larger loads and resulting broader peaks. The UV detector design can be a simple, single beam absorption unit or a more sophisticated double beam instrument with compensation for varying lamp intensity. A compensated detector can also be used in a version that permits simultaneous measurement at two wavelengths. Further extension of this concept can be an application of diode array or rapid scanning detectors, similar to those used in analytical chromatography. The drift during gradient elution may be countermeasured by the electronic module of the detector. Since the noise levels caused by turbulence are not significant when compared to the peak size and can also be countermeasured by the electronics of the detector, turbulence effects (Scott 1986) may not be considered critical in industrial detector design. A turbulent flow in the connecting tubing between the column and detector and between the detector and fraction collector is recommended to maintain the separation quality obtained on the column outlet, particularly if the connecting tubing is long (as may happen in some in-house designs).

Detectors can be obtained in a high pressure design (up to 1,500 psi or 100 bar), but a typical application does not require such high pressure. High pressure designs are also more costly. Safety measures should be undertaken (a pressure switch and a pressure relief valve) to protect the detector in case of flow path blockage (e.g., if a process valve actuator fails). The detector may give a simple electrical output signal to be interfaced with a recorder or a computer-based data acquisition system with the signal processing software, and may also have certain capabilities built-in, such as the processing of calibration data and the generation of a calibration curve. The latter can be generated from multiple measurements stored in the instrument memory. A computer-based system is recommended since it provides maximum capability of signal processing and data evaluation.

A novel approach to detector design and application may be to consider the use of a device based on fiber optics transmission. An example can be a miniature UV/VIS or fluorescence instrument, which can plug directly into the computer. The fiber optics cable brings the signal from a flow cell. Such an instrument may come with spectroscopy/peak analysis software, and, as a result, software development efforts can be reduced. For UV sensing the length of fiber optics can be several meters, thus facilitating system configuration. The multielement charge-coupled device (CCD) array is typically used for sensing. The flow cell can be designed with adjustable path length (by adjusting the ends of fibers using sealed ports). The control logic may be implemented in the same computer, using UV absorption data from the spectrophotometer.

Other types of detectors are seldom used in industrial chromatography. A refractive index (RI) detector could be applied in certain separations due to its modest cost and linearity of RI with protein concentration, although it is sensitive to temperature and flow pulsations (Scott 1986) and can only be used with isocratic separations (its readings are affected by changing salt concentration during gradient elution). A more general concept is that of a polarimetric detector (Yeung 1986), which may serve for the detection of chiral compounds. Even in complex mixtures the reading is related to the chiral purity of the compound. A fluorescence detector can detect molecules that can fluoresce (naturally or labeled with fluorescence marker). In special cases of preparative chromatography, the fluorescence detector can be used, as it is practiced in analytical chromatography. The fluorescence of protein molecules is due to tryptophan, tyrosine, and phenylalanine residues (Permyakov 1993). The phenylalanine emission spectrum has three peaks: 275 nm, 282 nm (major), and 289 nm (at peak width of about 30 nm with a shoulder above 300 nm); the tyrosine emission spectrum has a maximum peak at 304 nm (at a peak width of about 34 nm); and the tryptophan emission spectrum has a maximum peak at 353 nm that is rather wide (about 60 nm). Polar protein groups may quench the fluorescence of these residues. Histidine and arginine as well as hydroxyl groups are known to quench the fluorescence of chromophores. The fluorescence detector has very high sensitivity. Such high sensitivity is usually not required in industrial chromatography. The FT-IR detection technique (Yeung 1986), although used in protein spectroscopic studies (Strand and Jakobsen 1991) has not found application in industrial chromatography, due to problems caused by strong absorption by water molecules and difficult signal interpretation (complex deconvolution algorithms are needed for spectra analysis). This technique can identify distinct differences in the secondary structures of proteins. More information on detectors can be found in books by Scott (1986) and Yeung (1986). *Analytical Chemistry* publishes an annual review issue covering instrumentation methods, including detection techniques.

The distance between the major detector and the fraction collector should be minimized to reduce contained liquid volume and the detrimental effects of the flow velocity profile (longitudinal dispersion) in the outlet tubing. Since a sanitary multiport valve is difficult to fabricate, if many fractions are required, a compromise can be made and a combination of several multiport sanitary diaphragm valves can be arranged into a cluster. A major problem in such a cluster arrangement may be the size of valve actuators preventing tight valve configuration. Differences in flow path lengths between the fraction collection ports can be compensated by a computerized control system.

Monitoring and Controls

The typical process parameters measured and monitored in large-scale chromatography operations are as follows:

- Flow rate/volume in time
- UV absorption after the column
- Pressure
- Electrical conductivity
- pH

Other parameters may include temperature, refractive index, and fluorescence. Recorded parameters could include, in the simplest cases, flow/volume and UV absorption. For adequate process records, electrical conductivity and pH should also be included. If the process does not run in a controlled cold room environment, temperature levels should also be recorded for process documentation.

Transmitters and sensors should be of sanitary design regarding materials of construction, surface finishes, and cleanability under CIP conditions. The transmitter's long-term stability is very important;

it may facilitate maintenance and eliminate the need for frequent calibrations. Pressure combined with flow rate may provide useful information regarding the status of a chromatography column. Recommended pressure sensors should be of the integral, flow-through, tubular design, with pressure sensing by measuring the tube wall deflection. Such a design has a much better cleanability than the sanitary metal diaphragm sensors located in T piping nozzles. The accuracy of sanitary pressure transmitters is typically in the range of 0.2–0.5 percent full scale. Since the temperature of fluids affects their viscosity, the complete record should include pressure, flow rate, and fluid temperature.

A computer-operated system provides control flexibility, real-time data storage and documentation, data transfer and communications, process analysis, and optimization to the extent not possible to achieve by semimanual or PLC–controlled operations. Books by Astrom and Wittenmark (1990) and by Lang (1991) provide general design principles for computer-based control and instrumentation systems. Pump flow rates can be controlled on a feedback principle using flowmeters. Flowmeters should not operate at their minimum flow ranges because this is where accuracy is the lowest. The flowmeter-controller loop implemented in a computerized system can be used to maintain proper pumping system repeatability and to allow the collection of accurate run records. The actual flow rate is of interest, not the pump current set point and its relation to the calibration curve. Knowledge of pump performance parameters, such as motor speed/frequency and stroke length, may prove useful as data used in the automatic system diagnostics concept, since they can be related to flowmeter readings.

Existing systems can be easily upgraded by adding a flowmeter. A temporary step can be the addition of a clamp-on ultrasonic flowmeter, since it may not require any system configuration changes and is nonintrusive. However, its accuracy is about ± 1–2 percent and is lower than the typical magnetic or mass flowmeter accuracy (± 0.15–0.5 percent). It also requires a developed turbulent flow in pipe for proper measurements. Therefore, the final design configuration may be to use magnetic or mass instruments. The accuracy of flowmeters (given in percent of actual flow) typically decreases at flows below 10 percent of maximum flow. Guidelines on the application and installation of magnetic and mass flowmeters can be found in the work of Ginesi and Annarummo (1994). Van Laak (1993) reported results of a thorough evaluation and comparison of eight brands of magnetic flowmeters, depending on service conditions.

In the case of salt solution gradients, a rapid response conductivity probe is used after the mixing chamber for overall buffer delivery system monitoring, recording, and control. The low pressure, gradient-mixing system may require a well-tuned computer system to adjust the delivery valves in such a way that the smooth gradient is accomplished. Since an exact prediction of the performance of delivery valves may be difficult, an advanced concept adaptive control system (e.g., based on a neural network) may be applied. System identification techniques (Ljung 1987; Schwarzenbach and Gill 1992) can also be used to determine such system dynamic behavior.

A computerized system may employ these advanced control techniques, which might not be available using individual controllers, PLCs, or a combination of both. A computer can also serve very well as an operator interface. Simulated instrument panels can be displayed showing the trends of recorded parameters, dynamic displays of selected variables, numerical data, and alarms. A mimic diagram of the system can be displayed with dynamic fields showing variables of interest and the status and the performance of the system and its components. Screens can be divided into zones to show a variety of data. Large screens (at least 17 inch or 43 cm) with high resolution graphics are recommended, since they are able to show a large amount of information on a single screen (if possible, screen switching should be avoided in operational procedures).

Periodic column packing quality testing can be performed by using pulse tracer injection and the subsequent monitoring and analysis of the peak shape by a computerized system. The peak analysis program may automatically compute, display, and record parameters such as peak area, peak height, number of theoretical separation stages and stage height, peak asymmetry, and so on.

An additional advantage of the computerized system over the recorder- or integrator-based system is an ability to record, store, and analyze data from multiwavelength UV detectors (such as the diode array type). In addition to process control functions, the computerized system may provide numerous process analysis and optimization tools, which can be used in both process development and in production. Rigorous analysis of multiple chromatograms can be performed by overlaying them and comparing times, peak areas, absorbance levels at selected points, curve slopes, peak shapes (features such as peak tailing), shapes of the first and second derivatives, calculated resolution and reduced plate height, and so on. In the early stages of process development and start-up, the software analyzing peak overlap may aid in the decision where to cut the fractions between product and waste. Some of these parameters may become part of the permanent production record and provide much more information on process consistency than printouts of recorded chromatograms alone.

In addition to these functions, the computerized system may serve as a diagnostic tool to evaluate system performance. Deterioration of the chromatography column may be noticed earlier than by comparison of chromatograms if an algorithm combining flow rate, pressure drop, and peak shape is used. The media aging process may be observed by monitoring changes in peak tailing. Standardized column testing procedures (such as the calculation of the number of theoretical plates and resolution) performed after packing can be incorporated into the software as well. Expert systems have been proposed for use in the purification of proteins (Kenney 1990, 571–602) and they may be used as an aid in process development.

System Design and Integration

Hardware

System integration may not only mean assembly of the individual components into the working system, but also matching system performance to the intended separation. Development studies result in certain operational conditions to be pursued in the large scale.

The key parameters are chromatographic medium (stationary phase) and the selection of buffers. Other parameters follow–the column length and diameter, flow rates in each step and corresponding pressure drops, and column sample load. The flow rates and pressure rating would determine the selection of the pumping system, sensors, tubing and valves, and so on. The type of elution would determine whether simple buffer supply switching or a gradient elution system of different complexity is needed. Therefore, it is very important that the system design be conducted in close association with process development work performed in the bench or pilot scale (e.g., findings of process development should be considered during a conceptual phase of large system design). Such parallelism may shorten the time of moving from the development stage into the large-scale manufacturing stage and reduce the need for large-scale system adjustments, modifications, or redesign. The development team should also consider the capabilities of available, commercial, large-scale systems to avoid, if possible, the building of any unique, complex, process-customized systems with associated high costs and long development times.

Points to Consider for Custom and In-House Designs of Chromatography Systems

Since some users still assemble their chromatography systems in-house, there are certain factors to be considered when integrating the components into an operational system:

- Minimize overall tubing length, especially after the column. Select the tubing internal diameter after the column to maintain a turbulent or at least transitional flow regime (Re > 4,000).

- Collect fractions closely after the detector, using a cluster of valves.

- Pump selection is up to the user; for moderate pressure a double rotor lobe pump is sufficient. A flowmeter is recommended to work together with such a pump. Since aqueous solutions are used, a magnetic flowmeter of sanitary design is sufficient. If mass flowmeters are used, they should be of a drainable design. Ultrasonic flowmeters may not have adequate accuracy. Turbine flowmeters, even if they are claimed to be of sanitary design, should be avoided due to the presence of internal moving parts. Elevated pumping pressures call for a multihead diaphragm pump or a screw-type pump.

- The typical location of the pH and conductivity sensors is after the column in the vicinity of the UV absorbance detector. The conductivity sensor/transducer could also be located after the mixing chamber, prior to the column for strict control of gradient formation if a feedback control loop is implemented into the control system. If stepwise elution is used, the location may be prior to or after the column. If in a position after the column, its design should be of a flow-through type with no interference to the flow pattern. If there is an interference (a mixing volume involved), then the presence of such a sensor may affect adversely the quality of the separation. The same applies to the pH sensor/transducer, although its design may have an upper pressure limit, which may leave being located after the column as the only choice. For systems using monitoring/recording alone (no computations involved), the pH and conductivity sensors may be located after the column, close to the UV sensor, to avoid the time lag associated with liquid residence time in the column. pH/conductivity sensors after the column can be utilized for eluent monitoring, if there is a column regeneration scheme implemented into the control system, using the pH/conductivity measurements on the column outlet.

- Excessive length of the piping prior to the pump should be avoided. An adequate static liquid head should be maintained in front of the pumps to avoid cavitation.

- If a diaphragm pump is used, the location of the buffer feed reservoirs should not give a large liquid static head, since it can cause flow through the pump (by lifting the pump check valves) if the column is disconnected. Precautions would include operating procedures calling for the closing of the valves and/or a back-pressure valve located after the pump.

- Due to sample size, sample loading onto the column is done using a pump (main or dedicated), not by a combination of the multiport valve and a sample loop (as it is in small-scale separations). To monitor the amount loaded exactly, the sample may pass through a metering tank, or a system flowmeter can be used.

- The sensors and transducers should be of sanitary design. Transducers located in the T should be avoided. Instead, a flow-through type of transducer is recommended.

- Stacking the multiple columns (as practiced in gel filtration chromatography) requires careful design of the interconnecting piping systems to maintain the performance (HETP) of the whole stack close to the performance of a single column. A decline in performance can be due to the flow pattern in the piping and the presence of T pieces (used for cleaning, sampling, etc.), which add the mixing volumes to the flow path; valves located along the liquid path may also affect negatively the performance of a multicolumn unit. Valve design should ensure a liquid flow pattern closely resembling the pattern in the adjacent piping.

- The manufacturing plant environment requires watertight enclosures on control panels, transducers, instruments, elec-

tric motors, and actuators. Equipment for cold rooms should
be protected from internal condensation.

These points can also be useful for establishing the required system
specifications and in working together with equipment suppliers on
customizing the system design. Final skid design should be frame
based and on casters for easy movement. The frame dimensions
should be compatible with doors and open passages.

Controls and Software

The integration of controls and software with the hardware part
may require various levels of user involvement, mostly depending
on whether the system is assembled in-house or whether the processing skid is purchased from a vendor. In the first case the user
faces the lengthy task of developing the control concept and associated software. The user should closely collaborate with the vendor
during the skid design and preparation phases. Manufacturing
process control software may be expanded easily to control, monitor, and record cleaning and regeneration processes, as well as to aid
in calibration procedures. The flow, volume, pH, temperature, and
conductivity of cleaning/regeneration solutions are the parameters
most often monitored. Removal of contaminants from the column
can be monitored using the main UV absorption detector. Washing
steps may be monitored using UV, pH, and conductivity detectors.

CHROMATOGRAPHIC MEDIA AND THEIR USE

The term *media* (or *stationary phase* or *sorbents*) in liquid chromatography designates a solid particle on the surface of which
solutes can interact. With the advent of modern liquid chromatography, where high performances are expected in resolution, capacity, and speed, media for separation have been progressively refined.
Media design today is application oriented, and polymers and ligands used for media manufacturing are *a priori* selected as a function of the protein-media interaction. All the basic parameters of
solid particles, such as hydrophilicity or hydrophobicity, nonspecific
binding, porosity, and rigidity have been explored in depth; the
"general ideal sorbent" of the early age of protein chromatography
has been progressively replaced by the "specific ideal sorbent" in relation with the application and the purification step (see below).

Media classifications have been proposed based on chemical
composition, pore diameter, particle size, and specific properties, but

the one that is connected with the physicochemical structure is the distinction between aerogels and xerogels. Aerogels are incompressible structures that are not affected in their porous volume by the presence or the absence of solvent. Examples of aerogels are porous silica, porous glass particles, and to a certain extent polymethacrylates. Xerogels include media with shrinking and swelling properties as a function of the presence of solvents or solvent mixtures. Examples of xerogels are homogeneous cross-linked polysaccharides and polyacrylamides.

In spite of this unequivocal classification, there are examples of aerogel-xerogel hybrids with limited properties of shrinking-swelling. For more details see the review by Mikes et al. (1976). The chemical constitution of media and, more importantly, their surface characteristics are made to fit with the applications for which these media are designed. The separation of the constituents of complex mixtures is based on the differences in the protein–solid phase interaction of the individual components. Ion exchange, for instance, is one of the most common interactions used in separating proteins, which takes advantage of the difference in the total net charge of proteins at a given pH. Hydrophobic associations between low polar regions of proteins and hydrophobic ligands chemically attached to a polymer also constitute a valuable molecular interaction with the possibility of discriminating between proteins. More specifically, affinity chromatography uses biochemical ligands and is more focused on the biological properties of the proteins to separate than on physicochemical differences. Gel filtration takes advantage of differences between the molecular size of proteins and separates under a real molecular sieve effect. In practice, all of the mechanisms under which chromatographic separation of proteins occurs must be handled following known rules. Table 3.3 shows a summary of common experimental adsorption, elution, and regeneration conditions as a function of the molecular interaction mechanism.

Main Media Concepts for Liquid Chromatography

Early media for biological macromolecule separation were basically composed of highly hydrophilic polysaccharide gels obtained by chemical cross-linkage of dextran, a polymer of glucose with α-1,6 linkages. From this structure chemical derivatives were prepared for most known applications such as gel filtration (Stellwagen 1990, 343–357) and IEX (Wheelwright 1991). The tendency for these gels to shrink and swell when changing pH and ionic strength induced media suppliers to design more appropriate gel materials. Each

Table 3.3. General Physicochemical Conditions of Use for Media Applied to Protein Chromatography

Type of Chromatography	Common Adsorption Conditions	Common Elution Conditions	Regeneration Conditions
Cation-exchange	Low ionic strength, pH below protein pI	Increase ionic strength, increase pH	Acid/base washings, high concentration salts
Anion-exchange	Low ionic strength, pH above protein pI	Increase ionic strength, decrease pH	Acid/base washings high concentration salts
Hydrophobic	High ionic strength (ammonium sulfate)	Ionic strength decrease	Alkaline washings, organic acids, chaotropics, aqueous-miscellaneous solvents
Hydroxyapatite	Diluted phosphate buffers, pH 6.8	Increase phosphate buffer concentration	Sodium hydroxide
Gel filtration	Any ionic strength, any pH, low amount	Isocratic separation	Salt washings, diluted alkaline washings of sample
Affinity	Close to physiological conditions except special cases	pH changes, ionic strength changes, competitive elutions	Salt washings, specific displacement treatments
Reversed-phase	Hydroorganic mixtures	Organic modifiers (acetonitrile, methanol)	Solvents, glycols, urea, acidic solutions

media concept has been defined around a selected chromatographic property to confer special features.

The most successful organic-based media used in the past and still very popular today are agarose gels. Extracted from melted agar-agar, agarose generates stable gels as a result of intrachain and interchain hydrogen bondings. A three-dimensional network is then formed and is characterized by a large porosity constituted of a variety of interconnected pores of very different size. As an average, pores from agarose gels are generally larger than the size of the proteins, permitting a free diffusion of macromolecules with possible interaction with chain substituents. This kind of matrix shows a number of properties, permitting good acceptance as a candidate for chromatographic media. It was possible to obtain spherical particles with predetermined pores; the polysaccharide chains were reacted easily to introduce different chemical sites for protein adsorption. The lack of chemical and physical stability was solved by cross-linkage with bifunctional reagents. Polysaccharides are not stable in acidic conditions, but they tolerate alkaline washings that are used for cleaning purposes.

Agarose stationary phases possess medium and large pores, and they do not show nonspecific binding. They suffer, however, from compressibility under pressure, shrinkage when using solvents, a rapid decrease of dynamic binding capacity when increasing the flow rate, and sensitivity to acidic media. In spite of these limitations, agarose-based media are frequently used in small-, medium- and large-scale separations, and cover different techniques of liquid chromatography of proteins, such as gel filtration, ion exchange, hydrophobic, and affinity interactions. To avoid the chemical variability of natural extracted polymers like agarose, synthetic materials also have been used to make chromatographic media. All of these sorbents claim a good chemical consistency and pore size that are easy to control during polymerization processes. Small-pore as well as large-pore packing materials can be prepared using this technology. Chemical substituents were also introduced on monomers before and during the polymerization process for a better consistency of the final medium (Boschetti 1989).

The objective of synthetic stationary phases was to have mechanically improved media and to keep the pores as large as possible for a good mass transfer, even for very large macromolecules. Mechanical strength is proportional to the concentration of the polymer, while pore size diminishes as a function of the monomer concentration. High cross-linking ratios obtained with bifunctional monomers increase the bead hardness; however, they contribute to a decrease in the exclusion limit (Determann 1968, 17–19, 64–84). In this context, special polymerization processes were perfected to obtain "coagulated-like" structures with a random assembly of small particles yielding very large pores and small pores in the same network (Boschetti 1989). Elimination of sieving effects, stability in strong acidic media, increased volume stability toward pH, ionic strength changes, and resistance to medium pressure are the major advantages of this category of stationary phases. This type of media is formulated to have a hydrophilic surface characteristic.

The need to increase the resolution was approached by decreasing the particle size for a better separation efficiency. To stay as close as possible to theoretical separation predictions, monodisperse bead concepts have been developed (Ugelstad and Mork 1980). Monodispersity improved packing quality with acceptable back pressure with particles as small as 10 μm. Rigidity was also improved substantially to be compatible with back pressures generated by beads of 10–15 μm in diameter.

For very large production applications another concept has been developed associating rigidity, speed, and sorption capacity. The well-known advantages of soft polysaccharide material and the rigidity of silica beads with large pores were combined in a single medium (Tayot et al. 1978, 95–110). Dextran was introduced into the pores of silica beads and then cross-linked in place. This concept represents a big step forward in the large-scale application of chromatography in protein separation with columns as large as 1500 L and bed height of more than 1 meter.

High flow rates were achieved and many problems related to economics and productivity for the manufacturing of even low value biologicals were solved by use of this type of medium. Contrary to totally synthetic materials, where the polymer plays both the role of skeleton and active surface for chromatographic separations, in silica-dextran medium the roles of mechanical rigidity and interaction mechanism are played by two different entities.

The improvement of adsorption-desorption kinetics and the availability of interacting chemical groups for macromolecular solutes were at the basis of the introduction of another concept with so called "tentacular sorbents" (Muller 1990). Active groups are attached to linear, flexible, polymeric chains that increase the mobility of the interacting groups and facilitate the adsorption-desorption of macromolecules to be separated. This mode of action improves the resolution level when the pores of the polymeric network are large enough to allow the macromolecules to diffuse freely inside the beads.

Separation at high linear velocity was approached by another concept defined as "perfusive chromatography" (Afeyan et al. 1990). Extensively investigated in practice and also elucidated by theoretical models (Liapis and McCoy 1992, 1994, Liapis et al. 1995), it is based on the existence of very large pores where the convection of molecules dominates, bringing species to be separated very close to smaller diffusion pores. The factors involved are the flow around spheres and the driving force for intraparticular flow, particle internal characteristics (bead diameter and internal large and small pores), and fluid and solute characteristics (viscosity, density, diffusion coefficient). Mass transfer is improved and the dynamic sorption capacity is maintained almost constant over a wide range of linear velocities. Even if the total sorption capacity is limited as a consequence of reduced surface area per unit volume of the resin, the productivity per time unit can be increased using high flow rates (Fulton et al. 1992).

A combination of high dynamic binding capacity at high separation speed is at the basis of another recent concept defined as "hyperdiffusion chromatography," where incompressible macroporous structures are filled with soft hydrogels. The high sorption capacity is in this case obtained by a soft, three-dimensional gel well known at the early stages of chromatographic media development; the high speed is possible by the rigidity of the porous "shell," inside which the gel is distributed (Horvath et al. 1994; Boschetti et al. 1995). High capacity is understandable by the fact that interactions between the molecules to separate and the matrix is space-dependent rather than surface-dependent. Concerning the binding capacity of the soft gel itself, this is driven by the ligand density, which is controlled during the three-dimensional gel copolymerization process. Using this technology, a large variety of sorbents is obtainable, covering the different aspects and application of liquid chromatography. The softness and the flexibility of a gel are important features in keeping the ligand mobility high for better interaction kinetics with solutes. Table 3.4 summarizes the various media concepts with some of their main properties for the preparative separation of proteins where high levels of productivity, purity, and safety are required.

Media Features as a Function of Purification Steps

Downstream bioprocessing is composed of a series of operations starting from the crude extract and eventually isolating the biological of interest while removing any kind of impurity. It is generally

Table 3.4. Main Features of Media for Preparative Applications

Media Category	Composition	Main Properties
Nonuniform shape material, low cost	Fibrous cellulose	Usable in batch mode, low column flow rate
Hydrophilic gels in bead form	Dextran	Very high sorption capacity, limitations in flow rate due to compressibility
Improved polysaccharide gels	Cross-linked agarose	Large pores, moderate compression
Synthetic macroporous hydrophilic supports	Polymethacrylates, trisacryl, polyvinyl	Very large pores, moderate compressibility, stable in acids, nonbiodegradable
Gel-filled mineral porous material	Silica filled with dextran gels	Incompressibility, large pores, high sorption capacity
Matrix with convective pores	Polystyrene coated with hydrophilic polymers	Very large pores to allow convection of macromolecules
Tentacular sorbents	Porous synthetic particles with "active" polymeric tentacles	Rapid sorption-desorption kinetics, ligand availability
High diffusion material	Composite porous particles filled with viscoelastic synthetic gels	High sorption capacity at high flow rates, high resolution, incompressibility

admitted that downstream bioprocessing may represent from 50 percent to 80 percent of the overall production cost of a bulk biopharmaceutical, and an effort must be undertaken to reduce this cost. Savings are possible in the areas of raw material and consumables, labor, capital investment, and yields. It is relatively easy to compress all of these expenses, except capital investment and yields. These two items are tightly linked. Each purification step contributes some yield decrease due to product mass losses on the one hand and to biological activity reduction as a consequence of protein denaturation on the other hand.

Reducing the number of steps can result in very substantial savings in capital expenses and can provide higher overall yields. A reduction, for instance, of 15 percent in yield step after step (which is not uncommon in bioseparation) represents an overall yield loss of 62 percent for a bioprocess consisting of six steps. It is, therefore, logical that an appropriate means for reducing the downstream bioprocessing cost is to save yields by reducing the number of steps. A good practical compromise between cost and assurance of product quality is to have three to four steps, where each step corresponds to a choice of parameters in connection with the degree of purity. A bioprocess should consist of a capture phase or initial purification, a fine fractionation phase or intermediate purification, and a final polishing step. Crude biological material sources are from eukaryotic and prokaryotic cell cultures (using recombinant DNA technology) or from natural biological origin, such as biological fluids and organ extracts. At the capture stage concentration and selective extraction are generally required since the biological of interest is frequently diluted and constitutes a minor component among a number of other biological and chemical compounds. Both operations must, in fact, be performed at the earliest phase for economical reasons and to reduce the risk of denaturation.

Biochemical capturing technology traditionally involved precipitation, centrifugation, and/or filtration operations in order to obtain protein samples satisfying the requirements of subsequent liquid chromatography fractionation. These operations contribute significantly to concentrating and clarifying protein solutions; however, they are labor-intensive techniques with generally poor yields. Their selectivity for the target biological is low since they are based on physical and chemical principles. Direct capture with solid phases in batch, fluid, and expanded beds significantly improves the first purification stage. Solid phase media for expanded bed operations are derived from liquid chromatography with special particle size and appropriate density. With this material the expansion of a bed of solid phase medium can be achieved easily by introducing the feed stream through the bottom of the column at appropriate flow rates. The sample does not need to be clarified in a separate operation, thus saving a significant amount of time and labor. Very crude starting material containing living cells, such as bacteria, yeasts, and mammalian cells, as well as cell debris, can be processed. The characteristics of solid media to be used in expanded bed capture steps are a high density (to allow high linear velocities in expanded modes), a high porosity for easy mass transfer, and a modified surface chemistry to adsorb selectively the biological of interest. Special affinity chromatography media are, in fact, the most appropriate to achieve high levels of purity that can reach more than 50–70 percent. Today, such media are not yet popular, but they represent a big potential if they provide a high degree of selectivity with no, or limited, particle fouling. Expanded column design and operation was described in "Column Design."

The fine fractionation phase, following an effective capture phase, deals with a relatively concentrated protein solution, where the dominant component is the protein of interest. This purification phase is composed of one or a few steps, using less selective media such as ion exchangers and hydrophobic interacting stationary phases. The selectivity being limited, the required high resolution power can be achieved with media characterized by small particle size and narrow particle size distribution. If the sorption capacity of such media is high or very high, then the column dimensions can be reduced. Sorbents with such characteristics exist today. The purity that can be achieved at this stage could be as high as 95 percent in a single step, starting from a purity of about 50 percent. Critical contaminants, such as protein impurities, DNA, endotoxins, and viruses, are mostly eliminated at this stage.

Polishing is by definition the last purification stage, where traces of impurities are to be removed to comply with purity and safety standards. The impurities are generally composed of aggregates or oligomers of the same molecule, some possible degradation products, and leachables from earlier purification steps. As a final purification stage, the polishing step must be chosen on the basis of its ability to resolve compounds similar in their nature and behavior to the biological of interest. Media designed to polish protein solutions from their impurity traces are characterized by the ability to produce particularly high yields. Here, the value of the biological of interest is particularly high since it is a result of numerous, complex, and expensive manufacturing processes prior to this point. Most frequently, gel permeation media are good candidates to remove the last traces of impurities.

The size of particles that are necessarily used in packed beds should be relatively small for a better separation efficiency. Today, unfortunately, most of the gel permeation scalable media are not totally rigid and create unacceptable back pressures when used at large scale and when the particle size is below 40 μm. Reversed-phase media (RPM) could also be considered as adapted candidates for polishing purposes, unless they denature the proteins of interest. Figure 3.11 illustrates schematically what a purification bio-processing model should look like in order to be adaptable to most cases, providing the capture stage is very selective and involves the principle of affinity recognition. In the capture step affinity-based media frequently are a choice, while HIC and/or IEX are preferred for intermediate purification. Polishing is restricted to gel filtration or reversed-phase HPLC. Selective recognition between the medium surface chemistry and the protein to separate decreases over the bioprocessing steps. Efficiency of separation (with smaller rigid particles, for instance) is progressively increased for high resolution purposes. In this scheme, resolution level is supposed to be progressively higher over the steps.

Importance of Particle Shape, Size, and Porosity

Early designed sorbents consisted of irregular particles. The most popular example is the cellulose-based ion exchangers, which are

Figure 3.11. Schematic representation of a general model for downstream bioprocessing with a goal to minimize the number of steps, based on a rational choice of selectivity and efficiency for optimal resolution.

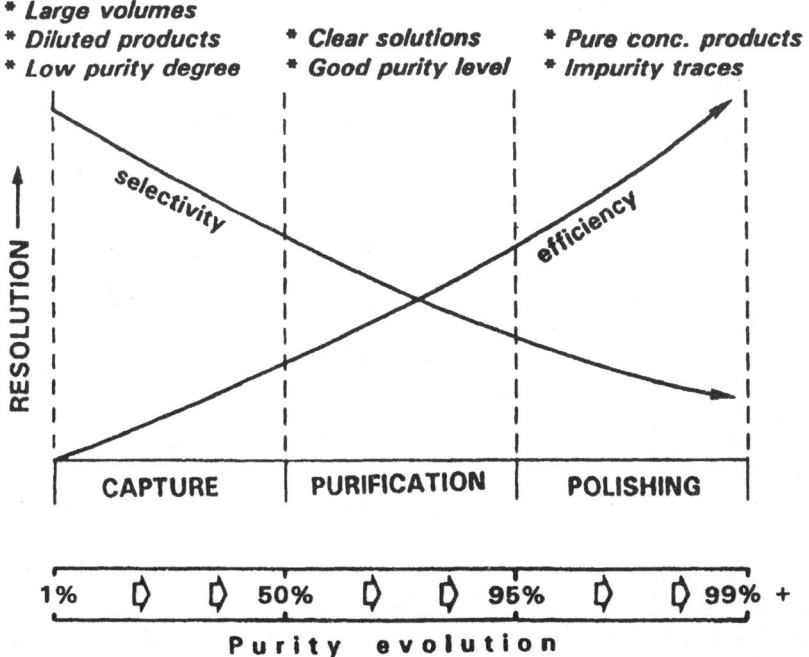

fiber shaped and are cut to have a length of about 100–300 μm. Other examples are dextran gels for IEX that were supplied in the past as irregular particles and porous silica that is available today in both irregular and spherical shapes. Irregular particles produce generally poor separation efficiency as a consequence of nonperfect column packings. Deformation of chromatographic peaks are observed in practice in preparative columns filled with irregular particles (Kaminski 1994). The bed void volume obtained with irregular particles is smaller when compared to spherical particles and generates higher back pressures, even if larger particles are used. These negative physicochemical consequences were at the origin of efforts made to obtain spherical cellulose and silica particles (Motozato and Hirayama 1984). The importance of physical shape of cellulosic material has been, for instance, discussed by James and Stanworth (1964); fiber-shaped particles seem, in fact, responsible for common disturbances, such as increased and nonuniform axial column diffusion and channeling phenomena that reduce dramatically the efficiency of the column bed.

Columns packed with spherical particles and, more specifically, with narrow diameter distribution beads provide high separation performance and generally show low back pressure. Particle size and particle size distribution impacts the chromatographic separation parameters of efficiency and dynamic binding capacity. It has a strong effect on back pressure and also on media cost. It is known that small particles provide a large number of plates for a given column length and, as a result, high column efficiency and resolution. The unavoidable tendency of an increase in back pressure can be limited by the use of rigid particles. Particle size also influences dynamic binding capacity when the flow rate is changed. The diffusion of solutes inside beads, where the interaction occurs, is time dependent—it takes longer to diffuse across a large diameter than a small one. Recommendations on how to select the size of media particles is, therefore, a very complex issue. Small particle size generally provides a higher dynamic capacity and a better resolution for protein mixtures, even for high separation velocities. A direct consequence of such a situation is a decrease of column size for a given load, yielding better separation properties with less packing material.

On the preparative scale, media with small particle size induce back pressures that are unacceptably high with soft and semirigid materials, which additionally influences the cost of the process. Particles of diameter smaller than 20 μm are generally expensive and represent a large capital investment, further affecting the purification process cost. Particles of diameter larger than 80 μm are much less expensive, but give lower performance. General economic models have been investigated to determine productivities of particles of different diameter, assuming that the sorbent life is within 100–300 separation runs (Peskin and Rudge 1992). With respect to cost considerations and for columns designed for preparative purposes, economic calculations based on productivity demonstrated that particles of 20–40 μm diameter have a definitive advantage over smaller particles. On the other hand, their advantage over particles of about 80–100 μm is essentially based on a time/performance ratio.

The porosity of media beads (porous volume and pore size) is also important for preparative applications in protein separation. Proteins are large macromolecules and must diffuse inside the medium network to reach all adsorption sites. The size of the pore must, therefore, be larger than the molecular size of the majority of the proteins. The exclusion limit for proteins expressed in kilodaltons is generally the parameter that is measured when dealing with soft gels, since the real pore diameter cannot be directly measured. Diffusion coefficients of proteins are within the range of 4.99–13.0 × 10^{-7} cm^2/sec depending on molecular weight and molecular shape (Creighton 1993). These values were established for water at 20°C at low protein concentrations. Diffusion time within the porous beads may not be estimated using the bead diameter alone and should include internal porosity characteristics as well (e.g., considering the tortuosity of pores). Small pores do not permit the protein to diffuse and restrict dramatically the sorption capacity, which is limited in this case to the external available surface of beads (pellicular particles). This situation, well suited for analytical purposes, is totally inappropriate for preparative and production applications. On the other hand, large or very large pores exceeding by far the protein size, do not offer specific benefits in terms of productivity at large scale where the linear velocity does not exceed 1–3 meters/hour. The only benefit is the possibility of running at very high velocities, but sacrificing the sorption capacity, which is the result of a limited surface area available for protein interaction.

Resolution Versus Packing Properties

Resolution is, in practice, defined as the ability of a given sorbent to separate two components. This is the result of the distance between two peaks related to the medium selectivity and their respective width related to the medium efficiency (Boschetti et al. 1974). Figure 3.12 represents the impact of these two parameters on resolution. *A* and *C* as well as *B* and *D* are separations obtained with the

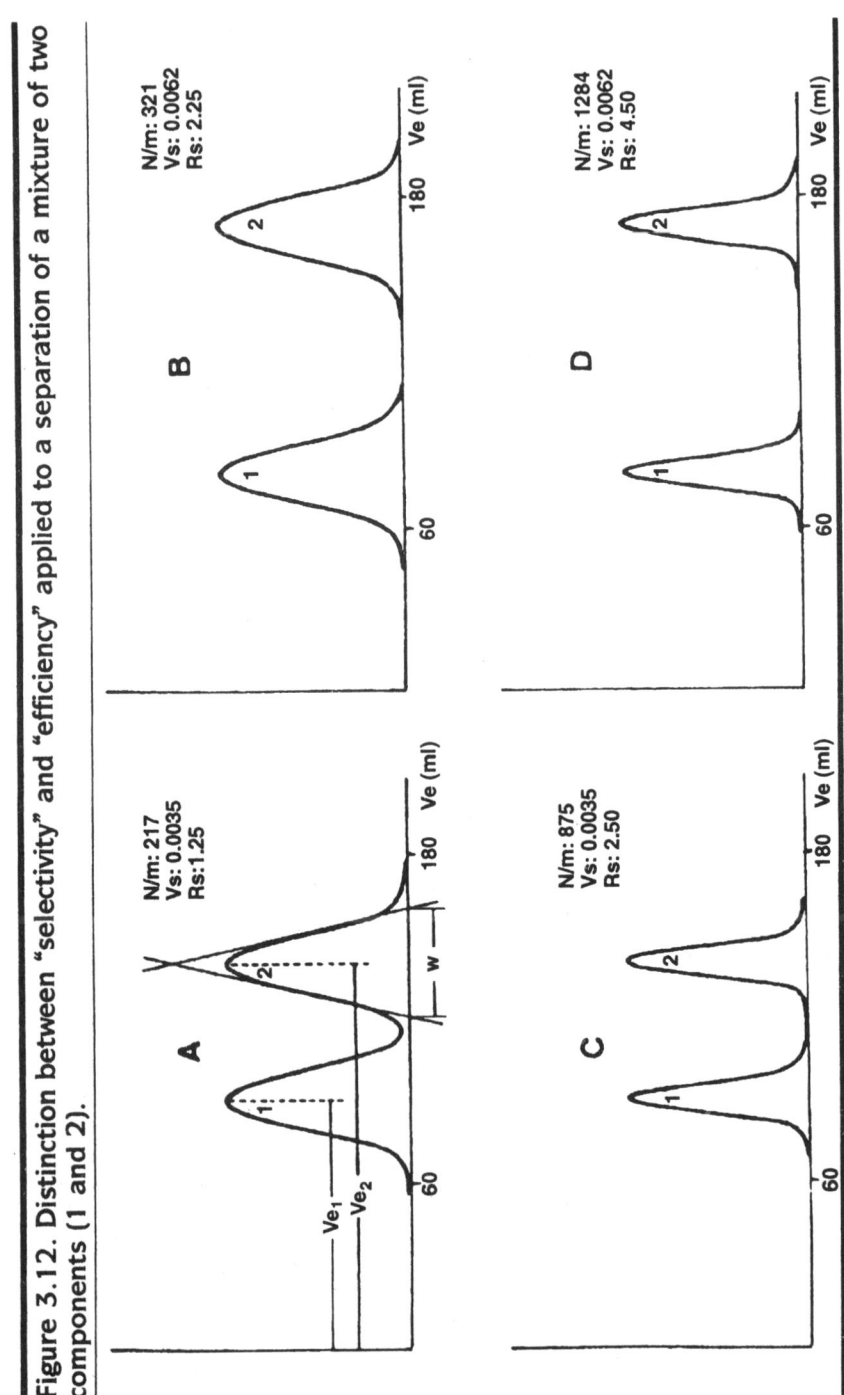

Figure 3.12. Distinction between "selectivity" and "efficiency" applied to a separation of a mixture of two components (1 and 2).

same sorbents (same selectivity, *Vs*), but the sorbents *C* and *D* are composed of smaller particles and give consequently higher separation efficiencies (higher number of plates, *N/m*). *A* and *B* as well as *C* and *D* are separations obtained with sorbents of different selectivity (selectivity of *B* is higher than *A*), but of similar particle size and consequently similar separation efficiency (peak width or *N/m*). Resolutions (*Rs*) for *B* and *C* are similar: the lower selectivity of *C* is compensated by its higher separation efficiency (*Ve* = elution volume).

Measurement of resolution is a common operation in protein separation by liquid chromatography and is used as a guide to optimize separation conditions. Some parameters related to resolution, such as flow rate, loading, temperature, and column geometry, are accessible to users so that they can modify and optimize the separation results. Other parameters more closely associated with media characteristics, which by definition are unaccessible to the user, could also have a significant impact on the resolution. Table 3.5 gives a picture of the situation. Parameters of importance are flow rate, particle size, and elution mode.

When increasing linear velocity, resolution decreases as a consequence of thermodynamic limitations. On the other hand, small particles provide a large number of plates, increasing dramatically column efficiency. With rigid media the back pressure generated when decreasing the particle size can be a secondary issue. Manufacturers of media generally balance between several parameters at a time; most of them are focused on selectivity (the chemical

Table 3.5. Main Parameters That Modify Resolution in Liquid Chromatography

Accessible and Modifiable by the User	Not Accessible to the User
pH of mobile phase	Type of sorption groups
Ionic strength of mobile phase	Site accessibility and density
Elution gradient slope	Particle size and distribution
Column geometry	Sorption capacity
Flow rate	Polymer properties
Temperature	Size of the pores
Loading volume and concentration	Nonspecific binding

structure of the sorption sites), the accessibility of pores, the flexibility of polymers, and the sorption capacity.

Media for Ion-Exchange Chromatography

Within the group of sorbents for protein separation, ion exchangers are most commonly used for large-scale applications. They are mostly composed of a polymeric porous structure, where electrically charged chemical groups are covalently attached. The mechanisms of ion exchange have been extensively described and are easily applicable to protein separations, since a protein is a polyelectrolyte with a dominant net charge modulated by the environmental pH. A wide variety of charged groups attached to a polymeric matrix are available on the market and are classified in two categories: cationic and anionic. Cationic groups are essentially represented by weak tertiary amino groups and strong quaternary amino groups. Anionic chemical groups include strong acidic residues, such as sulfonates, sulfates, and phosphates, and weak acids, such as carboxy groups. These chemical groups are covalently attached to a polymeric backbone through hydrocarbon chains of various length. The introduction of a chemically charged group is made by either chemical reactions with the polymeric chains (Peterson and Sober 1956) or by direct copolymerization of functionalized monomers (Mikes et al. 1979; Mikes et al. 1980; Girot and Boschetti 1981).

Sulfates are, in most cases, attached to polysaccharide sorbents and are typically used at pH below 7. Sulfonates are attached to both saccharidic polymer material and synthetic polymers. Carboxylates are obtained by alkaline reaction of chloroacetic acid on hydroxyl-containing polymers; they are widely used as cation exchangers in a more restricted range of pH than sulfonated media. Quaternary amino groups are well-known structures for strong cationic media; their high pK value allows their use in a wide pH range with, in a number of cases, the provision of higher selectivity in separating anionic proteins than media with tertiary amino groups. Diethylaminoethyl (DEAE) groups, very popular in protein separations, are complex structures resulting from the reaction between diethylaminoethyl chloride and a nonionic sorbent containing hydroxyl groups under alkaline conditions. Such chemical conditions induce secondary reactions on the monomer itself, generating oligo-DEAE chains. These complex structures with different pKs are characterized easily by titration curves; however, they do not modify the ion-exchange mechanism with proteins. In contrast to gel filtration media (see below), the matrix does not have a strictly defined pore size. Here the pores are generally large enough to avoid any possible molecular sieving effect during separation. Commercially available ion exchangers have various mechanical and chemical resistances and are based on natural, synthetic, and mineral composite materials. The type of group immobilized to the matrix determines the type and strength of the ion exchanger. There are a variety of groups that have been selected for use as ion exchangers (Table 3.6).

As far as preparative applications are concerned, productivity is an important aspect to consider. It is the result of the combination of sorption capacity and flow rate. The sorption capacity varies in a nonlinear fashion with the flow rate, and the extent of this variation depends considerably on media structure. Information on parameters related to the media itself that impact the productivity directly are not easily available from media manufacturers, and only limited data are published (Boschetti 1994). Some media sorbents undergo a small dynamic sorption capacity decrease with increasing flow rate; others show a rapid decrease in dynamic binding capacity with increasing flow rates. The loadability of an ion exchanger at a specified flow rate is a major feature with regard to productivity. Variations from sorbent to sorbent depend on the number of active sites, their availability to interact with the solute, and the total surface area available to large macromolecules. A compromise must be found between two extreme situations that are exemplified by pellicular-based sorbents with very high availability of ionic groups but very low sorption capacity, and dense polymeric networks with much higher surface area covered with numerous ionic sites but

Table 3.6. Functional Groups Used in Ion Exchangers

Anion Exchangers	Functional Group
Aminoethyl (AE)	$-OCH_2CH_2NH_3{}^+$
Diethylaminoethyl (DEAE)	$-OCH_2CHN^+H(CH_2CH_2)_2$
Quaternary aminoethyl (QAE)	$-OCH_2CH_2N^+(C_2H_5)CH_2CH(OH)CH_3$
Cation Exchangers	**Functional Group**
Carboxymethyl (CM)	$-OCH_2COO^-$
Phospho	$-PO_4H^{2-}$
Sulphopropyl (SP)	$-CH_2CH_2CH_2SO_3{}^-$

very low availability. The analysis of curves obtained by plotting the dynamic sorption capacity versus flow rate (Figure 3.13) are of major importance for the chromatographer to calculate the best productivity for a specific fractionation.

Resolution variations versus flow rate are also of importance when calculating the productivity of an ion exchanger, since when increasing the separation speed the targeted purity could not be achieved. It can be considered, however, as a general rule that highly selective ion exchangers (generally containing strong ionic groups) combined with high levels of dynamic capacity and pores large enough to have the proteins diffusing into the beads, constitute the best choice for large-scale applications. The media must not be limited in its flow rate characteristics. In a large-scale application, the productivity of an ion exchange medium is also a function of its ability to be regenerated properly so as to be used for numerous cycles.

Media for Hydrophobic Interaction Chromatography

Hydrophobic interaction chromatography is based on the association of lipophilic regions of certain amino acids constituting the

Figure 3.13. Variation of dynamic sorption capacity (DBC) of different ion exchangers with cationic groups as a function of the flow rate. Determinations of DBC were performed using breakthrough curves. Protein solution was bovine serum albumin at 5 mg/mL in 50 mM Tris-HCl buffer, pH 8.6. A: Q-HyperD; B: DEAE-Trisacryl Plus; C: cationic agarose beads.

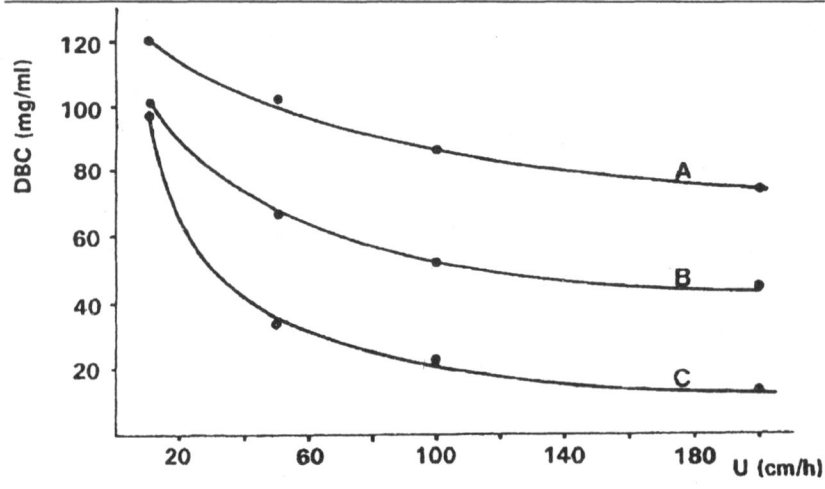

proteins and hydrophobic ligands immobilized on hydrophilic media. The hydrocarbon regions that are responsible for the hydrophobic character are either aliphatic or aromatic or both, and possess the common properties of excluding water and forming a hydrophobic association resulting in the rearrangement of water molecules. Hydrophobic interactions are relatively strong molecular associations that are dependent on the nature of the hydrophobic site structure and are influenced by salt concentration and by temperature. Numerous hydrophobic ligands have been described and coupled to an insoluble matrix for the separation of proteins and enzymes: butyl, octyl, and phenyl groups are the most popular. Pentyl, hexyl, dodecyl, octadecyl, and trityl groups have also been reported for a number of applications. The density of hydrophobic ligands in HIC media is lower than reversed-phase media, and the balance between hydrophilic and hydrophobic groups confers the appropriate binding capacity and specificity. Experimentally, HIC media can be synthesized by coupling hydrocarbon chains on an inert activated matrix. Matrices for hydrocarbon chain grafting are generally based on both agarose and hydrophilic synthetic copolymers where hydrophobic ligands are chemically attached via nonionic linkages. The most common way to immobilize these ligands is to use an oxyrane-activated matrix yielding ether bonds. More recently thioether linkages obtained by reacting oxirane-activated supports with thiols have been described (Maisano et al. 1985).

Phenyl-substituted sorbents are more often used with uncharacterized proteins. Their degree of hydrophobicity is intermediate, and the interaction occurs with aromatic residues of amino acids constituting the protein structure. Whereas phenyl groups are used for strongly hydrophobic proteins, aliphatic chains are chosen for weakly hydrophobic structures. For more information on HIC media, see specific reviews by Kennedy (1990, 339–343) and Wheelwright (1991). The adsorption of a protein by hydrophobic interaction is generally performed at high ionic strength. Elution of the adsorbed material is usually achieved by decreasing the ionic strength by using a linear or stepwise gradient. It can also be induced by the addition of detergents, urea, ethylene glycol, or chaotropic agents, such as potassium isothiocyanate or sodium perchlorate.

Media for Affinity Chromatography

Affinity media are prepared by attaching product-specific ligands on an inert porous matrix by means of a chemical reaction. The selection of specific ligands, the identification of the most appropriate immobilization chemistry, and the matrix choice are the most important parameters. The selection of the matrix is determined by a large pore dimension, a high rigidity, and the possibility of developing defined surface chemistry for ligand immobilization. The selection of all these parameters is the consequence of a rational approach to keep all the affinity molecular mechanisms free from side effects. The size of the media pores must be large enough to permit the free diffusion of macromolecules for a better interaction with the ligand active site. Inertness of the matrix is needed to avoid nonspecific binding, which would decrease the selectivity of affinity media. The matrix is also selected in order to have available chemical groups where ligands can be chemically attached after a preliminary treatment with a specific activating agent. These groups are most frequently hydroxyls. In special cases the matrix may contain amino, carboxy, or thiol groups for specific immobilization chemistries. Cross-linked agaroses and macroporous hydrophilic polymers are well known as basic matrices for the preparation of affinity media. The ligand immobilization process implies distinct phases called matrix activation and ligand immobilization. Depending on the molecular sizes of the ligand and the protein, a matrix with medium or large pore structure will be chosen. The choice of the activation reaction should consider the chemical composition of the matrix.

During coupling reactions in aqueous buffers, the activated sites compete with water molecules and may be hydrolyzed. This undesirable reaction decreases the potential coupling capacity of the support and may introduce nonspecific binding sites on the matrix. Depending on the nature of the activating agent, aqueous hydrolysis can produce chemical derivatives at the surface of the matrix that constitute possible sites for nonspecific adsorption. With certain activating agents, such as carbonyl-diimidazole and p-nitrophenyl-chloroformate, aqueous hydrolysis restores the initial structure of the matrix. After ligand coupling, unreacted groups must be capped with small hydrophilic molecules without damaging the matrix and the immobilized, biologically active ligand. In spite of the apparent complexity of affinity chromatography, large-scale applications are becoming more and more popular for the preparation of human injectables (Janson 1984; Lebing et al. 1994).

To help the user in the complex procedure of obtaining activated sorbents, a number of ready-to-use media are commercially available. As the combination possibilities are relatively large (type of porous matrix, activating agent, degree of activation, chemical link, etc.), ready-to-use affinity sorbents probably represent the largest list among chromatographic materials. For more details on matrix activation chemistries, specific procedures and applications, see Boschetti (1994), Mohr and Pommerening (1985), and Turkova (1978, 151–222).

Media for Molecular Sieving (Gel Filtration)

Gel filtration media for preparative applications are generally composed of natural, cross-linked polysaccharides (Mahuron 1979); synthetic, three-dimensional polymers (Barker et al. 1981); or a mixture of them (Haff and Easterday 1978; Boschetti et al. 1974). They are characterized by their exclusion limit and their selectivity range (Determann 1968), both of which are dependent on the gel pore size and on the pore size distribution. Generally, gel filtration is a limited resolution technique, where the selectivity between peaks is increased when the pore size distribution is very narrow. This situation explains why several media are necessary to cover, by zone overlapping, the total range of protein size (Andrewes 1965).

Regularity in polymer synthesis is the key to increasing the selectivity and batch-to-batch consistency. Such gel media are generally soft or semirigid, especially when designed for the separation of medium and large proteins. Unsubstituted agarose-based media are applied to the separation of very large macromolecules; dextran- and polyacrylamide-based media are used for small and medium-sized proteins.

Specific media with very low exclusion limits are used for desalting and buffer exchange. When the selectivity curve of gel permeation media is shallow with consequent large fractionation range, numerous protein peaks could be placed in the limited space between the void volume and the total column volume. The selectivity in this case is low. For similar column efficiencies (essentially similar particle size), the resolution is significantly lower with media showing shallow selectivity curves. Consequently, a large fractionation range must be compensated by small particle size to increase the separation efficiency in order to achieve acceptable resolution. Selectivity curves are, therefore, good "identity cards" of the general characteristics of gel filtration media (Figure 3.14).

Such curves are determined by plotting the log of the molecular mass of known proteins versus their K_{av}. Slopes of the curves indicate the selectivity of the gel filtration media: curve 2 is less selective than curve 1, because for two given molecules (m_1 and m_2), the K_{av} difference is lower. A similar exclusion limit, Ex.L. (curves 2 and 3), does not mean that the separation selectivity is the same.

$$K_{av} = \frac{V_e - V_0}{V_t - V_0}$$

Figure 3.14. Typical selectivity curves obtained in separating proteins by gel filtration.

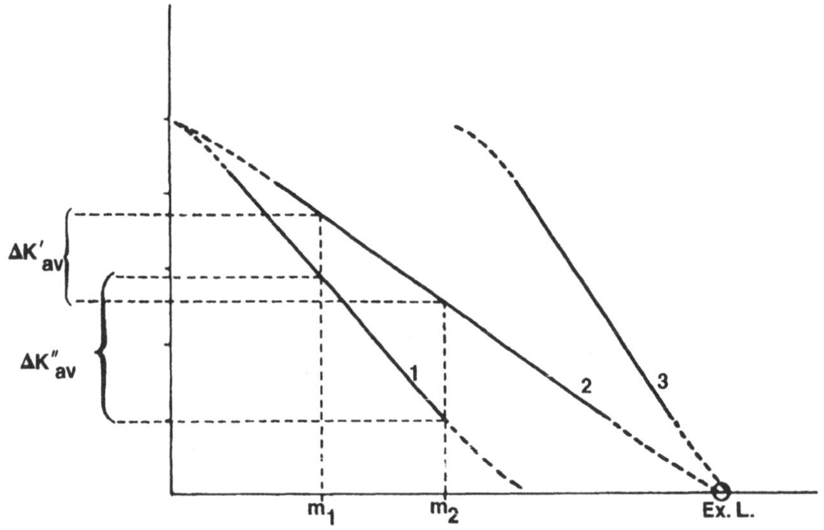

where V_e is the peak elution volume, V_t is the packed bed volume, and V_0 is the void volume.

Gel filtration media generally do not show nonspecific interaction with solutes. It is, however, described that some polymers under particular conditions of ionic strength and pH, show nonspecific adsorption disturbing the pure molecular exclusion separation mechanism (Belew et al. 1978). They may exhibit weak electrostatic interactions that are particularly evident at low ionic strength and when the pH is not neutral. These media can also show hydrophobic characteristics that can be minimized by decreasing the ionic strength or by adding small quantities of chaotropic substances. Gel filtration is not a very productive technology, but in a number of cases it is a very useful final purification/polishing step, where the remaining impurities consisting of traces of protein fragments, aggregates, and dimers are eliminated.

There are advantages linked to separation by molecular sieving chromatography. Samples to be injected into a column do not need to be dissolved in the same buffer used for the separation. Equilibration occurs inside the column without any modification in the separation mechanism. Gel filtration separation is independent of the pH and the ionic strength; it constitutes a clear advantage over other chromatographic separations. Since there are no adsorption-desorption phases, all of the separation cycle is performed with the same buffer and the column is automatically equilibrated for another cycle. If there are no nonspecific adsorptions, regeneration is also unnecessary.

In spite of all these advantages, running molecular sieving media at large scale requires modifications of the technology to increase its poor productivity. As a general rule, a cycle can be considered complete after a passage of a column volume of buffer. A second injection should consequently be performed after the passage of a column volume of buffer calculated from the first injection. Assuming that the excluded molecules appear after approximately one-third of the bed volume (void volume), the second injection could be effected when a volume of buffer corresponding to about 65 percent of the gel bed volume is passed from the sample injection. In case of the absence of products in the void volume, calculations should be accurately done in order to diminish even more the distance between sample injections (injection anticipation, see Figure 3.15).

In the space between the first injection point (Inj. 1) and the elution of the first peak (void volume Vo1, which corresponds at least to 30 percent of the bed volume) no events happen; this space can, therefore, be used partially or totally by anticipating sample injections. Injection 2 can be executed before the end of the first separation cycle (Inj. 2) in order to locate the Vo2 just after the conclusion of the first cycle (Inj. 1). Other injections (Inj. 3 and 4) follow the same rule of injection anticipation. The time saved per separation cycle and the buffer volume are represented by the distance between a given injection (e.g., Inj. 2) and the previous sample injection. Following these rules, it is possible to increase the productivity of a gel filtration column by at least 25 percent. The right side of the figure is a schematic view of two chromatographic profiles inside a column obtained following the principle of injection anticipation with their respective injections sequence and void volumes.

Gel filtration columns are characterized by a long length, frequently incompatible with soft gel media. To circumvent gel compression problems, portions of short columns can be stacked. This approach generates some difficulties that are associated with the complexity of the installation; however, it is possible to take advantage of this configuration by modifying the linear velocity individually from stack to stack and to use them in a more productive

Figure 3.15. Schematic representation of a gel filtration cycle, and a graphical explanation on how to increase productivity by anticipating the injections between runs.

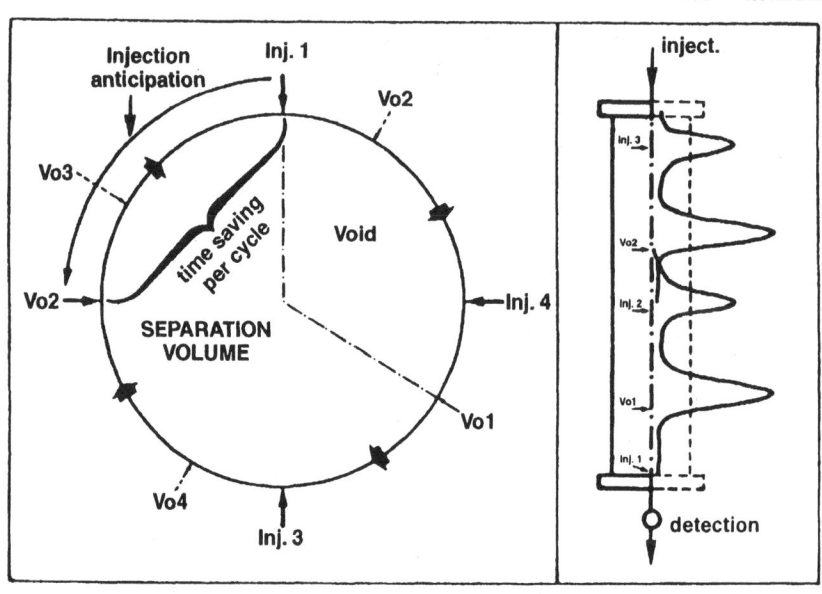

fashion than a regular column (see Figure 3.16). Each section can work independently, taking advantage of the two pumping systems (T-1 and T-2) and the set of valves. When the chromatographic cycles include a regeneration step (e.g., sodium hydroxide washing) it must be then buffer equilibrated. Both regeneration and reequilibration operations could be done under a rapid speed that justifies the use of an independent pumping system. To avoid time losses due to regeneration and reequilibration, each section can work independently and at different flow rates. Synchronization required between columns is managed using automated devices.

For instance, a column divided into three identical portions (or stacks) can be managed in such a way that the first portion is used for sample injection while the second portion is under reequilibration and the third is regenerated or washed. Each portion can thus run independently and at different speed.

Considering the nature of solutions—their volume and the flow rates—it is possible to give more flexibility to a gel filtration column than to any other chromatographic technique. Additionally, peaks

Figure 3.16. Preparative gel filtration setup consisting of a column divided in three sections.

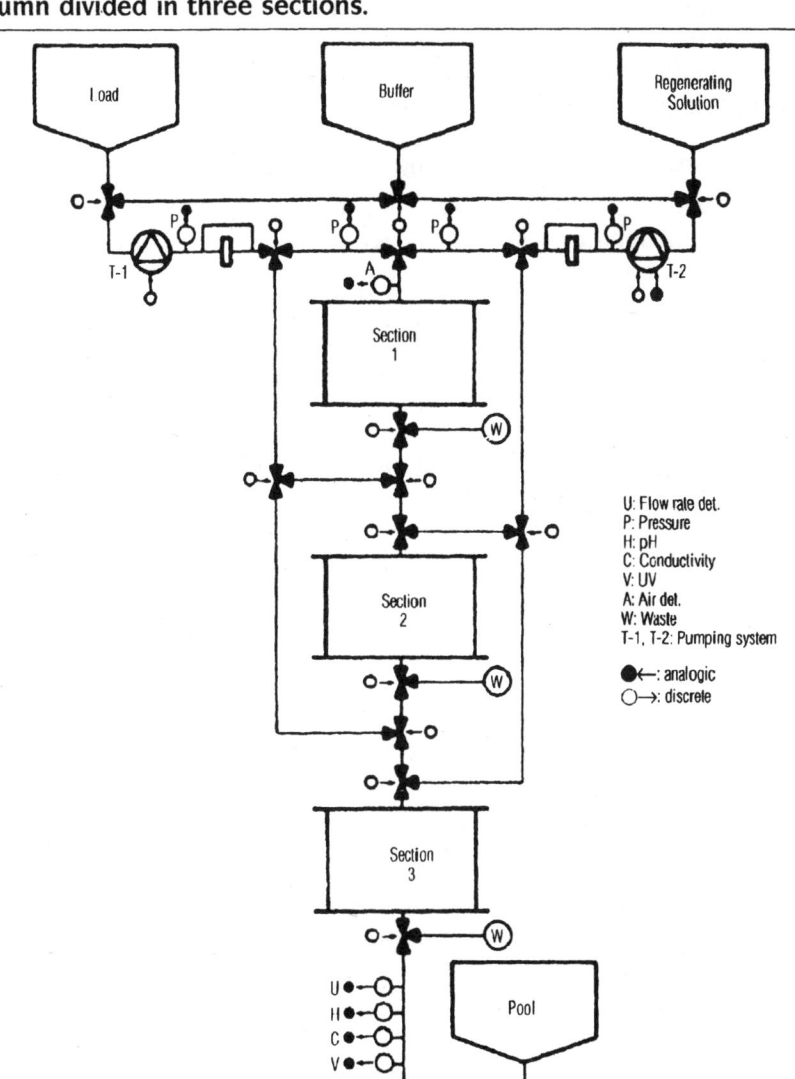

U: Flow rate det.
P: Pressure
H: pH
C: Conductivity
V: UV
A: Air det.
W: Waste
T-1, T-2: Pumping system

●←: analogic
○→: discrete

or portions of peaks could be recovered when needed between stacks, avoiding, in this case, unnecessary dilutions. Time savings are also possible by associating stack configurations with injection anticipation (discussed above).

Other Special Media Used in Bioseparation

Many unconventional media also are used in liquid chromatography for protein separation. Among them, hydroxyapatite, reversed-phase media, thiophilic sorbents, and solid phases to remove special chemicals deserve to be mentioned.

Hydroxyapatite Chromatography

Hydroxyapatite, which consists of a mosaic of complex, hydrated, calcium phosphate crystals, has been used for a long time in liquid chromatography. Solute–solid phase interactions are relatively complex and not completely elucidated (Gorbunoff 1990, 329–339). The crystal surface is essentially electronegative at neutral pH, and amino groups of the proteins interact easily with it. The lower the pH of the buffer, the higher the molarity of the buffer needed to desorb the protein. Proteins with high isoelectric points are eluted by displacement with phosphate ions, chloride gradients, or calcium ions. Free carboxyl groups of the proteins interact with calcium sites by complexation, and the desorption of a protein based on this mechanism is achieved by compounds forming strong complexes with calcium ions, such as phosphates and fluorides. In this case a simple increase of ionic strength using, for instance, sodium chloride is ineffective for protein desorption. The complexity of the molecular interaction associated with the difficulty to handle large quantities of hydroxyapatite without forming a large amount of fines explains the long-time reluctance to use this material. Today, particularly well-adapted hydroxyapatite sorbents are available, and this kind of separation is becoming more popular also at large scale. Advantages of hydroxyapatite are related to the specificity for some proteins, its ability to be treated with highly concentrated sodium hydroxide, its inertness toward biological degradation, and the absence of formation of toxic by-products.

Reversed-Phase Media

Reversed-phase media used extensively in the separation of fine chemicals are used more frequently at preparative scale for the purification of proteins of low or medium molecular size (Regnier and Gooding 1980; Wheelwright 1991) and peptides. These media are based mostly on silica of high surface area on which hydrocarbon chains (butyl, octyl, dodecyl, octadecyl, . . .) are chemically grafted. The interaction with proteins is essentially of hydrophobic nature, and hydroorganic mixtures are necessary to elute the solutes. The use of solvents is one of the major limitations of RPM due to the high cost of some pure solvents, solvent handling, disposal, and the need for an explosion-proof facility. Risk of protein denaturation should also be considered when using RPM. Large proteins are more susceptible to organic solvents than small proteins, explaining why these media are mostly limited to biological compounds of low molecular weight and peptides. One of the largest reported utilizations of RPM in bioseparation is the final purification of insulin (Kroeff et al. 1989). Other limitations to the extensive use of RPM in bioseparation are associated with hydrocarbon chain linkage that can contaminate the biological of interest and the high sensitivity of large surface silica to alkaline washings.

Thiophilic Media

Thiophilic sorbents were described more than a decade ago for protein purification (Porath et al. 1985) in general and for specific applications in antibody purifications (Schwarz et al. 1995). Different varieties of thiophilic media exist: aliphatic chains containing sulfur atoms and chains associated with heterocyclic compounds containing nitrogen and sulfur atoms. The mechanism of action of such material in protein separation is still incompletely elucidated; however, since it is mediated by salts, it seems that, among others, hydrophobic associations happen. Adsorption of proteins is generally obtained by using concentrated solutions of sodium, potassium, or ammonium sulfate; the elution is easily achieved by lowering the salt concentration and/or the pH.

The original ligand for thiophilic adsorption (Porath 1986) is as follows:

$$\text{Matrix–}SO_2\text{-}(CH_2)_2\text{–}S\text{–}(CH_2)_2\text{–}OH$$

Noper et al. (1988) modified the ligand to improve the specificity to achieve a one-step purification for monoclonal antibodies. They coupled the ligand to silica.

$$Si\text{–}(CH_2)_3\text{–}O\text{–}(CH_2)_3\text{–}O\text{–}(CH_2)_3\text{–}SO_2\text{–}(CH_2)_2\text{–}S\text{–}(CH_2)_2\text{–}OH$$

Thiophilic adsorption is an approach for creating generic ligands for protein purification. To what extent more rational approaches can be utilized in order to create a highly specific ligand is still an open question. Molecular modeling employing computational chemistry techniques may contribute to an explanation of how these types of ligands act.

Metal Chelate Chromatography

Metal chelating technique has recently received attention since it can target specific structures in proteins and, therefore, may have product-specific characteristics toward more than one product. Zinc and copper ions are frequently used. Zinc-containing media can be used with proteins having clustered groups of histidine or histidine-cysteine residues. For example, the enzyme carbonic anhydrase has a group of three histidine residues that are involved in zinc complexation (Christianson 1991). Hydrogen bonding is of importance for histidine-zinc interactions. In the case of cysteine, this is the sulfur atom, which interacts with zinc due to its size and polarizability (Chakrabarti 1989). In this technique the elution is carried by lowering the pH (Mohr and Pommerening 1985). A review of structural aspects of metal-protein interactions was given by Glusker (1991). The metal binding atoms are oxygen, nitrogen, and sulfur. The metal-binding oxygen atom occurs in aspartic and glutamic acids (carboxyl group) and in serine, threonine, and tyrosine (hydroxyl group); the metal-binding nitrogen occurs in histidine and tryptophan; and sulfur occurs in cysteine and methionine. Metal ions may form several complexing bonds with the surrounding residues and water molecules (e.g., in carboxypeptidase, zinc may form complexes with two histidines via nitrogen atoms, with glutamic acid via its two oxygen atoms, and with water [Glusker 1991]).

Other Stationary Phases

Dye-affinity chromatography media, Protein A sorbents, and media for immunoaffinity chromatography are also very important stationary phases useful for the preparative-scale purification of proteins. For reviews see Mohr and Pommerening (1985), Wheelwright (1991), and Boschetti (1994). Table 3.7 shows a review of affinity biological ligands (peptides and proteins) used for the purification of proteins and for diagnostics.

Proteins are sometimes extracted in the presence of nonionic detergents that must be removed during the final stage of purification. The possible presence of lipid-enveloped viruses necessitates an inactivating treatment involving nonionic solvent and detergent mixtures that must be removed during the bioseparation process. For whichever method is used, special media have been designed to deplete the protein solution from these undesirable chemical compounds. They are used as a "filter" since the proteins do not interact with the media during chromatography, but the solvents and detergents do (Guerrier et al. in press). Before and after purification, the proteins are collected in the flow-through and the medium is regenerated by using a water-miscible solvent, such as ethanol or isopropanol.

Future Development in Separation Media

The identified trend resulting from both technological progress and economical reasons is the reduction of the number of separation steps to obtain pure and safe therapeutic proteins. Any increases in media sorption capacity and speed may represent a significant improvement in productivity. Not only could a smaller column then be used with a lower amount of media, but also less numerous and smaller hardware will be needed in restricted manufacturing areas. Considering that liquid, large-scale chromatography is today an extrapolation of a laboratory analytical technique, modifications in the technology are anticipated. This kind of evolution will certainly impact the design of stationary phases. For example, fluidized and expanded bed technology, applied at the early stages, requires very dense and highly selective sorbents. High specificity means case-by-case surface design, and trends are already visible with the development of peptide or nucleotide libraries or specific chemical imprintings. Fast exchange kinetics (adsorption-desorption) are also one of the main features of these novel surface chemistries. Highly specific capturing phases would yield concentrated and relatively pure proteins that could be processed in much more effective solid phase separation systems, where the adsorption and gradient elution steps would be achieved by using sophisticated pumping systems or by centrifugation. Media beads will be in both cases small in size, thus increasing dramatically the separation efficiency and, consequently, the resolution.

Molecular Interactions

Liquid chromatography separations depend on the molecular interactions of molecules of interest and ligands of the stationary phase. Separation is also affected by the mobile phase composition and its pH. An interference from contaminants present in the stream is also possible. The separated molecules are large and their molecular weight range is from a few thousand (e.g., peptides), through tens of thousands (e.g., human growth hormone), to several hundreds of thousands (e.g., Factor VIII), or more. Traditional ligands used in IEX, HIC, and RPC are small when compared to the size of the

Table 3.7. Affinity Bioligands Used for the Purification of Recombinant Proteins and the Production of Diagnostics

Affinity Ligand	Affinity Tag or Type of Chromatography	Limits	References
Peptides			
Arg-Gly-Arg-Gly-Gly-Arg	Anhydrotrypsin	Coelution of contaminants	Hirabayashi and Kasai (1992)
Poly-Cys	Covalent chromatography	High cys concentration downregulates the expression rate	Person et al. (1988)
Poly-Phe	Hydrophobic interaction chromatography		Person et al. (1988)
Poly-His	Nickel-chelate chromatography	Decrease of pH may destroy protein	Hochuli (1990)
Proteins			
Glutathione-S-transferase	Glutathione		Davies et al. (1993)
Protein A binding domain	IgG		Samuelson et al. (1991)

Continued on next page.

Continued from previous page.

Affinity Ligand	Affinity Tag or Type of Chromatography	Limits	References
Glutamine-synthetase/ alkaline phosphatase β-galactosidase			Köhler et al. (1990, 1001–1004)
Streptavidin	Biotin		Sano and Cantor (1991)
Protein A/luciferase	IgG	Immunoassays	Lindbladh et al. (1991)
Protein A/ glutathione-S-transferase	Glutathione and IgG	Immunoprecipitation	Lew et al. (1991)

separated molecules. The affinity and, particularly, immunoaffinity ligands may be as large as the separated molecules. Protein chromatography techniques use protein surface characteristics (e.g., electrostatic charges [IEX] and hydrophobic areas [HIC] or specific residue configurations (affinity chromatography, metal-chelate, dye-specific, etc.). Only the reversed-phase technique, when in the unfolding mode, additionally utilizes the internal parts of protein molecules. Therefore, knowledge of the surface characteristics of the protein of interest may significantly aid in separation development. If the protein crystallographic structure is known at sufficient resolution, a molecular model can be built and surface residues identified; subsequently, the surface of the molecule can be evaluated. The next step can be a selection of a group of chromatographic techniques with consideration given to available ligand types. Figure 3.17 shows the comparison of the human growth hormone molecule with the new, long, hydrophilic Q-anion exchange and the traditional DEAE and CM ion exchange and butyl HIC ligands. All molecules were drawn using Hyperchem 4.0 molecular modeling software. The human growth hormone was drawn using the file from the Brookhaven Protein Data Bank. Ligand molecules spatial structures were optimized using the molecular mechanics force field (MM+).

Hydrophobic interaction and reversed-phase stationary phases use ligands that have hydrophobic characteristics. Hydrophobic attraction with the hydrophobic areas of the proteins depends on thermodynamics and is also related to the fact that water molecules form hydrogen-bonded clusters among themselves, while they may not form hydrogen bonds with the hydrophobic molecules or residues. Interestingly, the subject of hydrophobicity still remains controversial (Madan and Lee 1994). An accepted theory is that water molecule clusters usually involve three to six molecules; therefore, influence of the hydrophobic ligands on the surrounding water structure and on the hydrated protein with hydrophobic areas can possibly be evaluated. Figure 3.18 shows the butyl HIC ligand inside Jorgensen's "water box" model using Hyperchem 4.0. The hydrogen bonds are shown as dotted lines.

Recently Du et al. (1994) reported results of vibrational spectroscopy studies of water structures at hydrophobic surfaces. They found the presence of free (dangling) hydroxyl groups of water on the boundary between the hydrophobic surface and bulk water. The water structure near the surface is believed to assume an ordered hexagonal lattice. Such structure facilitates the presence of free hydroxyl groups. Since in these hydroxyl groups the hydrogen atoms

Figure 3.17. Human growth hormone molecule shown with the ion-exchange ligands (Q, DEAE, and CM) and the HIC ligand (butyl). Ligands are shown in sequence from top to bottom, at the left.

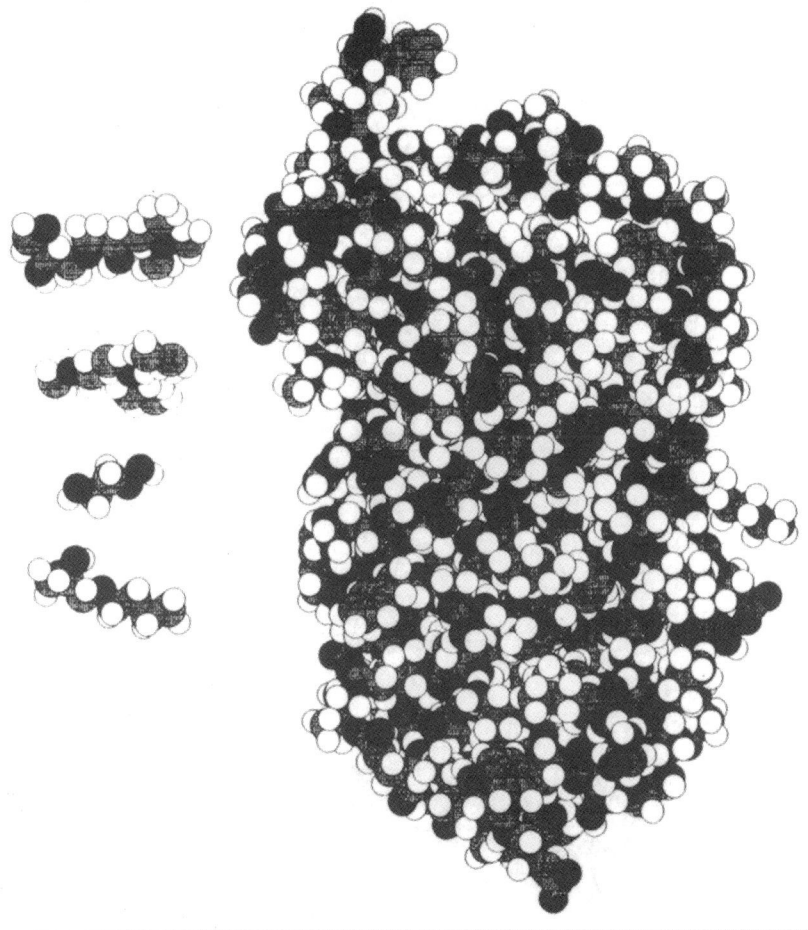

are exposed outside and oxygen atoms are closer to bulk water, they may not form hydrogen bonds with known hydrophobic structures such as $(CH_2)_n$ chains. If the solid surface is hydrophilic and only partly covered by hydrophobic alkyl chains, the water molecules may penetrate between the chains and induce their stretching (straightening).

Figure 3.18. The HIC butyl ligand placed in the "water box." Hydrogen bonds are shown as dotted lines. The hydrophobic part of the ligand does not form hydrogen bonds with the surrounding water molecules.

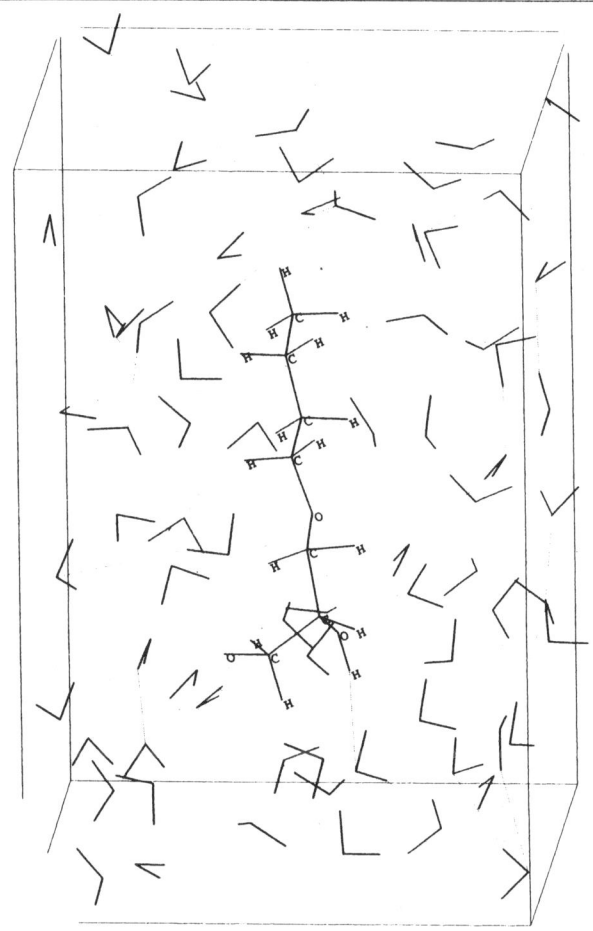

Molecular interactions among the proteins and traditional ion-exchange, hydrophobic interaction, and reversed-phase ligands are well described in literature. Molecular modeling may aid in exploring molecular interactions among biological macromolecules and more complex ligands, such as those used in affinity and product-specific separations (e.g., dyes, peptides, antibodies, and receptors).

The interactions between the ligands located on flexible tentacles and the surface residues of proteins may also be explored using this approach.

An important point in protein surface characteristics is its interaction with water. Mashimo and Miura (1993) conducted water structure investigations using microwave techniques and concluded that water may have two classes of structure. The local structure consists of 6 water molecules and the high order structure consists of 30 molecules. The last structure is similar to the ice lattice, although less ordered. How this proposed structure of water clusters may affect our understanding of protein-ligand interactions in chromatographic separations is yet to be seen.

OPERATIONAL CONSIDERATIONS

In the past chromatography systems have been frequently assembled by users with individual components coming from different vendors. Today, the user can work with vendors who can supply complete chromatography systems. Usually the vendors can customize their designs rapidly according to customer needs. Most of the hardware and controls testing can be done at the vendor's facility; therefore, system delivery can be matched with manufacturing site preparation. Site preparation may be standardized and requires certain floor space, air handling systems, floor and wall finishes, and utilities hookups. If the processing step requires low temperatures, a cold room or cold enclosure must be designed.

The needs of cold room operations may be reduced by the use of high flow resins and by shortening the purification time (such resins are described in "Chromatographic Media and Their Use"). The facility should assure separate areas of sufficient floor space to prepare buffers and cleaning/regenerating solutions. The handling of chromatographic packings should be performed in accordance with the manufacturer's recommendations (see also "Chromatographic Media and Their Use" and "Stationary Phase–Product Interaction Design and Operating Parameters in Large-Scale Chromatography").

The Purification Plant

Since the purification methods and the requirements are undergoing rapid development, a standardized outline of a purification plant for proteins is not available. Even the tube and pipe diameters, connectors, and so on are not standardized. In addition, there are still in use different measurement systems (metric and U.S.). Many purification plants are unique designs and are assembled using components from different manufacturers. It is also a strategy, especially of very large companies, to carry out the engineering using their own engineering departments to avoid giving away their production secrets to a contractor.

The unit operations involved are relatively simple. One is not confronted, for example, with very complicated mixing problems. Buffers and feedstocks are, in general, close to ideal Newtonian fluids. In most cases the eluents are aqueous solutions and are nontoxic, nonexplosive, and noncorrosive. The high aseptic design standards applied to the pharmaceutical industry must also be employed with the purification processes. These standards and the standards for production in open systems determine the design of a purification plant. The standards for the production of pharmaceuticals in open systems determine that the purification plant be equipped with air locks, systems providing clean air, established specifications for the surface of the floor and walls, and specific operator behavior. Typically, the purification areas are designed with air quality Class 10,000, with the number of air changes at 50 per hour, although separate areas may use higher air quality. The process piping for large chromatography separations can be routed behind the walls of the processing area with only connecting panels protruding inside. Chromatography skids are connected to these panels. Buffers, washing/cleaning, and sanitizing solutions are delivered from external tanks via the panels. Sample loading may be done locally to shorten the length of product-containing pipelines, but this decision depends on the plant layout. Plant operations may involve a concept of returning all spent liquids using the panels to waste tanks externally located, with only the product fraction being collected within the processing area. Pipelines are cleaned and sterilized in place using CIP systems and purified steam following standardized procedures.

The direction of the fluid stream is usually not reversed except for the packing procedure, where the column is sometimes operated from the bottom to the top in order to remove air bubbles. The velocity in the tube can be in laminar or turbulent range, while in the bed it is usually in the laminar range, and certain precision of the fluid delivery must be applied. The pressure drop is in the range of 1–3 bar for low pressure chromatography and reaches up to 50 bar in industrial-scale HPLC. One prerequisite is pulse-free liquid delivery, and pressure waves should be avoided. These pressure waves may occur during packing. When an adapter of large diameter is placed onto the column, a pressure wave may be induced if the adapter is lowered too fast. A crane with a high lift precision is essential in a purification plant.

The temperature requirements are not difficult to achieve and maintain. In most cases the processes are so robust that a temperature deviation of ± 5°C may have no effect on yield, purity, and peak position.

Validation of the process may have no apparent direct influence on the general design of the purification plant. However, assembly and validation of a system (hardware and process-controlling software) have a big impact on the records that must be made by the manufacturer, the parts for which are used for assembly and the design of the software.

At present chromatography is considered an "open" system (FDA 1987). A chromatography system cannot be completely sterilized, and in the sterilized portions the sterile conditions cannot be maintained over an extended period. It is very simple to sterilize tubes, pipes, valves, and so on, but it is rather complicated to sterilize the packed bed. In chromatography one can only autoclave the disassembled parts and to some extent the sorbents when they are kept in suspension. After sterilizing, the chromatography column must be packed under sterile conditions. Assuming that this is possible (it is not feasible), the system itself is not closed. The sealing of a chromatography column is not tight. The packing procedure is a very critical step in a sanitary operation. Column packing operations should, therefore, be performed in separate rooms with adequate air quality (HEPA–filtered air). Separate rooms for the packing of fresh columns and the unpacking of old columns are recommended.

Fraction collection may also be an open system. Adding sterile barriers to a fraction collector is possible, although rarely used. Also, a design of a double-sealed chromatography piston (movable column head) to improve the conditions of containment is not yet a common design. The introduction of media resistant to oxidizing conditions allows effective in situ chemical sterilization. Sodium hydroxide is only a weak sterilizing agent (Jungbauer and Lettner 1994), although it is an essential compound used in the chromatography of proteins. Sodium hydroxide effectively removes proteins, and lipid and cell wall components from the sorbents; it is also quite effective in the destruction of endotoxins. Peracetic acid, which is harmless in low concentrations and decomposes into acetic acid and water, is quite effective for the destruction of bacteria (Block 1991). Figure 3.19 shows inactivation kinetics of *Bacillus subtilis* using solutions of peracetic acid and peracetic acid and ethanol. Since

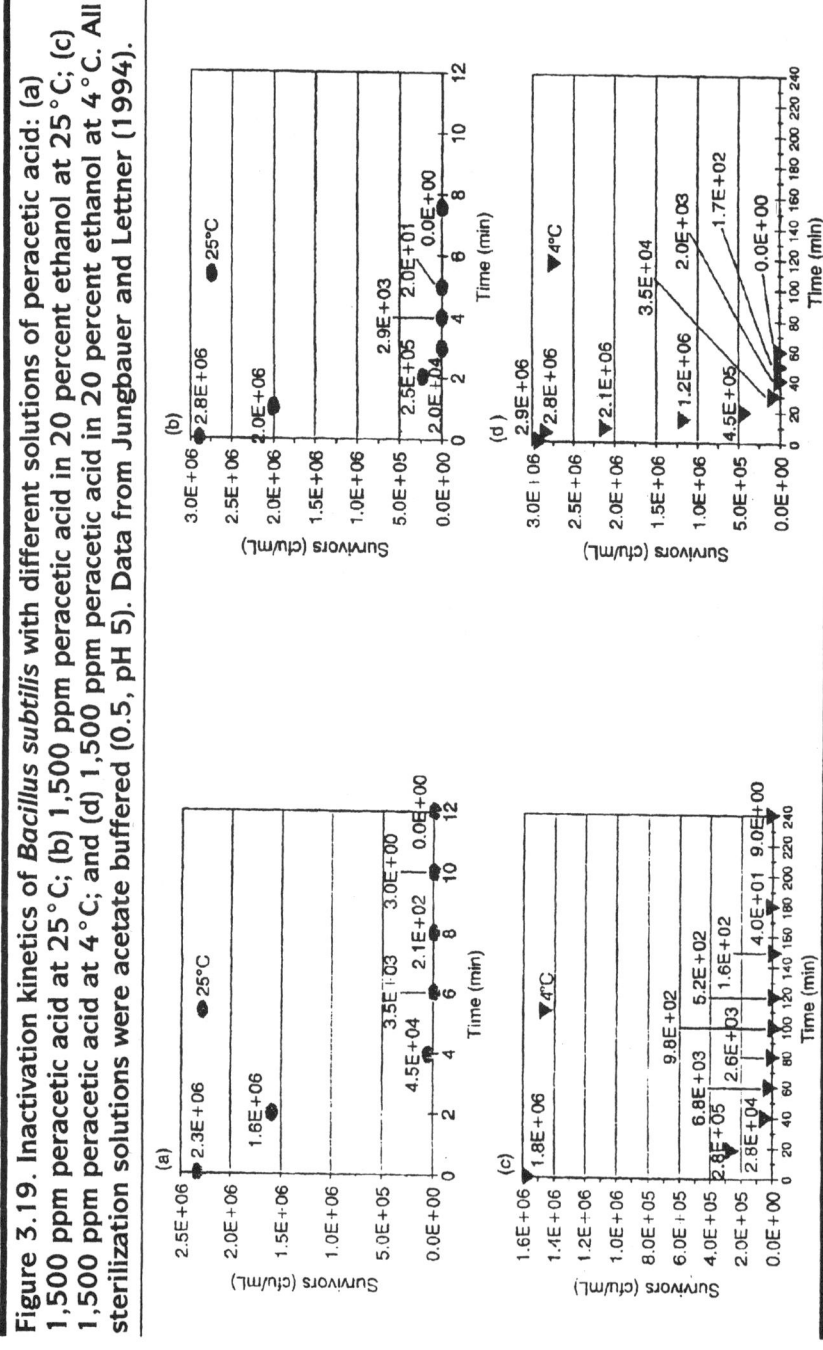

Figure 3.19. Inactivation kinetics of *Bacillus subtilis* with different solutions of peracetic acid: (a) 1,500 ppm peracetic acid at 25°C; (b) 1,500 ppm peracetic acid in 20 percent ethanol at 25°C; (c) 1,500 ppm peracetic acid at 4°C; and (d) 1,500 ppm peracetic acid in 20 percent ethanol at 4°C. All sterilization solutions were acetate buffered (0.5, pH 5). Data from Jungbauer and Lettner (1994).

peracetic acid decomposes rapidly, extended validation of the remaining sterilizing agents in the column is simplified. There are no harmful decomposition products formed. If one used NaOCl, an extensive validation of toxic by-products (chlorinated organic compounds) would be required. The reported lethality range of peracetic acid is at concentrations of 6–250 ppm for bacteria, at 25–83 ppm for yeast, at 100–150 ppm for fungi and bacterial spores, and 12–2000 ppm for viruses (Block 1991). Once in situ sterilization is possible, it may be possible to design a purification plant that meets the requirements for closed systems. Until now, the column design itself prohibits this goal, since presently designed columns have many potential dead-end spots. These dead-end spots protect microorganisms from being killed by sterilizing agents, since the agents may not reach these zones within a reasonable time.

General Concepts for Purification Plants

One must decide if the plant is used for the purification of a single product, or if the plant is considered to be a multiproduct facility. Since May 1994, the FDA has definitely allowed the purification of biologicals in a multipurpose plant (EFB 1995). High product costs and low market volumes are two of the driving forces used to produce valuable protein pharmaceuticals (valuable concerning the price and the benefit for mankind in order to cure very severe diseases) in multiproduct facilities. The worldwide demand for such products is often only hundreds of grams or a few kilograms. Building purification (production) plants for each protein pharmaceutical may not be justified. If certain precautions are taken into consideration, several pharmaceuticals can be produced in the same quality and with the same safety as in a plant dedicated for a single product.

Multipurpose (Multiproduct) Unit

In principle, there is no significant difference between a multiproduct manufacturing unit and a unit for the production of a single product. A multiproduct unit has more vessels, columns, and fraction collection devices than a unit dedicated only for one product. A very important rule is that a system is used only once in a production run. Changing the products requires validated cleaning and decontamination procedures for the system, piping, and vessels. Columns and packings are typically dedicated to the products and are moved in and out.

Operation Modes

Step Gradients Versus Linear Gradients

Both linear gradients and step gradients for elution are applicable for large scale. One advantage of stepwise elution over linear gradients is the sharpening of the peak. By using this technique, concentration factors up to 200 (Östlund et al. 1985; Jungbauer et al. 1989b) can be achieved. Especially at the initial purification stages, stepwise elution is recommended. The dilute protein solution can be concentrated this way. In addition, the step gradient can be simply produced. On the other hand, a stepwise elution is not always sufficient to obtain the required product purity, and linear gradients must be applied. When one takes into consideration the rules, which were described in "Process Development and Scale-Up," the linear gradient can be transferred into a larger scale without loss of resolution. Therefore, one should consider both linear gradients and step gradients for industrial chromatography applications.

Displacement Chromatography

In displacement chromatography the mixture, including the product of interest, is loaded onto the column and displacer, with high affinity to the media, displaces the adsorbed molecules on the principle of competitive adsorption/desorption. Due to differences between these competitive processes for various molecules in the initial mixture, the desorbed substances form bands moving in the form of a chain through the column. The bands of pure substances move along the column, with speed controlled by the movement of the displacer. Displacement chromatography is rarely used in large-scale industrial operations. Problems exist with the selection of displacers, and the simple UV detection technique may not be sufficient due to partial overlap of the elution bands (Freitag and Breier 1995). A fast analytical HPLC instrument may be used to monitor the bands.

Packed Bed Adsorption Versus Batch Adsorption

Traditionally, in blood plasma fractionation a batch adsorption in stirred tanks is carried out. The plasma or fractions of plasma may quickly foul chromatography media; at the time when chromatography media were introduced into the blood plasma fractionation industry, suitable rigid chromatography beads were not available. Process engineers in the biotechnology industry were somehow influenced by this traditional thinking. There is no reason why a protein solution should be adsorbed to a chromatography medium in a stirred tank. It also may not be wise to introduce another handling step into the unit operation. Due to the kinetics of batchwise adsorption, a 100 percent adsorption can never be achieved (Scopes 1994). A chromatography column can also be hypothetically seen as a series of small interconnected tanks. If only a fraction will adsorb in each virtual tank, repetitive adsorption will lead to a high recovery. After the adsorption process, the loaded suspension must be packed into a column for desorption. Otherwise, one will lose resolution and the advantage of the adsorption/desorption mode will be lost. Packed bed adsorption is the choice as long as the protein solution does not extensively induce fouling. Fouling is the partially irreversible buildup of layers of contaminants (lipids, carbohydrates, cell wall components, etc.) on the surface of the sorbent.

Packed Bed Adsorption Versus Expanded and Fluidized Bed Adsorption

When the protein solution induces fouling, a fluidized or expanded bed adsorption can circumvent this adverse effect. Fluidized or expanded beds can also be used for the processing of suspensions, such as cell homogenates and even fermentation broth (Gaillot 1990; Buijs and Weselingh 1980). During the adsorption step, the column is operated in an upward direction. Due to increased velocity, the bed expands, the beads start to fluidize, and the void fraction increases. This effect may lead to a lower dynamic capacity, but, on the other hand, fluidizing is a way to circumvent bed fouling. After the adsorption process is completed, the flow direction is usually reversed. The column is operated downwards in a packed bed mode. The unbound material is washed out and the product is eluted. In fluidized bed operation the bead size should be rather large, in order to have a stable bed and to accomplish fluidization at a reasonable flow velocity. However, the large particle diameter can be responsible for loss of resolution. Therefore, this mode is only suitable for initial stages in a purification procedure.

Simulated Moving Bed and Its Operation

A simulated moving bed system is composed of several columns (at least four) connected in series. The stationary phase is fixed in the different columns, and its flow is only simulated by shifting the injection and collection lines. Consequently, the profiles are continuously moving in the system, but the effluent concentration appears almost constant due to the shift of the collection lines (Fish et al. 1993). Simulated moving beds are not popular in the production of pharmaceutical proteins, although there were some investigations on peptide and protein purification (Hashimoto et al. 1988; Maki et al. 1987; Yamada et al. 1989). Very large applications are used in the food industry (for the separation of fructose and glucose).

Countercurrent Chromatography

Countercurrent chromatography (CCC) has a distinct feature among all chromatographic systems. The method does not utilize a solid support matrix. Countercurrent chromatography can be considered as a hybrid of two classical partition methods, countercurrent distribution and liquid partition chromatography. The method combines the benefits from both parent methods. A comprehensive overview of the method is given by Ito (1992). All existing CCC schemes have been derived from two basic systems: one is the hydrostatic equilibrium system and the other is the hydrodynamic equilibrium system.

Annular Chromatography

Annular chromatography (Fox et al. 1969) is a truly continuous chromatography, but there are no industrial applications of this technique at the present time. Sample solution is applied to a slowly rotating annular column. As the sample moves down the rotating bed, the components follow different helical paths. The various components leave the column at different points depending on their residence time in the column. Both sample application and the collection of fractions are performed continuously.

Stationary Phase–Product Interaction and Design and Operating Parameters in Large-Scale Chromatography

A user considers the following parameters when planning a large-scale purification step:

- Technique (separation principle) to be used
- Stationary phase to be used for separation
- Types of buffers involved
- Bed volume, bed height, column capacity (molecular loads for product and adsorbing contaminants)

- Liquid velocity, pressure drop, column diameter, and resulting flow rate

- Volume of product per batch to be processed, number of injections per batch

- Methodology of column washing, regeneration, and equilibration with associated liquid volumes

The method of elution (gradient or stepwise), which is the result of separation development using the selected stationary phase, determines system design and the types and volumes of liquids used for elution. The key step is the selection of the stationary phase, since it dictates most of the other parameters to follow. The stationary phase usually comes with instructions and recommendations from its manufacturer regarding capacities for standard proteins, particle sizes, flow velocities, pressure drops, acceptable pH range, agents recommended for cleaning and regeneration, methodology of packing, and data needed for validation. This information, combined with user's experience provides background for system design and final operating conditions.

The importance of stationary phase selection emphasizes the need for a thorough understanding of the molecular interactions between the stationary phase and molecule of interest, contaminants, and buffers. A user should have available thorough characteristics of the product molecule to be separated, including size (MW), primary through quaternary structures, charge (overall and possibly local) at the range of pH values, pI value, information on molecule stability within the pH range, information on the surface of the molecule (hydrophobic and hydrophilic areas), and the presence of structures that may interact with the known available ligands (structures binding to metals, dyes, peptides, etc.). If the molecule is glycosylated, information on the location and character of carbohydrates is also of importance, since it may affect the molecular weight, charge effects, and specific interactions with other molecules (e.g., lectins). If reversed-phase technology is considered, one should investigate the possibility of product molecule unfolding during the chromatography step and its effects on the final product structure and activity.

A thorough understanding of the stationary phase and the molecule of interest may facilitate the design of a separation step and lead to procedures based on molecular science principles. A practical laboratory approach frequently employed uses a methodology of packing columns with various stationary phases and then checking experimentally which phase will provide the better performance. In summary, the system is designed and its operating parameters are set around the separation based on the selected stationary phase, with a goal of providing the optimum conditions for product purification.

Handling of Chromatographic Media

Chromatographic media for protein purification, which are delivered either dry or as an aqueous slurry, must be adequately prepared before use.

Dry media must be hydrated; this operation is generally easy except with media having very high water regain or hydrophobic properties. Suppliers generally provide instructions on how to hydrate without creating physical and chemical damages. Some affinity dry media contain excipients to help the hydration operation. Common chemicals are sugars, polyalcohols, and polysaccharides; they must be removed completely by exhaustive repeated washings with appropriate buffers.

Media supplied in wet form are aqueous suspensions containing bacteriostatic agents. Sodium azide (0.01 percent to 0.04 percent w/v is the concentration range) and ethanol (about 20 percent v/v) are common chemicals used as preservatives for chromatographic media applied to biochemicals. They are either toxic or undesirable and must be removed totally prior to any purification run. Their elimination is not an easy task; to get rid of sodium azide, it is necessary to wash with high salted buffers of pH above 6; washing should be prolonged for 3–10 column volumes. This is also the case for ethanol, which in specific circumstances needs up to 20 column volumes in order to be completely washed out. Sensitive methods for the specific detection of these preservatives should be defined and validated case by case. The media preparation process requires equilibration with the right buffer to eliminate "fines" formed during transportation and/or handling.

The transfer of medium from drums, in which bulk media are delivered, to a large vessel or to a chromatographic column may not be an easy operation. When settled for a long time, dense medium may form a solid block that must be slurried without damaging the spherical particles. Mechanical agitation, used extensively to resuspend settled particles, may not be appropriate to put in suspension dense beads, such as hydroxyapatite and silica-based material. Specifically designed devices using a gentle water jet associated with a slurry aspiration could represent a convenient method for media suspension and transfer. Once slurried and before column packing, media should be degassed to avoid air bubble formation in the column bed. Various methods exist for degassing, such as sonication, applying a vacuum, and heating to the boiling temperature. The choice of method depends on the properties of the medium. All of these operations should preferably be performed once the media are already equilibrated with the buffer used for column packing.

As a general rule, biochromatography does not involve the use of organic solvents, unless special final cleaning and regeneration operations are needed (e.g., 60 percent ethanol–0.5 M acetic acid); however, some unconventional chromatographic operations, such as the elimination of detergents, the desorption of pigments, and lipid regeneration, may require aqueous-compatible solvents. Since RPC uses organic solvents, special explosion-proof features are required for the equipment and facility designs, including the resin handling and column packing operations.

VALIDATION

Validation is an essential part of process development and its implementation in manufacturing operations. General principles of pharmaceutical process and system validation also apply to production chromatography (Carleton and Agalloco 1986). The key elements in the validation process are the validation plan, identification of the validated system, the prequalification stage, qualification (hardware and software installation and operational qualification), system performance qualification, executing the protocol, ongoing evaluation, safety, and security. Since validation is not the major scope of this chapter, the reader may consult references for more details on the subject. An excellent book on the validation of chromatography systems and processes has been published by Sofer and Nystrom (1991) and followed with a paper by Weinberg et al. (1992). A recent series of references provides a summary of updated information on the subject of general validation (Akers et al. 1994 a and b; McEntire 1994) and on chromatography validation (Adner and Sofer 1994; Barry and Chojnacki 1994; Ng and Mitra 1994; Seely et al. 1994; Sofer 1994). Practical advice regarding validation of computer systems can be found in recent papers by Deitz and Herald (1993), George (1994), and Grigonis and Wyrick (1994).

Systems Validation

The validation plan includes the following elements: identification of personnel, a list of required documents, a list of critical parameters with an explanation of their nature, procedures to be used during the life of the system (including change procedures), and a description of the computer systems to be used (including the backup and recovery procedures).

The prequalification phase is performed prior to system installation. Documented evidence must be established showing that the process equipment and control systems are suitable for the job and would perform within the given range of parameters. When the equipment is being installed, the completeness of the shipment should be checked (this seems trivial, but it must be recorded). After identification and registering, the installation can be commenced.

The system qualification phase is divided into installation qualification (IQ) and operational qualification (OQ) procedures. Hardware IQ involves checking the function of equipment with the specifications and whether it has been properly installed. This work includes documented identification of all hardware components, verification of the functionality of components, and checking the electrical wiring, grounding, and shielding. More on an IQ for production chromatography systems can be found in the book by Sofer and Nystrom (1991). Computerized process control involves a separate issue of hardware and software validation. A typical approach to computer system validation has been the seven-step process, including planning, definition, selection, specification, development, integration and qualification, and ongoing evaluation. The reader should check the available references for more information (Grigonis and Wyrick 1994; Gruber 1994). System qualification includes hardware and software IQ. Software IQ involves verification of the proper installation of all software, and checking software documentation and version compatibility.

Hardware OQ is performed after completion of IQ. All system components must be tested in this phase. Inputs and outputs are executed and the performance of final control elements and sensors is examined. It must be demonstrated that if failure occurs, it occurs in a safe and predictable way. Software OQ involves verification of software module performance in accordance with the intended use. The testing of software modules may include simulation algorithms.

Some of these tasks can be performed and documented by the equipment vendor. The user may perform some of the IQ steps in collaboration with the supplier. Operational qualification steps, which are process specific, are usually performed by the user. Systems validation involves testing under normal operational and worst-case conditions. Testing involves the performance of basic system components, instrumentation (including calibration), and computer hardware and software.

The system Performance Qualification (PQ) follows and includes the integrated system performance regarding production specifications. Sample runs in a production environment are performed. The protocol execution follows the reviewed and approved procedures and includes establishing acceptance criteria for each function, exercising the system at its operational limits, analyzing data, reporting, and summary and conclusions.

Security procedures must be implemented to prevent unauthorized or unintentional changes in operation. Multiple access levels to the computerized system are an example, with the critical level being an access for allowing changes in system operational and control logic. The validated system is put into operation and the following phase is an ongoing evaluation. It includes validation of changes occurring in system design, operational procedures, and environment.

Hardware should be validated at regular time intervals prior to routine use and after repairs or system modifications. Software should be validated during and at the end of the development processes and after software updates. Computer software systems are often very complex and their development frequently lasts over many years. A description of software validation exceeds the scope of this chapter. A comprehensive overview and actual guidelines are published by Double and McKendry (1993) and Stokes et al. (1994). The user of chromatography systems should pay careful attention when a vendor offers validated software and should request the whole documentation, including the security concept, control/audit trail during development, and the inspection of an end-user system. The user may also request documented assurance that acceptable software development standards have been followed by qualified experts during the development and that the source code will be made available on request. A chromatography system can be validated according to what is known as modular validation and holistic validation (entire system). Usually one will use both concepts. The modular validation can be, for instance, the pump, UV detector, recorder, and valve-switching validation. A holistic validation can be the validation of sanitization, the packing procedure, and so on.

Media Validation

Validation of a chromatographic separation process also includes a media validation step. Packing validation consists of checking its performance repeatability, which is associated mostly with ligand density and column packing. Validation of ligand density in the media (affinity ligands, hydrophobic chemical chains, or ion-exchange groups) must be accomplished in small-scale experiments. Selective analytical methods can, in most cases, be defined to quantify the amount of ligand per media volume unit. The quantity of ligand present on the polymer surfaces could not, however, be easily determined over the cycles because of interference with nonspecifically adsorbed substances often present on the sorbent itself. A more direct way to validate the sorbent is to define, for example, the possible drift of sorption capacity or even the modification of the behavior of the separated protein over multiple cycles. The number of cycles is generally predefined and dictated by economic reasons. Irrespective to their nature and to their mode of coupling on the matrix, ligands can be lost little by little as a consequence of a natural or induced hydrolytic leakage during production runs. When this happens in large extent, shorter elution time and broader peaks are observed.

Partial progressive fouling and partial ligand inactivation may also be responsible for separation and capacity drifts, which must be validated using small-scale experiments under conditions similar to those defined for large scale. Resolution measurements between two model proteins might be a good way to detect chromatographic performance and the longevity of the medium. In such cases proteins must be chosen based on their purity, homogeneity, and availability. Polyclonal immunoglobulins are not an appropriate model because they are a mixture of antibodies with different properties, while monoclonals and pure proteins such as cytochrome *c*, chymotrypsinogen, and bovine serum albumin are good recommended models.

When a medium is extensively used, peak tailing, which is an indication of medium aging, could be a critical parameter, because it causes losses, dilutes the fractions, decreases the purity level, and increases the process time. Criteria of acceptable tailing phenomena must be fixed and taken into account; the measurement of the tailing factor must be performed cycle after cycle and limits of acceptance defined. The validation of media separation efficiency in preparative and large-scale chromatography is simply checked by determining the number of theoretical plates of a given column.

Such operations must be performed each time the column is packed. Calculations of theoretical plates are easily performed using the retention time and the width of a peak determined by the tangential method. Peak moments can also be used for the calculation of the theoretical plates; the mode of calculation can be very sensitive to peak tailing and baseline drifts.

Column packing quality is validated in practice by pulse experiments. Chosen substances should be of low molecular weight; linear flow rate should be low (no more than a few dozen cm per hour), and the amount of the tracer molecule should be very low. The molecule should be easy to detect and must not interact with the solid phase. All of these conditions are important, and making the choice of the ideal molecule is a difficult one. Sodium chloride is a useful substance to determine the number of plates; it is nontoxic, widely used in protein separation, and can be eliminated easily, but it is not recommended with ion exchangers. Acetone is also successfully used; however, when hydrophobic sites are present even at a limited extent, the results are not reliable. Amino acids and peptides are also used with different degrees of success. Table 3.8 shows differences in results when checking the number of plates of a given column with various molecules.

The user may expect to obtain from the vendor an extensive documentation file pertaining to the recommended use and validation of the chromatographic medium. Stationary phase manufacturers should provide the user with information contained in the FDA Master Files. The files include proprietary information on media production—their properties and methods of use. Regulatory Support Files are also available. In addition to the vendor's official documentation and the standardized validation procedures described above, users may need to perform a series of their own tests, which are process specific. This part may include DNA, virus, and endotoxin removal challenges, and compatibility with applied buffers and cleaning/regeneration solutions.

Cleaning Validation

In addition to the validation of stationary phase cleaning, regeneration, and sanitization steps, validation includes cleaning and sanitization of the system hardware, which is in contact with the product and buffers. In multiproduct plants the cleaning and decontamination validation may be of as much concern as the design of the plant itself. In order to ensure that cleaning is efficient, the design must obey some basic rules. The most important rule is the minimization

Table 3.8. Influence of the Solute Nature on the HETP Value Measured on a Column of Q-HyperD 10 μm of 4.3 mm Diameter and 100 mm Long

Molecule Used	MW (Da)	Rt (min:sec)	Adsorbance (nm)	HETP (mm)
Sodium chloride	58.5	2:58	ionic	0.169
p-nitroaniline	138.1	4:36	254	0.052
Glycine	75.1	1:42	210	0.415
Glycyl-glycine	132.1	2:36	230	0.058
Glycyl-glycyl-glycine	189.2	2:42	210	0.058
Phenylalanine	165.2	3:00	254	0.062
Phenylalanine ethyl ester	229.7	2:48	254	0.312
Uracyl	112.1	3:00	280	0.142
Histidine	209.6	2:48	225	0.182
Cinnamic acid	150.2	4:00	254	0.055
Benzoic acid	144.1	4:36	230	0.047
Tartaric acid	150.1	7:21	245	0.182

MW = molecular weight in Daltons, Rt = retention time in minutes and seconds, Adsorbance at wavelength in nanometers, HETP = height equivalent to a theoretical plate in millimeters. All determinations were performed in 0.1 *M* phosphate buffer, 0.5 *M* NaCl, pH 6.8 except for p-nitroaniline where 20 percent ethanol was present in the solution. Flow rate was 150 cm/hour.

of dead-end and holdup space. A valve, a bubble trap, or an in-line filter may create holdup volumes. This hold up is also partly responsible for the cleaning agents volume that is required to clean a system.

Additionally, the surface properties of the wetted parts determine the intensity of required cleaning. To ensure the absence of contaminants, reliable and validated cleaning procedures are required. If a very adhesive material is processed, a cleaning procedure consisting of several steps may have to be applied. Combinations of hot water, hot sodium hydroxide, and detergents will remove nearly all biogenic contamination. Since these conditions are not applicable for packed chromatography media, it is advisable in multiproduct plants to use separate chromatography columns and packings for each product. The vessels and peripheral equipment can be shared without further complications.

An analytical method with appropriate sensitivity and selectivity to test for residual contaminant levels is essential for validating equipment cleaning procedures. The presence of contaminants at the various steps within a pharmaceutical purification process typically has been determined by the use of either contaminant specific analyses (HPLC, immunoassays) or methods of general application such as total organic carbon (TOC), amino acid analysis, or total protein analysis (Strege et al. 1994). In addition to the sensitivity requirements, analytical methodologies must be compatible with the sample matrix itself. Currently, the preferred method of sampling is to swab equipment surfaces directly. This approach necessitates the employment of solubilizing solvents to wet the swab before sampling to facilitate the transfer of contaminants from the surface to the swab and to extract the contaminants from the swab into solution before determination. Formic acid (Strege et al. 1994) is a good agent for solubilizing contaminants derived from bacteria or animal cells. It solubilizes proteins, lipids (cell wall components), and carbohydrates. Formic acid is volatile and the extract from the swab can be concentrated by evaporation. After evaporation the solid material can be reconstituted in a much smaller volume. Using this procedure further increases sensitivity by a factor of 10–50.

SUMMARY

Large-scale industrial chromatography is the main technique used in the purification of biological pharmaceutical products. It is essential in accomplishing the required very high product purity levels. A good understanding of molecular interactions (molecule of interest, molecule-buffers, molecule-stationary phase, influence of contaminants) is required for the successful development of a high efficiency, chromatographic purification process. Studies of certain interactions (e.g., between molecule of interest and ligands) may involve molecular modeling using computational chemistry techniques in addition to bench experiments.

The most widely used large-scale chromatography techniques are ion exchange, hydrophobic interaction, gel filtration (size exclusion), and affinity. Reversed-phase technique is sometimes used, but it involves organic solvents, and the facility should be designed to meet safety requirements. Other techniques include metal-chelate, hydroxyapatite, thiophilic, and immobilized dyes. A separate field is an affinity chromatography using immobilized biomolecules (antibodies, receptors, proteins) with media individually tailored to the protein of interest.

The design of the separation process and its steps is based on the characteristics of the molecule of interest and the contaminants to be removed. The most important factor in the design of successful separation steps is the selection of the stationary phase. The following steps are system design and establishing its operating conditions, which depend on both stationary phase characteristics and performance. The stationary phase field is undergoing rapid development, with media characteristics continuously improving. In general, process media should be rigid, have uniform particle size and be spherical, have high dynamic binding capacity, and allow operation at high liquid velocities. Optimum particle size for nonperfusing process media has been found to be 20–40 μm, although smaller and larger particle sizes are also used. The media should not leak any ligands or support matrix components under processing and cleaning and regeneration conditions. High liquid velocity media for packed beds and expanded bed media have been recently introduced.

Process design considerations must include multiple physicochemical phenomena (hydrodynamics, kinetics, mass transfer, molecular interactions, surface chemistry) as well as process robustness and economics.

Large-scale industrial chromatography faces different requirements from the common, literature-referenced analytical- and laboratory-scale techniques. Chromatography conditions involve upper pressure limitation, imperfections of packing and flow distribution in large diameter columns, column overload, nonlinearity of adsorption, extracolumn dispersion, broad peaks, and reduced resolution of the separation.

Chromatography systems for multiproduct facilities should be designed with ease of cleaning and sanitization in mind. The columns and packings must be dedicated to the individual products, while tanks and certain hardware can be shared. Chromatography skids can be designed to pass requirements associated with product switching.

The use of modern process development aids (workstations and pilot systems combined with specialized software) is essential for a rapid move from the research stage into the manufacturing phase. Selected scale-up and process optimization approaches are very important in successfully translating the results of laboratory purifications into operational manufacturing processes. Scale-up procedures become complicated if the bead size and gradient slope change. Additional complication is introduced when scale-up involves change from gradient to step elution. There are software aids available to assist in scale-up and process development. If software packages can handle laboratory development work and the pilot and manufacturing scales, there are numerous benefits: uniformity of operational and regulatory documentation, easy data exchange, simplification of personnel training, and so on.

Modern purification processes are designed to minimize the number of purification steps. The approach has been to have three major steps: capture, purification, and polishing. The capture step leads to a consideration of product-specific ligands (affinity techniques) and direct capture of product from the cell culture or fermentation broths (expanded and fluidized bed technology). The purification stage may use ion-exchange and hydrophobic interaction techniques, and the polishing stage frequently uses gel filtration and sometimes reversed-phase techniques.

The consistency of performance of chromatography steps depends mostly on the performance of the chromatographic resin and ability to regenerate its characteristics during periodic cleaning and regeneration steps. The equipment (system combining hardware and software) shall assure maximal utilization of the resin separation capabilities and provide reliable and repeatable performance. Resin characteristics may be divided into external (particle shape, mean size and size distribution, presence of broken beads and fines) and internal (internal surface, porosity, pore characteristics and size distribution, type and number of active sites per surface unit) characteristics. External characteristics may affect packing uniformity and determine the flow in a packed bed. Internal characteristics determine intraparticle diffusion, binding, and elution. All of these parameters affect the overall stationary phase performance and, therefore, should be evaluated together.

Continuous improvements in resin characteristics and performance, and achieving better peak shapes and resolution impose more stringent requirements on the performance of chromatography systems. The quality of separation obtained by using an optimum resin/buffers environment must not be affected adversely by the performance of hardware. Hardware performance plays an important role in the implementation of the purification strategy. A key part of it is the control concept and the associated operational/control software.

Gradient elution procedures are more complicated than stepwise procedures; systems operating with gradient elution are more complex and require more attention (including adjustment and calibration) than the systems operating in a step mode.

The selection of a delivery system for liquids is crucial for system performance. Peristaltic pumps, although widely used in the past may not deliver adequate performance at back pressures higher than 25–30 psi (1.7–2.0 bar). Two-rotor lobe pumps and diaphragm pumps are usually the designs of choice. Lobe pump performance depends on system back pressure and, for this reason, such pumps should be coupled with a flowmeter. Diaphragm pumps may also be coupled with a flowmeter in order to avoid frequent adjustments and calibrations and to obtain a flow rate signal for recording and control purposes. Depending on the number of pump heads, a pulsation damper may be needed. The pulsation damper can be combined into a single design with a mixing and bubble trap chamber. For higher back pressures and smaller flow rates, the diaphragm pumps are preferred, while for larger flow rates and lower back pressures, twin rotor lobe pumps may be a better choice. Screw pumps may also be considered, since they provide pulseless flow and perform well under elevated back pressures.

Ultraviolet absorption detectors are most typical in industrial chromatography and the applied wavelengths are usually 280 nm and 254 nm. The technical requirements are less stringent for these detectors than for those used in analytical chromatography, due to much higher concentrations of molecules of interest and much broader peaks encountered in industrial chromatography. Other detectors play an auxiliary role in monitoring the process conditions (e.g., pH, conductivity). Rapid scanning or diode array UV detectors have not yet found their way into process chromatography. They allow obtaining an instant mapping of product and contaminant changes and, therefore, might provide not only a large amount of useful information on product and contaminants, but also an early warning of changes in the process. Absorbance of UV radiation at protein concentrations encountered in industrial purifications is very high and assures adequate peak detection. Therefore, other types of detectors (e.g., refractive index) are seldom used. Chromatography systems also include flow-through pH and conductivity sensors. Flow and pressure are also monitored.

Attention should be paid to the design of the sensors. They should fulfill a certain set of requirements: be of sanitary design (proper material selection and surface finish, lack of pockets and crevices), have no significant disturbance of flow pattern (no excessive mixing or stationary liquid volumes), have no moving parts, and be robust and resistant to external interferences (such as electrical noise or mechanical vibrations).

A computer-based control and recording system is recommended because of its flexibility and ability to perform complicated control and operational tasks. The recording capability of computers may be combined with certain software tools to be used in process consistency monitoring and analysis (e.g., by overlaying the chromatograms from many purification runs and performing deviation reporting and analysis).

Building unique, customized, chromatography systems should be avoided because of possible delays in bringing the system on-line and in product introduction, as well as the associated increase in capital and manpower expenditures. System manufacturers possess capabilities allowing the rapid adaptation of their typical designs to individual customer needs. Close collaboration between the user and suppliers of equipment and media in successful process development and its implementation into manufacturing is very important.

REFERENCES

Adner, N., and G. Sofer. 1994. Biotechnology product validation, part 3: Chromatography cleaning validation. *BioPharm* 7 (3):44–48.

Afeyan, N. B., N. Gordon, I. Mazsaroff, L. Varady, S. Fulton, Y. Yang, and F. Regnier. 1990. Flow-through particles for the high performance liquid chromatographic separation of biomolecules: Perfusion chromatography. *J. Chromatog.* 519:1–29.

Akers, J., J. McEntire, and G. Sofer. 1994a. Biotechnology product validation, part 1: Identifying the pitfalls. *BioPharm* 7 (1):40–44.

Akers, J., J. McEntire, and G. Sofer. 1994b. Biotechnology product validation, part 2: A logical plan. *BioPharm* 7 (2):54–56.

Andrewes, P. 1965. The gel filtration behavior of proteins related to their molecular weight over a wide range. *Biochem. J.* 96:595.

Arshady, R. 1991. Beaded polymer supports and gels. *J. Chromatog.* 586:181–197, 199–219.

Asif, M., N. Kalogerakis, and L. Behie. 1991. Distributor effects in liquid fluidized beds of low-density particles. *AIChE J.* 37:1825–1832.

Astrom, K., and B. Wittenmark. 1990. *Computer-controlled processes.* Englewood Cliffs, NJ: Prentice Hall.

Balakotaiah, V., and H.-C. Chang. 1995. Dispersion of chemical solutes in chromatographs and reactors. *Phil. Trans. R. Soc. Lond.* 351:39–75.

Baliga, J. 1994. Power semiconductor devices for variable-frequency drives. *Proc. IEEE* 82:1112–1122.

Barker, P. E., B. W. Hatt, and G. J. Vlachogiannis. 1981. Suitability of TSK-gel Toyo pearl packing for the gel permeation chromatography analysis of dextrans. *J. Chromatog.* 208:74.

Barry, A., and R. Chojnacki. 1994. Biotechnology product validation, part 8: Chromatography media and column qualification. *BioPharm* 7 (9):43–47.

Batchelor, G. 1972. Sedimentation in a dilute dispersion of spheres. *J. Fluid Mech.* 52:245–268.

Batchelor, G. 1982. Sedimentation in a dilute polydisperse system of interacting spheres, part 1: General theory. *J. Fluid Mech.* 119:379–408.

Batchelor, G. 1988. A new theory of the instability of a uniform fluidized bed. *J. Fluid Mech.* 193:75–110.

Batchelor, G., and C.-S. Wen. 1982. Sedimentation in a dilute polydisperse system of interacting spheres, part 2: Numerical results. *J. Fluid Mech.* 124:495–528.

Baumeister, E. et al. 1995. Determination of the apparent transverse and axial dispersion coefficients in a chromatographic column by pulsed field gradient nuclear magnetic resonance. *J. Chromatog.* 694:321–331.

Baur, J., E. Kristensen, and R. Wightman. 1988. Radial dispersion from commercial high-performance liquid chromatography columns investigated with microvoltametric electrodes. *Anal. Chem.* 60:2334–2338.

Belew, M., J. Porath, and J. Fohlman. 1978. Adsorption phenomena on Sephacryl S-200 superfine. *J. Chromatog.* 147:205.

Benenati, R., and C. Brosilow. 1962. Void fraction distribution in beds of spheres. *AIChE J.* 8:359–361.

Block, S., ed. 1991. *Disinfection, sterilization, and preservation,* 4th ed. Philadelphia: Lea & Febiger.

Bonnerjea, J., and P. Terras. 1994. Chromatography systems. In *Bioprocess engineering: Systems, equipment and facilities,* edited by B. Lyderson, N. D'Elia, and K. Nelson. New York: John Wiley and Sons, Inc.

Boschetti, E. 1989. Polyacrylamide gels to the service of bioseparation. *J. Biochem. Biophys. Meth.* 19:21.

Boschetti, E. 1994. Advanced sorbents for preparative protein separation purposes. *J. Chromatog.* 658:207.

Boschetti, E., R. Tixier, and R. Garelle. 1974. Determination of some parameters in gel permeation chromatography with polyacrylamide-agarose gels. *Sci. Tools* 21:35.

Boschetti, E., L. Guerrier, P. Girot, and J. Horvath. 1995. Preparative HPLC separation of proteins with HyperD. *J. Chromatog.* 664: 225–230.

Brink, R., D. Czernik, and L. Horve. 1993. *Handbook of fluid sealing.* New York: McGraw-Hill, Inc.

Bryant, C. et al. 1994. A review of expert systems for chromatography. *Anal. Chim. Acta* 297:317–347.

Buijs, A., and J. A. Weselingh. 1980. Batched fluidized ion-exchange column for streams containing suspended particles. *J. Chromatog.* 201:319–327.

Carleton, F., and J. Agalloco, eds. 1986. *Validation of aseptic pharmaceutical processes.* New York: Marcel Dekker.

Carlson, J., J. C. Janson, and M. Sparrman. 1989. Affinity chromatography. In *Protein purification: Principles, high resolution methods and applications,* edited by J. C. Janson, and L. Ryden. New York: VCH.

Ceulemans, J. 1991. Role of intermolecular interactions in chromatographic separations. In *Intermolecular forces,* edited by P. Huyskens, W. A. Luck, and T. Zeegers-Huyskens. Berlin: Springer-Verlag.

Chakrabarti, P. 1989. Geometry of interaction of metal ions with sulfur-containing ligands in protein structures. *Biochemistry.* 28:6081–6085.

Chase, H. 1986. Automated affinity separation processes. *J. Chem. Tech. Biotechnol.* 36:351–356.

Chase, H., and N. Draeger. 1992. Affinity purification of proteins using expanded beds. *J. Chromatog.* 597:129–145.

Christianson, D. 1991. Structural biology of zinc. *Adv. Protein Chem.* 42:281–355.

Clonis, Y. D. 1990. Large scale affinity chromatography. *Bio/technology* 5:1290–1293.

Coffman, J., K. Roper, and E. Lightfoot. 1994. High-resolution chromatography of proteins in short columns and adsorptive membranes. *Bioseparation* 4:183–200.

Corran, P. H. 1989. Reversed-phase chromatography of proteins. In *HPLC of macromolecules: A practical approach,* edited by R. W. A. Oliver. Oxford: IRL Press.

Creighton, T. 1993. *Proteins: Structures and molecular properties.* New York: W. H. Freeman.

Cretier, G., and J. Rocca. 1994. Gradient elution in preparative reversed-phase liquid chromatography. *J. Chromatog.* 658:195–205.

Cuatrecasas, P., M. Wilchek, and C. B. Anfinsen. 1968. Selective enzyme purification by affinity chromatography. *Proc. Nat. Acad. Sci. USA* 61:636–643.

Davies, A. H., B. M. Jowett, and I. M. Jones. 1993. Recombinant baculovirus vectors expressing glutathione-S-transferase fusion proteins. *Bio/technology* 11:933–936.

Davis, R., and A. Acrivos. 1985. Sedimentation of noncolloidal particles at low Reynolds numbers. *Ann. Rev. Fluid Mech.* 17:91–118.

Dean, P. D. G., and D. H. Watson. 1979. Protein purification using immobilized triazine dyes. *J. Chromatog.* 165:301–319.

Deitz, D., and C. Herald. 1993. Computer system validation and the software development process. *ISA Trans.* 32:65–73.

De Luca, J. et al. 1994. A study of the expansion characteristics and transient behavior of expanded beds of adsorbent particles suitable for bioseparations. *Bioseparations* 4:311–318.

Determann, H. 1968. *Gel chromatography.* New York: Springer-Verlag.

DiFelice, R. et al. 1991. Expansion characteristics of tapered fluidized beds. *AIChE J.* 37:1668–1672.

Double, M. E., and M. McKendry. 1993. *Computer validation compliance: A quality assurance perspective.* Buffalo Grove, IL: Interpharm Press.

Draeger, N., and H. Chase. 1991. Liquid fluidized bed adsorption of protein in the presence of cells. *Bioseparation* 2:67–80.

Du, Q., E. Freysz, and R. Shen. 1994. Surface vibrational spectroscopic studies of hydrogen bonding and hydrophobicity. *Science* 264:826–828.

EFB. 1995. Regulatory aspects of downstream processing. *EFB Newsletter* July.

Eon, C. 1978. Comparison of broadening patterns in regular and radially compressed large-diameter columns. *J. Chromatog.* 149:29–42.

Farkas, T., J. Chambers, and G. Guiochon. 1994. Column efficiency and radial homogeneity in liquid chromatography. *J. Chromatog.* 679:231–245.

FDA. 1987. *Use of aseptic processing and terminal sterilization in the preparation of sterile pharmaceuticals for human and veterinary use.* Rockville, MD: Center for Drug Evaluation and Research.

Firouztale, E., A. P. Scott, S. K. Dalvie, and G. M. Von Blohm. 1992. Experimental and theoretical study of key parameters of adsorption on reverse phase macroporous resins. *New Dev. in Biosep. AIChE Symp. Series* 88:25–33.

Fish, B., R. Carr, and R. Aris. 1993. Design and performance of a simulated countercurrent moving-bed separator. *AIChE J.* 39:1783–1789.

Fontana, M., and N. Greene. 1978. *Corrosion engineering.* New York: McGraw-Hill, Inc.

Foscolo, P., and L. Gibilaro. 1984. A fully predictive criterion for the transition between particulate and aggregative fluidization. *Chem. Eng. Sci.* 39:1667–1675.

Foscolo, P., R. DiFelice, and L. Gibilaro. 1989. The pressure field in an unsteady-state fluidized bed. *AIChE J.* 35:1921–1926.

Fox, J. B., R. C. Calhoun, and W. J. Eglinton. 1969. Continuous chromatography apparatus. *J. Chromatog.* 43:48–54.

Freitag, R., and J. Breier. 1995. Displacement chromatography in biological downstream processing. *J. Chromatog.* 691:101–112.

Fulton, P. S., A. J. Shahidi, N. F. Gordon, and N. B. Afeyan. 1992. Large scale processing and high throughput perfusion chromatography. *Biotechnology* 10:635.

Gaillot, F. P. 1990. Fluidized bed adsorption for whole broth extraction. *Biotechnol. Prog.* 6:370–375.

George, J. 1994. Lessons from the field: Real-life experiences in computer system validation. *Pharm. Technol.* 18 (11):38–50.

Gerstner, J., J. Bell, and S. Cramer. 1994. Gibbs free energy of adsorption for biomolecules in ion-exchange systems. *Biophys. Chem.* 52:97–106.

Ginesi, D., and C. Annarummo. 1994. Application and installation guidelines for volumetric and mass flowmeters. *ISA Trans.* 33:61–72.

Girot, P., and E. Boschetti. 1981. Physicochemical and chromatographic properties of new ion exchangers. I. CM-Trisacryl. *J. Chromatog.* 213:389.

Glusker, J. 1991. Structural aspects of metal liganding to functional groups in proteins. *Adv. Protein Chem.* 42:1–76.

Goldshan-Shirazi, S., and G. Guiochon. 1992. Comparison of the various kinetic models of non-linear chromatography. *J. Chromatog.* 603:1–11.

Gooding, K., and F. Regnier. 1990. *HPLC of biological macromolecules.* New York: Marcel Dekker, Inc.

Gooding, K. M., and M. N. Schmuck. 1983. Purification of trypsin and other basic proteins by high-performance cation-exchange chromatography. *J. Chromatog.* 266:633–642.

Gorbunoff, M. J. 1990. Protein chromatography on hydroxyapatite columns. In *Guide for protein purification,* edited by M. P. Deutscher. New York: Academic Press.

Goto, M., T. Imamura, and T. Hirose. 1995. Axial dispersion in liquid magnetically stabilized fluidized beds. *J. Chromatog.* 690:1–8.

Grigonis, G., and M. Wyrick. 1994. Computer system validation: auditing computer systems for quality. *BioPharm* 7 (7):22–31.

Groundwater, E. 1985. Guidelines for chromatography scale-up. *Lab Practice* (Feb):17–22.

Gruber, M. 1994. Use of structured design and development in the validation of application software. *ISA Trans.* 33:125–131.

Gu, T., G. Tsai, G. Tsao. 1993. Modeling of nonlinear multicomponent chromatography. *Adv. Biochem. Eng./Biotechnol.* 49:46–71.

Guerrier, L., I. Flayeux, E. Boschetti, and M. Burnouf-Radosevich. In press. Specific sorbent to remove solvent-detergent mixtures from virus-inactivated biological fluids. To be published in *J. Chromatog.*

Haff, L. A., and R. L. Easterday. 1978. Sephacryl gels: Physical properties and evaluation of performance in gel filtration. *J. Liquid Chromatog.* 1:811.

Harr, M. 1977. *Mechanics of particulate media.* New York: McGraw-Hill, Inc.

Hashimoto, K., S. Adachi, and Y. Shirai. 1988. Continuous desalting of proteins with a simulated moving-bed adsorber. *Agric. Biol. Chem.* 52:2161–2167.

Hearn, M. T. W., A. N. Hodder, and I. Aguilar. 1988. High-performance liquid chromatography of amino acids peptides and proteins. *J. Chromatog.* 443:97–111.

Hirabayashi, J., and K. Kasai. 1992. Arginine tail method, an affinity tag procedure utilizing anhydrotrypsin agarose. *J. Chromatog.* 597:181–187.

Hochuli, E. 1990. Purification of histidine fusion proteins by metal chelate chromatography. In *Proceedings of the 5th European Congress on Biotechnology,* 8–13 July, in Copenhagen. Proceedings edited by C. Christansen, L. Munck, and J. Villadsen, and published by Munksgaard International Publisher (Copenhagen).

Horvath, J., E. Boschetti, L. Guerrier, and N. Cooke. 1994. High performance protein separation with novel strong ion exchangers. *J. Chromatog.* 679:11–22.

Ito, Y. 1992. Countercurrent chromatography. In *Journal of chromatography library,* vol 51A, edited by E. Heftmann. Amsterdam: Elsevier.

Jack, G. et al. 1987. The automated purification by immunoaffinity chromatography of the human pituitary glycoprotein hormones thyrotropin, follitropin and lutropin. *J. Chem. Tech. Biotechnol.* 39:45–58.

Jaffrin, M., and A. Shapiro. 1971. Peristaltic pumping. *Ann. Rev. Fluid Mech.* 3:13–36.

James, K., and D. R. Stanworth. 1964. The effect of the chemical and physical nature of the exchanger. *J. Chromatog.* 15:324.

Jandera, P., and J. Churacek. 1985. *Gradient elution in column liquid chromatography.* Amsterdam: Elsevier.

Janson, J. C. 1984. Large scale affinity purification: State of the art and future prospects. *Trends in Biotechnol.* 2:31–38.

Janson, J. C., and P. Hedman. 1982. Large-scale chromatography of proteins. In *Advances in Biochemical Engineering,* vol. 25, edited by A. Fiechter. New York: Springer-Verlag.

Janson, J. C., and L. Ryden. 1989. *Protein purification: Principles, high resolution methods and applications.* Weinheim, Germany: VCH.

Johansson, B., and P. Wnukowski. 1992. Hydrodynamic stability of the liquid fluidized bed of small particles: An experimental study. Poster presented at the Annual AIChE Meeting, 1–6 November, in San Diego, CA.

Johnston, A., Q. Mao, and M. Hearn. 1991. Analysis of operating parameters affecting the breakthrough curves in fixed bed chromatography of proteins using several mathematical models. *J. Chromatog.* 548:127–145.

Jordan, J., and H. Pardue. 1992. Experimental evaluation of theoretical response equations for an unsegmented flow system with a well-stirred mixing chamber. *Anal. Chim. Acta* 270:195–204.

Jungbauer, A. 1993. Preparative chromatography of biomolecules. *J. Chromatog.* 639:3–16.

Jungbauer, A., and H. Lettner. 1994. Chemical disinfection of chromatography resins. *BioPharm* 7 (June):46–56.

Jungbauer, A. et al. 1989a. Comparison of Protein A, Protein G and copolymerized hydroxyapatite for purification of human monoclonal antibodies. *J. Chromatog.* 476:257–268.

Jungbauer, A. et al. 1989b. Pilot scale production of a human monoclonal antibody against human immunodeficiency virus HIV-1. *J. Biochem. Biophys. Methods* 19:223–240.

Kaltenbrunner, O., and A. Jungbauer. In press. Adsorption isotherms in protein chromatography: Combined influence of protein and salt concentration on adsorption isotherm. To be published in *J. Chromatog.*

Kaminski, M. 1994. Reasons for nonuniformity of bed structure in wet packed preparative liquid chromatography columns. *Isolat. & Purificat.* 2:1.

Kato, Y. 1987. High-performance hydrophobic interaction chromatography of proteins. *Adv. Chromatog.* 26:97–115.

Kato, Y. 1989. Aqueous size exclusion chromatography. In *Size exclusion chromatography,* edited by B. Hunt, and S. Holding. New York: Chapman and Hall.

Katti, A., and G. Guiochon. 1992. Fundamentals of nonlinear chromatography: Prediction of experimental profiles and band separation. *Adv. Chromatog.* 31:1–118.

Kennedy, R. M. 1990. Hydrophobic chromatography. In *Guide to protein purification,* edited by M. P. Deutscher. New York: Academic Press.

Kenney, A. 1990. Automation in protein purification: The use of expert systems for control of process chromatography. In *Separation processes in biotechnology,* edited by J. Asenjo. New York: Marcel Dekker.

Knox, J., and J. Parcher. 1969. Effect of column to particle diameter ratio on the dispersion of unsorbed solutes in chromatography. *Anal. Chem.* 41:1599–1606.

Knox, J., G. Laird, and P. Raven. 1976. Interaction of radial and axial dispersion in liquid chromatography in relation to the infinite diameter effect. *J. Chromatog.* 122:129–145.

Koch, D., and J. Brady. 1985. Dispersion in fixed beds. *J. Fluid Mech.* 154:399–427.

Köhler, K., A. Veide, and S. O. Enfors. 1990. Purification of beta-galactosidase fusion proteins by partitioning in aqueous two-phase systems. In *Proceedings of the 5th European Congress on Biotechnology,* 8–13 July, in Copenhagen. Proceedings edited by C. Christiansen, L. Munck, and J. Villadsen, and published by Munksgaard International Publisher (Copenhagen).

Kopaciewicz, W., and F. Regnier. 1983. Mobile phase selection for the high-performance ion-exchange chromatography of proteins. *Anal. Biochem.* 133:251–259.

Kramer, A. et al. 1993. Simultaneous synthesis of peptide libraries on single resins and continuous cellulose supports: Examples for the identification of protein, metal and DNA binding peptide mixtures. *Peptide Res.* 6:314–319.

Kroeff, E., R. Owens, E. Campbell, R. Johnson, and H. Marks. 1989. Production scale purification of biosynthetic human insulin by reversed-phase HPLC. *J. Chromatog.* 461:45–61.

Kuperman, V. et al. 1995. A new technique for differentiating between diffusion and flow in granular media using magnetic resonance imaging. *Rev. Sci. Instrum.* 66:4350–4355.

Kurnik, R. et al. 1995. Buffer exchange using size exclusion chromatography, countercurrent dialysis and tangential flow filtration: Models, development and industrial application. *Biotechnol. Bioeng.* 45:149–157.

Labrou, N., and Y. Clonis. 1994. The affinity technology in downstream processing. *J. Biotechnol.* 36:95–119.

Ladish, M. R., R. L. Hendrickson, and E. Firouztale. 1991. Analytical and preparative-scale chromatographic separation of phenylalanine from aspartame using a new polymeric sorbent. *J. Chromatog.* 540:85–101.

Lameloise, M.-L., and V. Viard. 1994. Choice of a tracer for external porosity measurement in ion-exchange resin beds. *J. Chromatog.* 679:255–259.

Lang, T. T. 1991. *Computerized instrumentation.* New York: John Wiley and Sons, Inc.

Laurent, T. C., and J. Killander. 1964. A theory of gel filtration and its experimental verification. *J. Chromatog.* 14:317–330.

Lebing, W. R., D. J. Hammond, J. E. Wydick, and G. A. Baumbach. 1994. A highly purified antithrombin III concentrate prepared from human plasma fraction IV-1 by affinity chromatography. *Vox Sang* 67:117.

Lee, J. S., and K. Ogawa. 1994. Pressure drop through packed bed. *J. Chem. Eng. Japan* 27:691–693.

Levenspiel, O. 1962. *Chemical reaction engineering.* New York: John Wiley & Sons, Inc.

Levenspiel, O. 1979. *The chemical reactor omnibook.* Corvallis, OR: OSU Book.

Lew, A. M., D. J. Beck, and L. M. Thomas. 1991. Recombinant fusion proteins of protein A and protein G with glutathione S-transferase as reporter molecules. *J. Immunol. Meth.* 136:211–219.

Lewis, R. V., A. Fallon, S. Stein, K. D. Gibson, and S. Udenfried. 1980. Supports for reversed phase high performance liquid chromatography of large proteins. *Anal. Biochem.* 104:153–159.

Liapis, A. 1989. Theoretical aspects of affinity chromatography. *J. Biotechnol.* 11:143–160.

Liapis, A. I., and M. A. McCoy. 1992. Theory of perfusion chromatography. *J. Chromatog.* 599:87.

Liapis, A., and M. McCoy. 1994. Perfusion chromatography. Effect of micropore diffusion on column performance in systems utilizing perfusive adsorbent particles with a bidisperse porous structure. *J. Chromatog.* 660:85–96.

Liapis, A. et al. 1995. Perfusion chromatography. The effects of intraparticle convective velocity and microsphere size on column performance. *J. Chromatog.* 702:45–57.

Lindbladh, C., K. Mosbach, and L. Bülow. 1991. Preparation of a genetically fused protein A/luciferase conjugate for use in bioluminescent immunoassays. *J. Immunol. Meth.* 137:199–207.

Ljung, L. 1987. *System identification. Theory for the user.* Englewood Cliffs, NJ: Prentice Hall.

Madan, B., and B. Lee. 1994. Role of hydrogen bonds in hydrophobicity: The free energy of cavity formation in water models with and without the hydrogen bonds. *Biophys. Chem.* 51:279–289.

Magnico, P., and M. Martin. 1990. Dispersion in the interstitial space of packed columns. *J. Chromatog.* 517:31–49.

Mahuron, D. 1979. Stability of Sepharose CL-6B column in 6 M guanidine-HCl. *J. Chromatog.* 172:394.

Maisano, F., M. Belew, and J. Porath. 1985. Synthesis of new hydrophobic adsorbents based on homologues of uncharged alkylsulfide agarose derivatives. *J. Chromatog.* 321:305.

Maki, H., H. Furuda, and H. Morikawa. 1987. The separation of glutathione and glutamic acid using a simulated moving-bed adsorber system. *J. Ferment. Technol.* 65:61–70.

Mant, C., and R. Hodges. 1991. *High-performance liquid chromatography of peptides and proteins: Separation, analysis and conformation.* Boca Raton, FL: CRC Press.

Mashimo, S., and N. Miura. 1993. High order and local structure of water determined by microwave dielectric study. *J. Chem. Phys.* 99:9874–9881.

Matthew, J. et al. 1985. pH-dependent processes in proteins. *CRC Crit. Rev. Biochem.* 18:91–197.

McEntire, J. 1994. Biotechnology product validation, part 5: Selection and validation of analytical techniques. *BioPharm.* 7 (5):68–80.

Melander, W. R., D. Corradin, and C. Horvath.1984. Salt-mediated retention of proteins in hydrophobic-interaction chromatography. *J. Chromatog.* 317:67–85.

Mikes, O., P. Strop, and J. Zbrozek. 1976. Chromatography of biopolymers and their fragments on ion exchange derivatives of the hydrophilic macroporous synthetic gel Spheron. *J. Chromatog.* 119:339.

Mikes, O., P. Strop, J. Zbrozek, and J. Coupek. 1979. Ion exchange derivatives of Spheron. II. Diethylamino ethyl-Spheron. *J. Chromatog.* 180:17.

Mikes, O., P. Strop, M. Smirz, and J. Coupek. 1980. Ion exchange derivatives of Spheron. III. Carboxylic cation exchangers. *J. Chromatog.* 192:159.

Mohr, P., and K. Pommerening. 1985. *Affinity chromatography: Practical and theoretical guide.* New York: Marcel Dekker, Inc.

Moks, T. et al. 1987. Large scale affinity purification of human insulin-like growth factor I from culture medium of *Escherichia coli. Biotechnology* 5:379–382.

Motozato, Y., and C. Hirayama. 1984. Preparation and properties of cellulose spherical particles and their ion exchangers. *J. Chromatog.* 298:499.

Muller, W., 1990. New ion exchangers for the chromatography of biopolymers. *J. Chromatog.* 510:133.

Nadgir, V. M., and Y. A. Liu. 1983. Studies in chemical process design and synthesis, Part V: A simple heuristic method for systematic synthesis of initial sequences for multicomponent separations. *AIChE J.* 29:926–934.

Narayanan, S. 1994. Preparative affinity chromatography of proteins. *J. Chromatog.* 658:237–258.

Narayanan, S. R., and L. J. Crane. 1990. Affinity chromatography supports: A look at performance requirements. *Tibtech* 8:12–16.

Ng, P., and G. Mitra. 1994. Removal of DNA contaminants from therapeutic protein preparations. *J. Chromatog.* 658:459–463.

Noar, P., and R. Shinnar. 1963. Representation and evaluation of residence time distributions. *I&CE Fundamentals* 2:278–286.

Noper, B., F. Kohen, and M. Wilchek. 1988. A thiophilic adsorbent for one-step high-performance liquid chromatography purification of monoclonal antibodies. *Anal. Chem.* 180:66–71.

Östlund, C., P. Borwell, and B. Malm. 1985. Process-scale purification from cell culture supernatants: Monoclonal antibodies. *Develop. Biol. Standard* 66:367–375.

Pahlman, S., J. Rosengreen, and S. Hjerten. 1977. Hydrophobic interaction chromatography on uncharged sepharose derivatives. *J. Chromatog.* 131:99–108.

Permyakov, E. 1993. *Luminescent spectroscopy of proteins.* Boca Raton, FL: CRC Press.

Person, M., M. G. Bergstrand, and K. Mosbach. 1988. Enzyme purification by genetically attached polycysteine and polyphenylalanine affinity tails. *Anal. Biochem.* 172:330–337.

Peskin, A. P., and S. R. Rudge. 1992. Optimization of large scale chromatography for biotechnological applications. *Appl. Biochem. Biotech.* 34:49.

Peterson, E. A., and H. A. Sober. 1956. Chromatography of proteins. I. Cellulose ion exchange adsorbents. *J. Am. Chem. Soc.* 78:751.

Pharmacia. 1995. Large scale column chromatography: The case for fixed end pieces. *Downstream* 18:10–12.

Porath, J. 1986. Salt-promoted adsorption: Recent developments. *J. Chromatog.* 376:331–341.

Porath, J., F. Maisano, and M. Belew. 1985. Thiophilic adsorption–a new method for protein fractionation. *FEBS Lett.* 185:306–310.

Porsch, B. 1994. Some specific problems in the practice of preparative high-performance liquid chromatography. *J. Chromatog.* 658:179–194.

Regnier, F. E., and K. M. Gooding. 1980. High performance liquid chromatography of proteins. *Anal. Biochem.* 103:1.

Rice, R., and B. Heft. 1991. Separations via radial flow chromatography in compacted particle beds. *AIChE J.* 37:629–632.

Rippel, G., E. Alattyani, and L. Szepesy. 1994. Characterization of stationary phases used in reversed-phase and hydrophobic interaction chromatography. *J. Chromatog.* 668:301–312.

Rodbard, D. 1976. Estimation of molecular weight by gel filtration and gel electrophoresis. In *Methods of protein separation,* edited by N. Catsimpoolas. New York: Plenum Press.

Roper, K., and E. Lightfoot. 1995. Separation of biomolecules using adsorptive membranes. *J. Chromatog.* 702:3–26.

Rounds, M. A., and F. E. Regnier. 1984. Evaluation of a retention model for high-performance ion-exchange chromatography using two different displacing salts. *J. Chromatog.* 283:37–45.

Rounds, M. A., W. Kopaciewicz, and F. E. Regnier. 1986. Factors contributing to intrinsic loading capacity in silica-based packing materials for preparative anion-exchange protein chromatography. *J. Chromatog.* 362:187–196.

Sadana, A. 1992. Inactivation of proteins and other biological macromolecules during chromatographic methods of bioseparation. *Bioseparation* 3:145–165.

Sadana, A., and A. Beelaram. 1994. Efficiency and economics of bioseparation: Some case studies. *Bioseparation* 4:221–235.

Salles, J. et al. 1993. Taylor dispersion in porous media: Determination of the dispersion tensor. *Phys. Fluids* 5:2348–2376.

Samuelson, E., H. Waldenstein, M. Hartmanis, T. Moks, and M. Uhlen. 1991. Facilitated in vitro folding of human recombinant insulin-like growth factor I using solubilizing fusion partner. *Bio/technology* 9:363–366.

Sano, T., and C. S. Cantor. 1991. A streptavidin-protein A chimera that allows one-step production of a variety of specific antibody conjugates. *Bio/technology* 9:1378–1381.

Sarker, M., and G. Guiochon. 1994. Study of the packing behavior of radial compression columns for preparative chromatography. *J. Chromatog.* 683:293–309.

Sarker, M., and G. Guiochon. 1995. Study of the packing behavior of axial compression columns for preparative chromatography. *J. Chromatog.* 702:27–44.

Schlichting, H. 1979. *Boundary layer theory.* New York: McGraw Hill, Inc.

Schwartzenbach, J., and K. Gill. 1992. *System modelling and control.* New York: Halsted Press.

Schwarz, A., F. Kohen, and M. Wilchek. 1995. Novel heterocyclic ligands for the thiophilic purification of antibodies. *J. Chromatog.* 664:83–88.

Scopes, R. 1994. *Protein purification: Principles and practice.* New York: Springer Verlag.

Scott, R. 1986. *Liquid chromatography detectors.* Amsterdam: Elsevier.

Seely, R. et al. 1994. Biotechnology product validation, part 7: Validation of chromatography resin useful life. *BioPharm* 7 (7): 41–48.

Shoikhet, K., and H. Engelhardt. 1994. A photometric flow measurements method for characterisation of HPLC pumps. *Chromatographia* 38:421–430.

Slemon, G. 1994. Electrical machines for variable frequency drives. *Proc IEEE* 82:1123–1139.

Sofer, G. 1994. Biotechnology product validation, part 4: Clearance of impurities from protein and peptide biotherapeutics. *BioPharm* 7 (4):46–50.

Sofer, G., and L. Nystrom. 1989. *Process chromatography.* San Diego: Academic Press.

Sofer, G., and L. Nystrom. 1991. *Process chromatography: A guide to validation.* San Diego: Academic Press.

Stellwagen, E. 1990. Chromatography of immobilized reactive dyes. In *Guide to protein purification,* edited by M. P. Deutscher. 343–357, San Diego: Academic Press.

Sternberg, J. 1966. Extra column contributions to chromatographic band broadening. In *Advances in chromatography,* vol. 2, edited by J. Giddings, and R. Keller. New York: Marcel Dekker, Inc.

Stokes, T., R. C. Branning, K. G. Chapman, H. Hambloch, and A. J. Trill. 1994. *Good computer validation practices: Common sense implementation.* Buffalo Grove, IL: Interpharm Press.

Straetkvern, K., A. J. Raae, K. Folkvord, B. A. Naess, and J. M. Aasen. 1991. Optimization and scale up of the adsorption fractionation of cod pyloric caeca deoxyribonuclease using axial and radial flow columns. *Bioseparation* 2:81–93.

Strand, S., and R. Jakobsen. 1991. The application of FTIR spectroscopy to the study of proteins in solution. *Am. Lab.* May:28–31.

Strege, M. A., J. J. Dougherty, W. R. Green, and A. L. Lagu. 1994. Total protein analysis of swab samples for the cleaning validation of bioprocess equipment. *BioPharm.* 7 (November):40–41.

Sulk, B., G. Birkenmeier, and G. Kopperschläger. 1992. Application of phase partitioning and thiophilic adsorption chromatography to the purification of monoclonal antibodies from cell-culture fluid. *J. Immunol. Meth.* 14:165–171.

Szepesy, L., and G. Rippel. 1994. Effect of the characteristics of the phase system on the retention of proteins in hydrophobic interaction chromatography. *J. Chromatog.* 668:337–344.

Tayot, J. L., M. Tardy, P. Gattel, R. Plan, and M. Rumiantzeff. 1978. Industrial ion exchange chromatography of proteins on DEAE-dextran derivatives of porous silica beads. In *Chromatography of synthetic and biological polymers,* edited by R. Epton. Chichester, UK: Ellis Horwood.

Timperley, D., R. Thorpe, and J. Holah. 1992. Implications of engineering design in food industry hygiene. In *Biofilms: Science and technology,* edited by L. Melo et al. Amsterdam: Kluwer.

Truei, Y. H. et al. 1992. Large-scale gradient elution chromatography. *Adv. Biochem. Eng./Biotechnol.* 47:1–45.

Turkova, J. 1978. *Affinity chromatography.* Amsterdam: Elsevier Scientific Publishing Company.

Ugelstad, J., and P. C. Mork. 1980. Swelling of oligomer-polymer particles: New method of preparation of emulsions and polymer dispersions. *Adv. Colloid Interf. Sci.* 13:101.

van Laak, F. A. 1993. Application limits of electromagnetic flowmeters: What do we really know about them? Evaluation of eight different makes. *ISA Trans.* 32:247–275.

Vetter, G. et al. 1993. Know your diaphragm pump internals. *Chem. Engng.* Nov: 130–136.

Vissers, J. et al. 1995. Colloid chemical aspects of slurry packing techniques in microcolumn liquid chromatography. *Anal. Chem.* 67:2103–2109.

Vorauer, K., M. Skias, A. Trkola, P. Schulz, and A. Jungbauer. 1992. Scale-up of recombinant protein purification by hydrophobic interaction chromatography. *J. Chromatog.* 625:33–39.

Wainer, I., and T. Noctor. 1993. Molecular biochromatography: An approach to the liquid chromatography determination of ligand-biopolymer interactions. *Adv. Chromatog.* 33:67–96.

Wang, T. et al. 1990. Packing of preparative high-performance liquid chromatography columns by sedimentation. *J. Chromatog.* 523: 23–34.

Watanabe, E., S. Tsoka, and J. Asenjo. 1994. Selection of chromatographic protein purification operations based on physicochemical properties. *Ann. N.Y. Acad. Sci.* 721:348–364.

Weinberg, S. et al. 1992. Up to code: Validating a chromatography system. *Bio/Technology* 10:870–872.

Wheelwright, S. 1991. *Protein purification: Design and scale up of downstream processing.* Munich: Hanser Publishing.

Whitley, R. D., J. M. Brown, N. P. Karajgikar, and N. H. L. Wang. 1989. Determination of ion exchange equilibrium parameters of amino acid and protein systems by an impulse response technique. *J. Chromatog.* 483:263–287.

Whitley, R. D., J. A. Berninger, N. Rouhana, and N. H. L. Wang. 1991. Nonlinear gradient isotherm parameter estimation for proteins with consideration of salt competition and multiple forms. *Biotechnol. Prog.* 7:544–553.

Wilhelm, A., and J. Riba. 1989. Scale-up and optimization in production liquid chromatography. *J. Chromatog.* 484:211–223.

Wisniewski, R. 1988. Design objectives for aseptic seals. *Proceedings of the Bioprocess Engineering Symposium of the American Society of Mechanical Engineers,* 27 November–2 December, in Chicago, IL.

Wisniewski, R. 1992. Principles of the design and operational considerations of large scale high performance liquid chromatography (HPLC) systems for proteins and peptides purification. *Bioseparation* 3:77–143.

Wu, S. L., A. Figuero, and B. L. Karger. 1986. Protein conformational effects in hydrophobic interaction chromatography. *J. Chromatog.* 371:3–27.

Wu, D., and R. R. Walters. 1992. Effects of stationary phase ligand density on high-performance ion-exchange chromatography of proteins. *J. Chromatog.* 598:7–13.

Yamada, M., S. Adachi, and Y. Shirai. 1989. A simulated moving-bed adsorber with three zones for continuous separation of L-phenylalanine and NaCl. *J. Chem. Eng. Japan* 22:432–434.

Yamamoto, S., K. Nakanishi, and R. Matsuno. 1988. *Ion-exchange chromatography of proteins.* New York: Marcel Dekker.

Yamamoto, S., N. Nomura, and Y. Sano. 1990. Predicting the performance of gel-filtration chromatography of proteins. *J. Chromatog.* 512:77–87.

Yamamoto, S., K. Nakanishi, R. Matsuno, and T. Kamikubo. 1983. Ion exchange chromatography of proteins: Prediction of elution curves and operating conditions. *Biotechnol. Bioeng.* 25:1465–1483.

Yang, V. C., and R. Langer. 1985. pH-dependent binding analysis: A new and rapid method for isoelectric point estimation. *Anal. Biochem.* 147:148–155.

Yang, B. L., and S. Goto. 1993. Affinity purification by tapered bed. *J. Chem. Eng. Japan* 26:752–754.

Yeung, E. 1986. *Detectors for liquid chromatography.* New York: John Wiley and Sons.

Yun, T., and G. Guiochon. 1994. Modeling of radial heterogeneity in chromatographic columns: Columns with cylindrical symmetry and ideal model. *J. Chromatog.* 672:1–10.

4

LYOPHILIZATION OF PROTEIN PHARMACEUTICALS

John F. Carpenter

Department of Pharmaceutical Sciences, University of Colorado

Byeong S. Chang

Amgen, Inc.

There are numerous unique, critical applications for proteins in human healthcare. Many protein drugs are already on the market, and over 200 candidate proteins and peptides are currently in clinical trials (Geisow 1992; Wang and Pearlman 1993; Talmadge 1993). However, even the most promising and effective protein therapeutic will not be of benefit to human health, if its stability cannot be maintained during packaging, shipping, long-term storage, and administration. For ease of preparation and cost containment by the manufacturer, and ease of handling by the end user, an aqueous protein solution is often the preferred formulation. Unfortunately, water fosters protein degradation by providing a medium for molecular movement and conformational perturbations, as well as serving as a reactant in chemical degradation pathways (e.g., hydrolysis).

Because the free energy of stabilization for a native protein is only about 50 ± 15 kJ/mol (Jaenicke 1991), proteins are readily denatured (often irreversibly) by the many stresses arising in solution, such as heating, agitation, freezing, pH changes, and exposure to denaturants (Arakawa et al. 1993). In addition, various chemical modifications of amino acid side chains can occur relatively rapidly in aqueous solution (Manning et al. 1989, In press). These physico-chemical modifications often result in undesirable by-products, including soluble and insoluble aggregates, and inactive and/or antigenic species. Such alterations may not only compromise the clinical efficacy of the protein drug, but may also increase the risk of adverse side effects (e.g., Thornton and Ballow 1993). Thus, the inherent instability of the protein, and/or the logistics of product shipping, storage, and use, often preclude preparation of the protein as an aqueous solution (Pikal 1990a,b). Also, simply preparing stable frozen protein formulations, which is a relatively straightforward process, is not a desirable alternative. Shipping and storing products at subzero temperatures are not technically and/or economically feasible in many markets.

The practical solution to the protein stability dilemma is to remove the damaging component—water. Lyophilization (freeze-drying) is the method most commonly used to prepare dehydrated proteins. In this process the product is first frozen at atmospheric pressure. Then water is removed by reducing the chamber pressure of the lyophilizer and collecting the water as ice onto a condenser. Theoretically, lyophilized proteins should have the desired long-term stability at ambient temperatures. Such stability would allow the product to be handled conveniently and distributed to a wider market, including those markets in Europe that do not guarantee refrigerated delivery.

However, as will be described in this review, without the proper insight into the lyophilization process and how it affects proteins, it is not a simple task to remove water by freeze-drying, without damaging the protein. Recent infrared spectroscopic studies have documented that the acute freezing and dehydration stresses of lyophilization can induce protein unfolding (Prestrelski, Tedeschi, et al. 1993; Prestrelski, Arakawa, et al. 1993, 1994 [148–169], Dong et al. 1995). Unfolding can not only lead to irreversible protein denaturation, if the sample is rehydrated immediately, but can also reduce storage stability in the dried solid (Chang, Beauvais, et al. in preparation; Prestrelski et al. 1995). Thus, when one is trying to prepare a lyophilized protein product, one must develop a formulation that stabilizes the protein during freezing, the lyophilization cycle itself, and subsequent storage of the dried solid. Simply obtaining a native protein in samples rehydrated immediately after lyophilization is not necessarily indicative of adequate acute stabilization, nor is it predictive of storage stability. Many proteins unfold during lyophilization but readily refold if rehydrated immediately (cf. Prestrelski,

Tedeschi, et al. 1993; Dong et al. 1995). Without directly examining the structure of the dried solid (using infrared spectroscopy, as described below), it is not possible to know whether an unfolded protein with poor storage stability is present or not. Finally, even if the protein is native in the dried solid, this may not be adequate if other crucial physical factors—the glass transition temperature and the residual moisture of the dried solid—are not optimized.

To develop a protein formulation that has both acute and long-term storage stability, it is crucial that the specific conditions (i.e., pH, specific stabilizing ligands) for optimum protein stability be established *and* the appropriate nonspecific stabilizing additives (i.e., those excipients that generally stabilize any protein) be incorporated into the formulation. For acute stabilization the appropriate excipients must be chosen to protect the protein during *both* the freezing and drying steps (Carpenter et al. 1993; Prestrelski, Arakawa, et al. 1993). For storage stability, in addition to providing acute protection, the excipients must also form an amorphous solid (i.e., a glass) with the protein, and, hence, provide an environment that is restrictive to physical and chemical degradation (Franks 1990; Franks et al. 1991; Roy et al. 1990). Furthermore, the glass transition temperature of this amorphous solid varies inversely with the sample residual moisture, which is then greatly influenced by the lyophilization cycle itself (e.g., final product temperature). Therefore, the lyophilization cycle parameters can also greatly affect the storage stability conferred by a given formulation.

Finally, in addition to protein stability, a lyophilized pharmaceutical product must also have acceptable cake morphology and dissolution properties. Often the most desired cake has a strong, porous structure, formed from a crystalline bulking agent, into which is incorporated the protein/stabilizer amorphous phase. Therefore, additives must also be selected, and the lyophilization cycle designed, such that freeze-drying takes place without the collapse of the amorphous phase of the cake. Finally, the formulation must maintain protein stability and cake integrity during a rapid and efficient lyophilization cycle (i.e., without the need for excessively rigid control of cycle parameters such as chamber pressure and shelf temperature [Pikal 1990a; Chang and Fischer 1995; Nail and Gatlin 1993, 163–233]).

Optimizing the protein and cake stability during the lyophilization cycle appears and can be a daunting, complicated process. However, as will be documented, achieving these goals can be relatively straightforward if the underlying physical principles are understood and a rational approach is taken. In general, for long-term storage stability of dried proteins, it appears that only four criteria must be met:

1. Acute lyophilization-induced unfolding must be minimized and, ideally, the protein should be native in the dried solid.

2. The dried powder must have a glass transition temperature that is higher than the desired storage temperature.

3. The residual moisture must be relatively low (i.e., $\approx < 0.01$ g H_2O per g dried solid).

4. Specific formulation conditions (e.g., pH) must be developed to inhibit chemical degradation pathways, which might arise even in native proteins.

The purpose of this review is to provide an overview of the principles that must be followed, and how essential physical data are obtained and used to meet these criteria. In addition, in order to provide a rational basis for choosing excipients, a description will be given of the mechanisms for protein stabilization by additives.

At this point it is important to note that the principles and mechanisms to be discussed should be generally applicable to any protein. However, obtaining a stable lyophilized formulation of a given protein may not necessarily be as straightforward as it appears based on the generalizations provided in this review. Each protein has unique physicochemical characteristics, which produces its unique "personality." Sometimes this personality manifests itself as a protein that "cooperates fully" during formulation development. At other times the protein seems to be a "spoiled child who follows or breaks the rules in an apparently illogical pattern of frustratingly inconsistent behavior." Interestingly, with such a "recalcitrant" protein, once the problems are analyzed carefully, often one learns that the protein did follow the rules, but the patterns of consistent behavior were too complicated to discern during the initial phases of the research. Currently, it is not possible to predict if a protein will fall into one of these extremes or somewhere in between, which in a way is beneficial to the careers of formulation scientists. If all that was needed to obtain stable proteins was the purchasing of a "kit of magic excipients" or simply following a single, simple recipe, then there would not be much need for highly skilled protein stabilization experts in the industry or for further advances in the field from basic researchers. Since this is not the case, there is a great need to increase the fundamental understanding of protein formulation and to document by case studies the applicability of general rules to individual proteins.

Since the purpose of this chapter is to outline the main principles that are important, at least as a starting point for guiding the development of stable lyophilized protein products, there will *not* be an exhaustive review of all of the published studies, many of which are excellent, on acute and storage stability of lyophilized proteins. There will not be an in-depth exploration of some of the rigorous physical mechanisms and theories that govern the design of lyophilization cycles (e.g., the connection between sample collapse temperature and glass transition temperature $[T_{g'}]$ of the frozen sample). Excellent reviews of these issues are already available (see MacKenzie 1975 [277–307], 1976; Pikal 1990a; Pikal and Shah 1990; Nail and Gatlin 1993). Instead, selected examples from the literature will be used to illustrate the theoretical and practical elements of developing an optimally stable, lyophilized protein product.

This chapter will consider, in order, the following individual topics, with special consideration of how the individual areas are interrelated and impact on each other:

- The first topic will be how to design an econonical lyophilization cycle that results in the desired cake properties and residual moisture. As described, an important part of this process is the use of differential scanning calorimetry to obtain essential physical data (i.e., $T_{g'}$ and eutectic crystallization temperatures of formulations) that dictate the cycle parameters.

- Consideration will then be given to how to design formulations that stabilize proteins during both freezing and drying, and the mechanisms for stabilization by additives. An introduction to the use of infrared spectroscopy to monitor protein conformation directly in frozen and dried samples will also be provided. Although this method is just beginning to be used in commercial formulation development, it should soon become an invaluable part of this process, because structural information about the protein during lyophilization and storage is crucial.

- In the final section the optimization of formulations for long-term storage stability will be discussed. A major part of this discussion will focus on the impact of the physical properties of the dried solid (i.e., T_g and protein conformation) on protein stability. These physical properties are directly dependent on both the design of the lyophilization cycle and the choice of stabilizing additives.

Therefore, the intention is for the reader to gain an understanding of how long-term storage stability in the dried solid is inseparable from, and ultimately dictated by, both acute stabilization and lyophilization cycle parameters.

DESIGN OF FREEZE–DRYING CYCLES

The efficient and consistent production of a stable, freeze-dried, protein product, contained in a mechanically strong and rapidly dissolvable cake, is the ultimate objective during the development of a freeze-drying cycle. The freeze-drying cycle must be controlled easily for greater reproducibility, with the utility to correct rapidly any problem arising. Also, the drying process must be fast enough so that it does not slow down overall manufacturing. Finally, the cost of freeze-drying should be reasonable compared to other production operations. The goal is to design the fastest and most robust (i.e,. results in acceptable product quality even with variations in operating parameters) cycle, which consumes the least amount of energy and does not compromise product quality.

Obtaining this goal can appear difficult because many variables in the freeze-drying process can affect the stability of the protein, and the structure and dissolution properties of the dried cake. The choice of values for the operating parameters of the cycle must be based on sound physical characterization of the formulation and understanding of how these parameters impact the final product. As described below, if cycle parameters (e.g., sample temperature) are not controlled with reference to formulation properties, such as glass transition temperature of the amorphous material in the frozen state, there can be unacceptable collapse of cake structure, excessive residual moisture, and/or uneven moisture distribution.

This section will outline how the various aspects of the protein formulation and lyophilization cycle itself are interrelated and how they impact on achieving the goals noted above. First, the steps involved in the freeze-drying cycle will be defined. Next, the key physical properties of the formulation, how they dictate cycle control and how they can be measured will be discussed. Then the specific considerations for each step of the process and how key parameters must be controlled will be discussed. Finally, some of the practical limitations of lyophilizers will be considered. This basic overview will not cover other rigorous physicochemical aspects of freeze-drying (e.g., effect of vial on mass and heat transfer rates). For more details the reader is directed to earlier reviews and original papers (e.g., MacKenzie 1976; Nail 1980; Pikal 1985, 1990a; Pikal et al. 1983, 1984; Pikal and Shah 1990; Franks 1990; Nail and Gatlin 1993).

The Freeze-Drying Cycle

The freeze-drying cycle can be divided into three main steps: freezing, primary drying, and secondary drying (MacKenzie 1976; Pikal 1990a; Nail and Gatlin 1993). Typically, samples are placed in glass vials and frozen, either prior to being placed into the lyophilizer or on the lyophilizer shelves. In a frozen sample there are ice crystals and nonice phases composed of unfrozen water, amorphous solids (including the protein), and/or crystalline additives. When the pressure is reduced, primary drying commences as ice crystals are sublimed. The unfrozen water entrapped in the amorphous solid is more difficult to remove. Therefore, after primary drying, the product temperature must be increased to facilitate this stage of the process, which is called secondary drying. The final temperature achieved during secondary drying is the most important factor in determining the residual moisture in the dried cake. In general, residual moisture is related inversely to the final temperature.

For some formulations, annealing steps, during which samples are maintained at a given temperature, are also used to crystallize excipients. For example, prior to primary drying, crystallization of a bulking agent (e.g., glycine) is accomplished by warming the frozen formulation above the devitrification temperature (i.e., the temperature where a metastable glass component crystallizes, T_d) of the compound of concern. Annealing might also be used during the latter stage of secondary drying to complete the crystallization of excipients that have remained partially amorphous. This step assures that undesired crystallization and release of moisture does not arise in an uncontrolled fashion during subsequent shipping and storage.

Optimization of Formulations

The composition of the formulation dictates how a cycle must be designed in order to achieve the desired final cake and residual moisture. The formulation can include the protein product, stabilizers, buffer, isotonifier, bulking agent, and other additives necessary for specific therapeutic uses. Although the stability and the specific delivery of the protein are the major objectives when the formulation is developed, it is also very important to optimize the formulation for a successful, efficient, freeze-drying process. The two most important factors to be considered are the role of the bulking agent and the effect of formulation on the undesirable processes of sample collapse and melt-back.

A bulking agent is often required in lyophilized protein formulations to retain the dried powder in the container. Without a bulking agent, the small mass of protein that is often used in a dose can be blown out of the vial as the sample is dried. The bulking agent also plays an important role in forming a rigid cake structure. With crystalline bulking agents, such as mannitol and glycine, the amorphous protein fraction is dispersed between the rigid crystal structure. Amorphous bulking agents, such as polymers or sugars, can also maintain cake integrity if the glass transition temperature of the amorphous excipients is higher than the shipping and storage temperatures. Finally, the bulking agent(s) often can serve as protein stabilizers. However, with crystalline bulking agents, an additional amorphous excipient (e.g., sucrose) is usually needed to protect the protein during the dehydration step (see below).

Collapse can occur during primary drying if the product exceeds a characteristic temperature, which is a unique property of each formulation, but can be influenced by product manipulations. Collapse is the loss of the microscopic and macroscopic structure (e.g., porous network with high surface area) of the amorphous phase created during freezing (MacKenzie 1975, 1976; Pikal and Shah 1990; Nail and Gatlin 1993). Above the characteristic temperature, which is associated with a glass transition, there is sufficient product mobility such that the amorphous phase cannot maintain its structure. The result is sample consolidation and the loss of pores created by sublimed ice crystals and, hence, a reduction in the product surface area. Collapse can result in a cake appearance that the consumer may find unacceptable for a pharmaceutical product. Besides unacceptable appearance, various undesirable properties result from the collapse of the cake during freeze-drying. As a result of decreased surface area for water removal during secondary drying, the final product tends to retain a higher moisture content than the product dried without collapse, and the residual water may be distributed unevenly through the sample. Also, slower reconstitution is generally experienced with the collapsed product, due to the loss of porosity and resultant reduction in powder surface area. Finally, there has been some speculation that the collapse of a cake may perturb protein structure, but no supporting data are available yet.

As ice is sublimed during primary drying, collapse is prevented by maintaining the structural integrity of the maximally freeze-concentrated amorphous phase that surrounds the ice crystals (MacKenzie 1975; Franks 1990; Pikal and Shah 1990). Below its glass transition temperature (T_g'), this amorphous phase exists as a "glass," which is a hard and brittle material, and in which available thermal energy is insufficient to allow large-scale motion. However, as the temperature is raised above T_g', there is a dramatic increase in the motion in this fraction, which results in viscous flow. The characteristic temperature at which this motion begins has been found to correlate strongly with the temperature at which the frozen cake undergoes collapse (refer to Pikal and Shah [1990] and MacKenzie [1976] for a detailed explanation).

Factors besides T_g' can affect the collapse temperature. The reader is directed to the seminal paper by Pikal and Shah (1990), in which they explain in detail that the collapse temperature will increase as the sublimation rate is increased, and that for a given sublimation rate, the collapse temperature may increase as the surface area of the frozen solid is increased. Despite these complicating factors, in general, during primary drying it is sufficient to maintain the sample temperature below the T_g' of the formulation to prevent the collapse of the cake (MacKenzie 1975, 1976; Pikal and Shah 1990; Pikal 1990a; Nail and Gatlin 1993). To provide a margin of safety, which accounts for such factors as interval variations in product temperature and sublimation rate, the product temperature in the reference vials is usually maintained at least 2–5°C below the T_g' of the formulation.

The choice of temperature needed to avoid collapse must be balanced with the practical/economic need to dry samples as rapidly as possible. As described in detail later, the rate of sublimation correlates inversely with sample temperature. To allow reasonable drying, the T_g' of the formulation should not be lower than about -40°C, where, with the 2–5°C safety margin, drying can take more than a week. Also, some lyophilizers may not be capable of achieving the appropriate sample temperature, if the T_g' is too low. To obtain the desired fastest drying without the risk of collapse, amorphous excipients that have a high T_g' should be chosen. The formulation T_g' is based on the mass averaged T_g' values of each of the amorphous components. Therefore, T_g' can be increased by increasing the weight fraction of excipients with higher T_g' or by including additional excipients that have higher T_g's (Chang and Randall 1992). Ideally, the excipient chosen to increase $T_{g'}$ will also serve as a protein stabilizer (e.g., disaccharides). With most materials, and specifically documented in detail with carbohydrates, it has been found that the higher the molecular weight, the higher the $T_{g'}$ of the compound (Levine and Slade 1988a,b, 1992 [83–221]).

Also, proteins have a relatively high $T_{g'}$ of $\approx$ -10°C (Chang and Randall 1992). Therefore, if the protein constitutes a large fraction of the formulation, then excipients with lower $T_{g'}$s can be chosen for protein stabilization. However, a relatively large amount of stabilizer may be required to protect the protein sufficiently. Concomitantly, the $T_{g'}$ of the formulation is lowered, and drying time is increased. This provides an example of one of the compromises that must be considered in protein lyophilization. Nondrug proteins (e.g., serum albumin) can be used to increase the protein content of the sample, but this can complicate subsequent analysis of the protein drug.

Excipients with very low T_g's (e.g., sorbitol, $T_{g'}$ = -43.5°C) are difficult to freeze-dry and should be avoided. Also, crystalline bulking agents, such as glycine, can remain, at least partially, amorphous during the initial freezing. Because such materials have a very low $T_{g'}$ ($\approx$ -50°C) and are often used at relatively high weight fractions, they can predominate and lead to a very low formulation $T_{g'}$. As will be described below, this difficulty can be avoided by using a presublimation annealing step to crystallize the excipient fully, such that it no longer affects the amorphous phase.

Finally, another approach is to include additives that crystallize and give the cake a rigid macroscopic structure. Then collapse of the amorphous fraction will only be manifested on a microscopic scale in the regions between crystals. This approach is only recommended in cases where other options fail, because even microscopic collapse can lead to the adverse effects noted above.

In contrast to collapse, melt-back is due to the eutectic melting of crystalline agents in the frozen formulation (MacKenzie 1975, 1976; Nail and Gatlin 1993). Although collapse proceeds with the freeze-drying front at a slow pace, eutectic melting occurs rapidly throughout the frozen portion of the product (MacKenzie 1975). To prevent melt-back during primary drying, the product temperature must be kept below the eutectic melting temperature (T_e) of the crystalline component(s) of the formulation. Additives with low eutectic melting temperatures (e.g., the T_e for calcium chloride is -51°C) are particularly difficult to lyophilize and should be avoided in protein formulations (Chang and Randall 1992). Fortunately, the

T_e for commonly used bulking agents, mannitol and glycine, are usually higher than the $T_{g'}$ of the amorphous phase and, hence, the latter value is predominate in cycle design.

Prior to attempting to lyophilize a protein formulation, the $T_{g'}$ and the T_e of the formulation must be known. Detailed information on the physical properties of various individual additives is available in the literature (Levine and Slade 1988 a and b; Chang and Randall 1992; Her and Nail 1994). However, since the actual transition temperature of a given excipient will be influenced by the total sample composition, it is crucial that these values be obtained for each formulation. The transition temperatures can be determined with any of several thermal analysis techniques, including differential scanning calorimetry (DSC), differential thermal analysis, thermomechanical analysis, electrical thermal analysis (Her et al. 1994), and freeze-drying microscopy (reviewed in Nail and Gatlin 1993). Presented here will be some examples of the usefulness of DSC in obtaining the data needed to determine the key parameters of the lyophilization cycle (see Chang and Randall 1992; Her and Nail 1994). Differential scanning calorimetry was selected because it is a method that is used most often for this purpose and because it is capable of determining all of the needed physical values.

Figure 4.1 shows thermograms of three different excipients that are commonly used in freeze-dried protein formulations. The first thermogram (a) is for a sucrose solution, which serves as an example of a glass-forming additive, that was frozen by cooling to –60°C and then warmed at 10°C/minute. The data were obtained during the warming scan. Glass-forming additives tend to remain amorphous during product freezing and warming until the characteristic $T_{g'}$ is reached. At this point the sample undergoes a glass transition, which appears as a second order transition to a new baseline in the thermogram. The value used for the $T_{g'}$ is calculated as the midpoint of this transition. For the current data the $T_{g'}$ occurs at –32°C. Continued warming results in ice melting, which is indicated by the large endothermic transition around 0°C. With glass-forming solutes, such as sucrose, the material will reform the glassy phase upon recooling (i.e., the glass transition is reversible). Therefore, the glass transition can be detected during repeated scans of the same sample in the calorimeter. Finally, it is important to note that the value for $T_{g'}$ will increase as the warming rate is increased (Her and Nail 1994). However, Her and Nail have shown that for rates ranging from 2°C/min to 20°C/minute, the variation in $T_{g'}$ for a number of individual excipients is only about 4°C. Usually, a warming rate of

Figure 4.1. Differential scanning calorimetry thermograms of frozen solutions commonly used in protein formulations: (a) sucrose solution with glass transition signal; (b) glycine solution with glass transition and devitrification signals; (c) glycine solution, after warming through devitrification and recooling, with eutectic melting signal; (d) KCl solution with eutectic melting signal. All thermograms were recorded during warming at 10°C/minute.

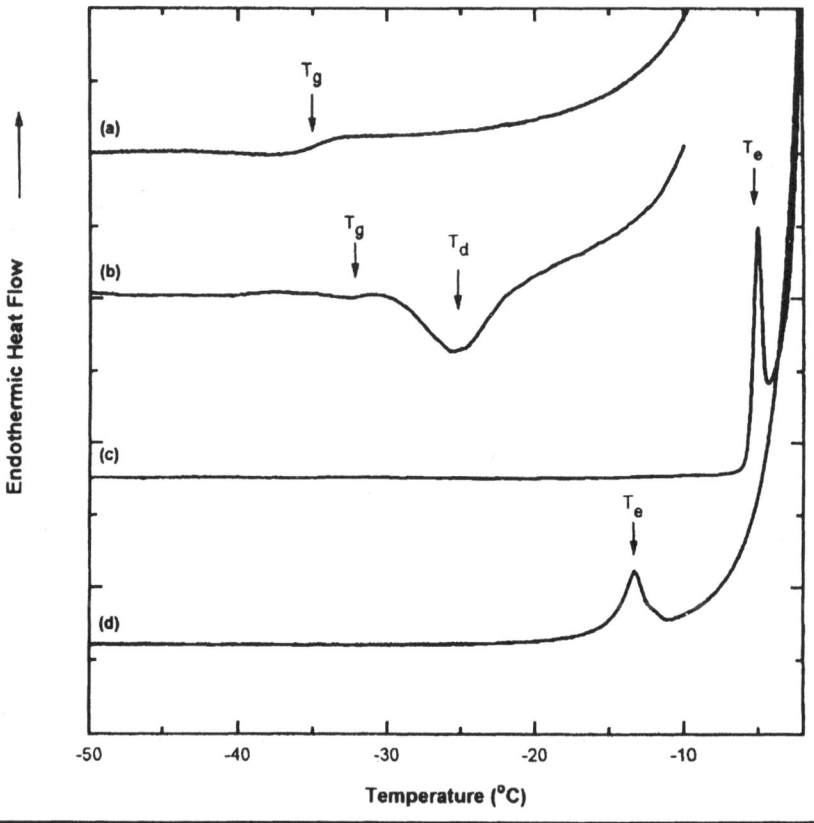

10°C/minute has been used to determine $T_{g'}$ for protein formulations to be lyophilized.

The second thermogram is for glycine (b), which represents a class of additives that form a metastable glass during freezing. In this case during subsequent warming, the unstable amorphous fraction will go through a glass transition, which is followed by devitrification (i.e., solute crystallization [MacFarlane 1987]). With glycine the glass transition $T_{g'}$ occurs at -37°C. Devitrification is indicated by the exothermic peak at -25°C. As warming is continued, the sample passes the eutectic melting temperature of the crystalline solute, which for this scan is indicated by the endothermic transition having an onset at -15°C.

Since additives such as glycine have a relatively low $T_{g'}$ and often are included as bulking agents, it is desirous to crystallize the solute prior to the initiation of primary drying. The data from DSC can be used to determine the appropriate protocol for this treatment. Crystallization is induced in the lyophilizer by slowly warming the frozen formulation through the devitrification temperature and holding the temperature below the eutectic melting temperature for several minutes. To determine the duration of this annealing period necessary to foster maximum crystallization, this process can be mimicked in the calorimeter. After the annealing process, the sample is recooled and then heated through the eutectic melt. An example for glycine is shown in (c). The area of this endothermic melt peak can be determined; it serves as a measure of the amount of crystalline excipient present after annealing. Increasing durations of annealing can be tested until no increase in endothermic melt area is detected. A precaution for the annealing process is that the crystallization of some additives (e.g., mannitol), can result in the breakage of glass containers due to the solute expansion. Breakage can be avoided by filling to less than one-third of the vial capacity.

After the annealing protocol is established, the calorimeter is then used to determine the $T_{g'}$ of the amorphous phase remaining after excipient crystallization. Since a material with a very low glass transition temperature has been removed from the amorphous phase, the $T_{g'}$ should be higher after the annealing process. In the calorimeter the sample is annealed and then recooled. The $T_{g'}$ is then determined during a subsequent warming scan.

Finally, the DSC characterization of the thermal behavior of KCl (d) provides an example of an additive that crystallizes during the freezing process. The thermogram shows the eutectic melting peak obtained as the frozen sample is warmed. Disodium phosphate, a component of sodium phosphate buffer, is another salt that crystallizes during freezing. In contrast, monosodium phosphate, the other component in phosphate buffer, is a glass-forming salt. Differential crystallization results in an amorphous fraction containing the predominantly monosodium phosphate and a significant pH drop during the freezing process (van den Berg 1959; van den Berg and Rose 1959). Inclusion of other glass-forming additives, such as sucrose, can be useful in minimizing the crystallization of excipients, including disodium phosphate (Chang and Randall 1992).

Optimization of the Freezing Step

The manner in which a sample is frozen greatly affects the size of ice crystals formed and, hence, the capacity to remove water from the frozen sample once a vacuum is applied. The freezing protocol also affects the morphology of the final cake. Samples are routinely placed in glass vials and onto the lyophilizer shelf, and then frozen by either cooling from ambient temperature or cooling rapidly on a prechilled shelf. The former treatment leads to supercooling and results in relatively homogeneous, small ice crystals. In contrast, with the latter method, nucleation and ice formation is initiated at the bottom and proceeds to the top of the vial. The result is the formation of larger ice crystals, with varying sizes.

Supercooling is defined as cooling a sample below its equilibrium melting temperature without the formation of ice. Supercooling can be achieved in a lyophilizer by equilibrating the product just above the melting temperature and then cooling slowly through this point. Samples can also be supercooled by slowly reducing the product temperature from ambient. The rate of the formation of ice nuclei in a supercooled solution is greater than that for ice crystal growth. Thus, there is a relatively homogenous distribution of ice nuclei just prior to ice crystal formation. Once ice crystal formation begins, freezing takes place instantaneously throughout the product, with the formation of numerous small ice crystals and the uniform distribution of the product throughout the container. Usually, the greatest degree and uniformity of supercooling throughout the container are obtained at moderate cooling rates ($\approx 1^{\circ}C$/min). The advantage of having some degree of supercooling is the consistency of product throughout the vials, which includes moisture content, crystallinity of excipient, and distribution of product. In addition, the increased surface area of the amorphous phase remaining after ice crystals are removed by sublimation improves the rate of secondary drying (MacKenzie 1976; Pikal 1990b; Nail and Gatlin 1993). However, if ice crystals are excessively small, the pathways for water vapor removal from the cake become restricted, thus slowing sublimation. Therefore, excessive supercooling should be avoided.

Another approach is to freeze the product so that the growth of ice crystals occurs faster than the nucleation. The vials can be frozen by loading onto a shelf that has been prechilled (e.g., at –50°C), or by immersion into a cold medium (e.g., liquid nitrogen). Ice crystal growth starts at the colder bottom of container and progresses to the warmer top of the container. This freezing approach leads to larger ice crystals than those seen with the supercooling method. Larger ice crystals create a better path for water vapor removal from ice; therefore, the sublimation rate is faster. However, there may be inconsistent distribution of the product, crystallization of excipients, and composition of the amorphous fraction throughout the container. Such heterogeneities can lead to variation in product stability and cake quality in different regions of the vial.

Usually, the most desirable freezing process leads to a moderate degree of supercooling. For example, product vials are loaded on a shelf that is preequilibrated at a temperature slightly above the equilibrium melting temperature (e.g., 0°C). After all the vials are equilibrated at this temperature, the temperature of the shelf is reduced at a moderate rate (e.g., 1°C/min) down to –40 to –50°C. Samples will usually freeze with the desired degree of supercooling (e.g., ≈ –20°C).

Presublimation Annealing

After freezing is completed, the frozen product can be treated thermally to facilitate the drying process and to improve product appearance. As noted above, such treatment can be used to crystallize excipients, such as mannitol and glycine. Another use of thermal treatment is to increase the size of ice crystals for faster primary drying. In this case the frozen product is warmed to a relatively high subzero temperature (e.g., –10 to –5°C), at which point a process termed *migratory recrystallization* takes place. Thermodynamically, small ice crystals have a higher interfacial free energy and are less favorable than larger crystals (see Knight et al. [1984, 1988]; and Knight and Duman [1988] for a detailed explanation). The overall free energy of the system is lowered by the growth of large crystals at the expense of small crystals, which shrink and disappear. This process is kinetically inhibited at relatively low temperatures. However, if the temperature is raised sufficiently, there is sufficient kinetic energy for water molecules to move from small to larger crystals. The redistribution of water molecules can take place without an increase in the total fraction of water as ice. This approach is particularly useful when drying products formulated with slow-drying amorphous additives that have relatively low T_g's.

Optimization of Primary Drying

Optimization of Process Parameters

The optimum lyophilization cycle will have the shortest primary drying time, while the product temperature is maintained at the safest level below the maximum allowable temperature (e.g., $T_{g'}$ or T_e). Parameters that are controlled to achieve this goal include shelf temperature, chamber pressure, and duration of primary drying. The shelf temperature affects product temperature by heat transfer with the product in the vial. The chamber pressure affects product temperature by modulating evaporative cooling and by controlling the thermal transfer between the vial and the shelf (Nail 1980). The completion of primary drying should be determined accurately in order not to waste energy by excessive duration of the process, while at the same time avoiding premature transition to secondary drying.

Equation 4.1 can be used to represent the drying rate during the primary drying (Pikal 1990a; Pikal et al. 1983).

$$dm/dt = \frac{P_0 - P_c}{R_p + R_s} \qquad (4.1)$$

where dm/dt = rate of sublimation, g/cm^2/hr; P_0 = vapor pressure of ice at the product temperature, μm Hg; P_c = chamber pressure, μm Hg; R_p = product resistance (cm^2 μm Hg hr g^{-1}); and R_s = stopper resistance (cm^2 μm Hg hr g^{-1}).

An example using a formulation with a $T_{g'}$ of –20°C will illustrate how this equation can be employed to maximize the sublimation rate. Figure 4.2 shows the relationships between chamber pressure, shelf temperature, product temperature, and sublimation rate. Attempting to increase the sublimation rate by simply reducing chamber pressure (P_c) will actually result in a decreased rate, because of the concomitant decrease in product temperature and ice vapor pressure (P_0). For example, starting with condition "A" shown in Figure 4.2, reduction of the chamber pressure to 140 μm Hg will result in a reduction of the product temperature to –25°C (condition "B") and in a decrease in the sublimation rate from 0.16 to 0.11 g/cm^2/hr. On the other hand, increasing chamber pressure at a given shelf temperature increases the sublimation rate, due to increased product temperature. In this example increasing the chamber pressure to 420 μm Hg (transition to condition "C") results in faster sublimation rate of 0.19 g/cm^2/hr, due to an increase in the

Figure 4.2. Effect of shelf temperature and chamber pressure on the sublimation rate of ice during primary drying of IL-1ra formulations. Data taken from Chang and Fischer (1995).

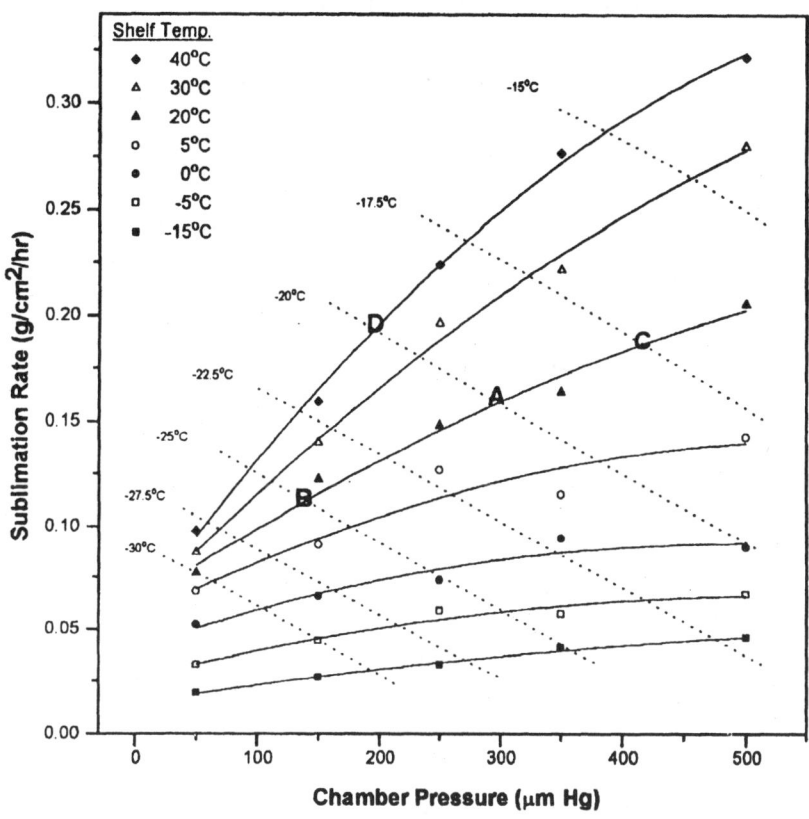

product temperature to $-17.5°C$. However, this increase of product temperature above T_g, will cause collapse. By examining isothermal curves of product temperature, it can be seen that the combination of high shelf temperature and low chamber pressure provides a higher sublimation rate than the combination of low shelf temperature and high chamber pressure. In the current example the maximum sublimation rate, without collapsing the product, can be found when the process is changed from condition "A" ($P_c = 300$ µm Hg and shelf temperature = 20°C) to condition "D" ($P_c = 195$ µm Hg and shelf temperature = 40°C), where sample temperature is maintained at −20°C. Thus, the most efficient drying can be achieved when shelf temperature is set as high as possible, within the allowance of system and product stability, and product temperature is maintained below the maximum allowable temperature by reducing chamber pressure.

Determination of the Completion of Primary Drying

Accurate determination of the completion of primary drying is important because a premature transition to secondary drying may result in collapse. Conversely, maintaining primary drying conditions after sublimation is completed does not provide further drying of the product and is a needless waste of time and energy. The completion of primary drying can be monitored in four ways (Nail and Gatlin 1993).

1. As the sublimation of ice and the resultant product cooling are completed, the product temperature starts to increase and equilibrate to the shelf temperature.

2. A chamber pressure rise test can be employed. The chamber is temporarily isolated from the vacuum pump by closing a valve. If sublimation is not complete, there will be a rise in chamber pressure due to water vapor from the product.

3. Vials may be withdrawn from the drying chamber, via a sample extractor, without disturbing the vacuum, and weighed to determine the completion of sublimation.

4. The moisture content in the drying chamber can be monitored by analyzing the gas composition with mass spectrometry or other methods. A rapid drop of moisture content indicates the completion of primary drying.

Optimization of Secondary Drying

At the completion of primary drying, the product temperature must be increased to start secondary drying, during which the unfrozen water contained in the amorphous fraction and/or adsorbed to crystalline material is removed by evaporation (Pikal et al. 1990). A highly porous cake structure is advantageous for secondary drying, because the rate of drying will increase as the surface area of the material containing the unfrozen water is increased. At least for the model systems they employed, Pikal et al. (1990) found that the rate of secondary drying was independent of chamber pressure up to

200 μm Hg. Thus, there usually is not a need to alter the pressure from that used during primary drying.

The main parameter to be controlled is product temperature, which is usually raised by increasing the shelf temperature, if a relatively low shelf temperature was employed during primary drying (e.g., $\approx$ < 20°C). For model systems Pikal et al. (1990) found that the product water content during the initial phase of secondary drying far exceeded the equilibrium water content, which was calculated from sorption isotherm data and partial pressure of water in the drying chamber. However, additional evaporation and a reduction in water content can be obtained by increasing the product temperature. The T_g and, hence, the collapse temperature of the partially dried product will increase as water is removed by evaporation. To avoid collapse, however, the rate of increase in product temperature must be slow enough so that sufficient moisture can be removed by evaporation to increase the T_g to a value greater than the product temperature. The safest method is to increase the product temperature as slowly as possible. However, an unnecessarily slow transition will delay the drying process. In practice, the optimum rate must be determined empirically by essentially a "trial and error" process. In a series of experiments, the warming rate is progressively increased until a rate fast enough to lead to collapse of the final dried cake is noted. Then a slightly slower warming rate is employed in the final cycle. Progress in this determination can be hastened if a sample extractor is employed to remove samples from a given run for analysis without breaking chamber vacuum (Pikal et al. 1990).

In addition to the rate of warming, the final product temperature and the duration of product exposure are important factors in secondary drying, because they determine the final moisture content of the product. The final product temperature, which is primarily determined by the shelf temperature, is more critical, assuming sufficient drying time is given (e.g., Pikal et al. 1990). For example, completion of secondary drying at 30°C will reduce residual moisture content more than that seen at 20°C, even if the final duration of drying is longer at the lower temperature. Therefore, if a drier product is desired, as usually is the case, it is recommended to raise the secondary drying temperature rather than to extend the drying time (Pikal et al. 1990). In practice, the most rapid way to determine the optimum duration of secondary drying is to employ a sample extractor to remove samples during the course of this step. Then residual moisture can be analyzed by the Karl Fischer titration or by thermogravimetric analysis.

Single-Step Freeze-Drying Cycle

The complexities and empirical determination of optimum parameters associated with cycles employing arbitrary primary and secondary drying phases can be avoided with a single-step cycle. In this approach the shelf temperature is set for the final product temperature desired during secondary drying. The product temperature for primary drying is maintained below the maximum allowable temperature by setting the chamber pressure properly (Chang and Fischer 1995). Heat loss by the sublimation of ice keeps the product frozen during primary drying. As the sublimation of ice is completed and the heat loss at the sublimation front diminishes, the product temperature in this region will naturally begin to rise and secondary drying will proceed. Collapse is usually avoided because the increase in T_g due to evaporative water loss occurs more rapidly than the increase in product temperature. The final product temperature will equilibrate with the shelf temperature. There are numerous advantages to this approach. The combination of high shelf temperature and low chamber pressure provides faster sublimation as demonstrated in Equation 4.1 and Figure 4.2. Also, it is not necessary to wait for the last vial in a lot to complete primary drying before starting secondary drying, which eliminates the need for external control of the transition. Simplifying the process by eliminating a controlled step reduces the opportunity for operator error and manufacturing deviations. Finally, since the product temperature is controlled not by the shelf temperature but primarily by the chamber pressure, this approach will be useful for containers that have poor thermal transfer from the shelf (e.g., prefilled syringes).

A precaution for this single-step drying cycle is that some products may collapse during the transition from primary drying to secondary drying, if the temperature gradient between the shelf and sample at the end of primary drying is too great, resulting in an excessively fast warming rate. Such a problem cannot be predicted theoretically and must be tested for by experimentation with the formulation of interest. Also, with some formulations it may not be possible to set the shelf temperature to the secondary drying temperature and still maintain a sufficiently low product temperature by decreasing chamber pressure. Finally, the extent to which pressure affects product temperature can be dependent on the physical parameters of the lyophilization system, such as the contact resistance to heat transfer, the capacity of the condenser, and the rate of mass transfer (Nail and Gatlin 1993). However, in general, the advantages of the single-step system make it an important alternative to consider.

High Temperature Annealing

Annealing of the dried powder at the end of secondary drying may be necessary for some formulations in order to complete the crystallization of excipients (e.g., mannitol) that form metastable glasses. Without annealing, there can be a risk of crystallization and a release of associated moisture during storage, which may significantly reduce the storage stability of proteins. By assuring complete crystallization, storage stability can be more consistent between lots and between individual vials within a lot. Annealing can be accomplished by raising the shelf temperature above the devitrification temperature, while the product is still at the low pressure used during secondary drying. Analogous to annealing of the frozen product prior to primary drying, DSC can be used to determine the appropriate annealing temperature and if such a step is needed for a given formulation. Since most dried proteins do not denature or precipitate during such relatively short-term heating to as high as 100°C (Bell et al. 1995), there is little risk of damaging the protein acutely.

Functional Limitations of Lyophilizers

A key parameter that must be determined for each lyophilizer is the lowest shelf temperature that can be obtained while the condenser is at its minimum operating temperature. This shelf temperature will determine the capability of the lyophilizer to dry formulations with lower collapse temperatures. However, it is not necessary to compare directly the lowest shelf temperature to the collapse temperature of each formulation, because the product temperature during primary drying is generally lower than the shelf temperature, due to sublimation cooling. Also, the lowest obtainable condenser temperature must be known. Sublimation will only occur at product temperatures that are greater than the condenser temperature. Similarly, the lowest chamber pressure that a lyophilizer can maintain is also critical, because this parameter will dictate the lowest product temperature at which there can be sublimation. Active sublimation can only occur when the chamber pressure is lower than the vapor pressure of ice at the product temperature (Pikal 1990a; Pikal et al. 1983; Nail and Gatlin 1993). For example, assuming that the vapor pressure of ice is not affected by the formulation, pressures less than 29.6 μm Hg and 96.6 μm Hg are necessary for drying products at -50 and -40°C, respectively.

The maximum cooling and heating rates are useful information for the design of freezing, annealing, and temperature ramping processes. The maximum mass transfer rate for water vapor from product to condenser is also important because it must be considered when optimizing the volume of drying product, sublimation rate, and heat transfer (Nail and Gatlin 1993). Slow mass transfer may become a rate-limiting step for the overall freeze-drying process. In such a case, increasing the sublimation rate may not be a useful approach for accelerating drying.

Finally, the precision of control for individual parameters must also be considered. Variations in shelf temperature, chamber pressure, and condenser temperature during the freeze-drying of a fully loaded shelf should be determined to assure that a safe and consistent cycle is developed.

ACUTE STABILIZATION OF PROTEINS DURING FREEZING AND DRYING

Most of the early research on acute protein stabilization during lyophilization was with labile enzymes, which were found to be irreversibly inactivated to varying degrees after rehydration. As such, attempts at improving the recovery of activity were focused on the entire process of lyophilization and rehydration. It was not known at what point(s) during the process that damage arose and that stabilizers were operative. More recently, using infrared spectroscopy, documentation has shown that unprotected proteins are unfolded (nonnative) in the dried solid and that stabilizers prevent unfolding. Finally, recent experiments have demonstrated that proteins must be protected during both the freezing and drying steps to obtain a native protein in the dried solid. This is because the structure of many (if not most) proteins is perturbed by freezing. Freezing-induced structural transitions for many proteins may be reversed by thawing and, thus, often are not detected during formulation development. However, during lyophilization, the protein would not have an opportunity to refold, and any attempt at protection during subsequent dehydration would be futile.

If developing a formulation conferring acute stabilization is to be more than the empirical screening of additives, a clear understanding of the mechanisms by which additives protect during *both* freezing and dehydration is imperative. This mechanistic insight provides a rationale for choosing stabilizers for each stress, for finding that some compounds (e.g., sucrose) protect during both freezing and dehydration, whereas others only protect during one stress, and for determining if freezing contributes to lyophilization-induced damage to a given protein. Since the mechanisms of protection during freezing and drying are different, knowing the relative contributions of these stresses to protein damage can be crucial in choosing the appropriate stabilizers for a given protein. To give the background needed for these decisions, this section will describe protection during the entire lyophilization/rehydration process, the two mechanisms proposed for stabilization by additives during the dehydration step, the use of infrared spectroscopy to study structural changes, evidence that the protein must be protected during both freezing and drying, and the mechanism for protection of proteins by solutes during freezing.

Protein Stabilization During Lyophilization/Rehydration

Most studies on the protection of proteins during the entire process of lyophilization and rehydration have tested the capacity of nonspecific stabilizers (i.e., those that will generally protect any protein) to prevent irreversible protein denaturation (i.e., aggregation) and inactivation. However, for practical purposes, the first step in increasing the resistance of a given protein to lyophilization-induced damage is to choose the specific conditions that provide the greatest stability to that protein. In general, any factor that alters protein stability in solution will tend to have the same qualitative effect, at least, during the freezing step of lyophilization. The pH and specific ligands that confer optimum stability often are known from purification protocols and/or earlier efforts at designing a liquid formulation. For example, the stability of many enzymes during freeze-thawing is altered by the presence of substrates, cofactors, and/or allosteric modifiers (e.g., Chilson et al. 1965). Even for nonenzyme proteins, specific ligands can be important components of the formulation. For example, the stability of fibroblast growth factors is greatly increased in the presence of heparin or other polyanionic ligands (reviewed in Chen et al. [1994]).

However, many labile proteins are not adequately stabilized by specific solution conditions. Of the nonspecific stabilizers that have been tested, sugars have been shown to stabilize the most proteins during lyophilization and have been known to have this property for the longest time. To our knowledge, the first published report is the 1935 paper by Brostreaux and Eriksson-Quensel, in which they described the protection during dehydration/rehydration of several proteins by sucrose, glucose, and lactose. Subsequent detailed comparisons of sugars documented that disaccharides usually provide the greatest stabilization (e.g., Carpenter et al. 1987; Arakawa et al.

1993; Isutzu et al. 1991). Both reducing and nonreducing disaccharides are effective for acute protection. However, during storage reducing sugars (e.g., lactose and maltose) can degrade proteins via the Maillard reaction (protein browning), a process that can be accelerated at intermediate residual moisture contents (Hageman 1992, 273–309; Isutzu et al. 1991). Therefore, the choice of disaccharides is limited to the nonreducing sugars, sucrose and trehalose. Since trehalose currently is not used in any FDA–approved parenteral product, sucrose is usually the first choice for commercial formulation.

Although the data are much more limited, polyvinylpyrrolidone (PVP) and bovine serum albumin (BSA) have also been shown to protect a few tetrameric enzymes (i.e., asparaginase, lactate dehydrogenase [LDH], and phosphofructokinase [PFK]) during lyophilization and rehydration (Hellman et al. 1983; Anchordoguy and Carpenter, unpublished observations). Polyvinylpyrrolidone and BSA will form a glass during lyophilization and should then partition with the labile protein into the amorphous phase of the dried sample. Sugars must also form a glass to protect proteins during freeze-drying. Solutes that crystallize during lyophilization usually do not protect proteins, and in some cases (e.g., with crystalline mannitol) have been shown to confer additional damage (Carpenter and Crowe 1989; Carpenter et al. 1993; Izutsu et al. 1991, 1993). It is important to note, however, that substantial stabilization has been achieved with solutes (including buffer salts) that alone crystallize, but in combination interfere with each other's crystallization (Pikal et al. 1991). In such systems (e.g., mannitol plus glycine), the amorphous fraction can protect the protein. Izutsu and colleagues have recently demonstrated approaches to inhibit solute crystallization, to which the reader is directed for further information (Izutsu et al. 1993, 1995). Most importantly for the purposes of this discussion, they found that inhibition of crystallization always correlated with an increase in the protection of the protein during lyophilization. Again, stabilization is ascribed to the fraction of the solute remaining amorphous.

The nature of the protective interaction of amorphous solutes with the protein during dehydration is a subject of controversy in the literature. There are, at least, two nonexclusive mechanisms proposed, which will be discussed in detail later. One group contends that the formation of an amorphous solid is all that is needed for the preservation of proteins in dried samples. Carpenter et al. (1987, 1993, 1994) have argued that within this glassy matrix, *sugars* (note:

this mechanism was originally proposed *only* for sugars and is not meant to explain protection of proteins by all stabilizers) prevent dehydration-induced denaturation by hydrogen bonding to the protein in the place of the water that is removed. Currently, it appears that neither of these mechanisms alone is sufficient to explain fully acute stabilization during lyophilization, because both mechanisms focus only on the effect of stabilizers during the terminal stress of dehydration. Both mechanisms essentially ignore the freezing step. Finally, no matter what the nature of the interaction of the additive with the dried protein, the most important factor is that the additive(s) prevent unfolding during *both* freezing and dehydration. As will be described in detail below, infrared spectroscopy is the only means by which this data can be obtained for any protein and, hence, should be viewed as an essential tool for the protein formulation researcher. In the following sections each of these mechanistic and practical viewpoints will be considered.

Stabilization by the Amorphous Additive Mechanism

Proponents of this mechanism state that proteins are mechanically immobilized in the glassy, solid matrix during dehydration (e.g., Franks et al. 1991). The restriction of translational and relaxational processes is thought to prevent protein unfolding, and spatial separation between protein molecules (i.e., "dilution" of protein molecules within the glassy matrix) is proposed to prevent aggregation. Although it is clear that protective additives must partition with the protein into the amorphous phase of the dried sample, simply forming a glassy solid does not assure protein stabilization. First, if all that were needed to prevent damage to a protein is the formation of a glass, then the protein by itself should be stable. Clearly, this is not the case, since many proteins are grossly damaged in the dried solid (Prestrelski, Tedeschi, et al. 1993; Prestrelski, Arakawa, et al. 1993; Prestrelski et al. 1994; Dong et al. 1995), but all proteins should form an amorphous phase during dehydration (Angell 1995). In some cases adding another protein (e.g., BSA), which should simply add the mass of the final protein glass, confers protection.

One might further qualify the mechanism by proposing that the requisite mechanical restriction to unfolding and aggregation can only be achieved if another amorphous compound is present to provide immobilization and spatial separation of the protein drug molecules. However, then the question becomes: What amount of additive is sufficient to provide the desired physical properties of the dried solid, which are not achieved with the protein alone? This question has not been answered or addressed in the literature. However, it is expected that, in general, the capacity of an additive to protect a protein specifically during dehydration should depend on the final additive to protein mass ratio. This observation could lend support to a glass transition mechanism, because the mass ratios between all compounds in the dried solid is a key criterion governing the influence of the compounds on each other's crystallization (e.g., with glycine and mannitol). Also, spatial separation and immobilization of the protein within the glassy matrix would be favored as the mass ratio of additive to protein is increased. However, as discussed later, the importance of this mass ratio has also been argued to support the water replacement mechanism for the stabilization of proteins during dehydration.

Several studies have also shown that formation of a glassy phase by an additive, even when it is used in large excess relative to the protein, is not a sufficient condition for the acute stabilization of proteins during lyophilization. For example, studies have shown that formulations of 100 mg/mL interleukin-1 receptor antagonist, prepared with sucrose concentrations ranging from 0–10 percent (wt/vol), all formed a glass during lyophilization and all had T_g of $66 \pm 2°C$ (Chang et al. in preparation). Yet only in formulations containing ≥ 5 percent sucrose was lyophilization-induced unfolding prevented. Tanaka et al. (1991) have found that the capacity of carbohydrates to protect freeze-dried catalase decreased with increased carbohydrate molecular weight. Dextrans were the largest and least effective of all the carbohydrates tested; the larger the dextran molecule, the less it stabilized catalase. Although they did not determine whether their dried samples were amorphous, it is well known that as the molecular weight of the carbohydrate is increased, the glassy state is formed more readily (Levine and Slade 1988 a and b, 1992). In addition, more recent studies have shown (Randolph, Zhang, Prestrelski, Arakawa, and Carpenter, unpublished data) that PFK was not protected, and LDH was inactivated further by dextran during freeze-drying and rehydration. Differential scanning calorimetry documented that the dried samples were amorphous. Therefore, in conclusion, although it is necessary for stabilizing additives to remain amorphous to protect proteins during lyophilization, glass formation alone does not appear to be sufficient for the acute protection of dried proteins.

It has been suggested that polymers, such as dextran, fail to protect proteins because they phase separate from the protein during the freeze-drying process (Pikal 1994, 120–133). The dried solid could contain two or more amorphous phases. As Pikal (1994, 120–133) has stated, it is crucial that the stabilizing additive not only remain amorphous, but also form a single phase with the protein. Phase separation of protein-polymer solutions has been used as a method to fractionate protein preparations. Although visible separation does not occur prior to freezing in the systems tested, the increased concentration of all solutes during freezing could provide conditions favorable to phase separation (Randolph and Carpenter, unpublished observation). Then during subsequent dehydration, the polymer would not be available to protect the protein. Polymers, such as dextrans, could provide many desirable properties (e.g., high T_g) to the freeze-dried formulation. Therefore, it is essential that future research address the theoretical and practical aspects of protein-polymer phase separation and develop the mechanistic insight to prevent this phenomenon during lyophilization. Also, as part of this effort, it is important to discern why other polymers (e.g., PVP and BSA) that protect labile proteins apparently do not phase separate from the protein during lyophilization.

Stabilization by the Water Replacement Mechanism

There are several studies supporting the contention that sugars protect labile proteins during drying by hydrogen bonding to polar and charged groups as water is removed and, thus, preventing drying-induced denaturation of the protein. For example, in early studies using solid-state Fourier-transform infrared (FT-IR) spectroscopy, it was found that the band at 1583 cm^{-1} in the spectrum for lysozyme, which is due to the hydrogen bonding of water to carboxylate groups, is not present in the spectrum for the dried protein (Carpenter and Crowe 1989). However, when lysozyme is dried in the presence of trehalose or lactose, the carboxylate band is retained in the dried sample, indicating that the sugar is hydrogen bonding in the place of water. Similar results have been obtained with α-lactalbumin and sucrose (Prestrelski, Tedeschi, et al. 1993). More recently, it has been documented that the carboxylate band can be titrated back to its solution intensity by freeze-drying lysozyme in the presence of increasing concentrations of either trehalose or sucrose (Allison and Carpenter, unpublished observations). This effect correlates directly with an increased inhibition of protein unfolding in the presence of increasing amounts of sugar.

Two other recent studies on enzyme preservation provide further support for the water replacement mechanism. Tanaka et al. (1991) have found that the capacity of a saccharide to protect catalase during freeze-drying is related inversely to the size of the saccharide molecule. They suggest that as the size of the saccharide increases, steric hindrance interferes with hydrogen bonding between the saccharide and the dried protein. In support of this contention, recent experiments have shown that the carboxylate band is only minimally detectable in the infrared spectrum of lysozyme freeze-dried in the presence of dextran (Barberi, Randolph, and Carpenter, unpublished observation). In addition, in the system employed by Tanaka et al. (1991), inactivation of the catalase during lyophilization/rehydration was constant across a wide range of initial protein concentrations. Therefore, they could vary either protein or saccharide concentration independently. They found that the degree of stabilization was based on the saccharide to protein mass ratio, which is to be expected if protection is due to the hydrogen bonding of the saccharide to the protein in the dried solid.

Some of the most compelling evidence for the water replacement hypothesis comes from studies on the effects of freeze-drying on a model polypeptide, poly-L-lysine (Prestrelski, Tedeschi, et al. 1993). This peptide assumes different conformations in solution, which have been well characterized with FT-IR spectroscopy, depending on pH and temperature. At neutral pH poly-L-lysine exists as an unordered peptide. At pH 11.2 the peptide adopts an alpha-helical conformation. Poly-L-lysine assumes a β-sheet conformation in the dried state, regardless of its initial conformation in aqueous solution. The preference for β sheet in the dried state appears to be a compensation for the loss of hydrogen bonding interactions with water. The β sheet allows for the highest degree of hydrogen bonding in the dried sample. If poly-L-lysine is freeze-dried in the presence of sucrose, the original solution structure is retained in the dried state, because sucrose hydrogen bonds in place of water.

Stabilization of Multimeric Enzymes by Polymers

Hellman et al. (1983) found that PVP acutely stabilized the tetrameric enzyme, L-asparaginase, during freeze-drying and rehydration. It has recently been shown that PVP and BSA stabilize tetrameric PFK and LDH during freeze-drying (Anchordoguy and Carpenter, unpublished data). Increased recovery of activity after rehydration can also be realized with LDH by simply increasing the initial concentration of the enzyme. The water replacement mechanism cannot explain such acute protection of proteins by polymers. Steric hindrance should minimize the ability of PVP or BSA to hydrogen bond effectively to the charged and polar groups on the surface of the dried protein. Also, as has already been described, polymer-induced stabilization cannot be ascribed just to the formation of a glassy phase with proteins during the dehydration step.

With multimeric enzymes, adding bulky polymers or increasing enzyme concentration also decreases inactivation during freeze-thawing (reviewed in Carpenter et al. [1994, 134–147]). Such results suggest that these conditions could also increase protein stability during lyophilization by protecting during the freezing step. Alterations in quaternary structure (i.e., dissociation) appear to be important in freezing-induced inactivation of multimeric proteins. First, simply reducing the temperature can foster dissociation of many multimeric proteins. The chilling lability is due to a disruption of hydrophobic interactions at the monomer-monomer contact sites (Bock and Freiden 1978). Secondly, Chilson et al. (1965) demonstrated that dissociation can be induced during freeze-thawing and that stabilizers inhibit dissociation. The recovery of enzyme activity correlated directly with the degree to which dissociation was inhibited. They employed a mixture of two LDH isozymes (i.e., rabbit muscle and porcine heart LDHs) that can be separated electrophoretically on native gels and identified by activity staining. Hybrid tetramers are formed during freeze-thawing. These hybrids arise because freezing induces dissociation; upon thawing nondenatured monomers can reassociate into the hybrid tetramers, as well as homotetramers. Stabilizers prevent the formation of hybrid tetramers and, thus, prevent freezing-induced dissociation.

Employing this model, it has been found that both PVP and BSA prevent hybrid formation during both freeze-thawing and lyophilization/rehydration (Anchordoguy and Carpenter, unpublished data). More importantly, dissociation and its inhibition were operative almost exclusively during the freezing step of the process. Thus, to obtain active tetramers upon rehydration, the initial freezing-induced dissociation must be inhibited.

Finally, it has been shown that polymers (e.g., polysucrose, 70 kDa) can inhibit unfolding of a monomeric protein, ribonuclease A (Krielgard and Carpenter, unpublished observation), during freeze-drying. However, even in this case it appears that, at least part of, the protective action of the polymer is manifested during the freezing step. As described later, there are several other lines of evidence documenting the importance of the freezing step in lyophilization-induced damage.

Infrared Spectroscopic Studies of Lyophilization-Induced Structural Changes

Until recently, the only way to assess the capacity of an additive to stabilize a protein during lyophilization was to measure activity and/or structural parameters after rehydration. Due to a lack of appropriate methodology to detect conformational changes of proteins under various physical conditions (i.e., in the dried solid, as well as in aqueous solution), freezing- and drying-induced changes in protein structure were unknown. To confound matters further, it was proposed in the protein chemistry literature that dehydration did not alter a protein's conformation (Rupley and Careri 1991). Such a claim was clearly counter to the known contributions of water in the formation of the native, folded protein (Kuntz and Kauzman 1974; Edsall and McKenzie 1983). Also, it was difficult to reconcile the finding that proteins could be inactivated and aggregated irreversibly after rehydration with the contention that protein structure was not perturbed by dehydration.

Reconciliation of this apparent dilemma was provided by FT-IR spectroscopy, which can be used to study protein secondary structure in any state (i.e., aqueous, frozen, dried, or even as an insoluble aggregate). Prior to describing the recent lyophilization studies, the method and considerations for data processing and interpretation must first be introduced (see review in Dong et al. [1995]). Fourier-transform infrared spectroscopy has long been used for the quantitation of protein secondary structure and for studies of stress-induced alterations in protein conformation (e.g., Susi and Byler 1986; Surewicz and Mantsch 1988; Byler and Susi 1986). Structural information is obtained by analysis of the conformationally sensitive amide I band, which is located between 1600 cm^{-1} and 1700 cm^{-1}. This band is due to the in-plane C=O stretching vibration, weakly coupled with C-N stretching and in-plane N-H bending (Krimm and Bandekar 1986; Susi and Byler 1986; Byler and Susi 1986). Each type of secondary structure (i.e., α-helix, β-sheet, β-turn, and disordered) gives rise to a different C=O stretching frequency (reviewed in Dong and Caughey [1994]), and, hence, has a characteristic band position, which is designated by wavenumber, cm^{-1}. Band positions are used to determine the secondary structural types present in a protein. The relative band areas (determined by curve fitting) can then be used to quantitate the relative amount of each structural component. Therefore, an analysis of the infrared bands in the amide I region can provide quantitative as well as qualitative information about protein secondary structure (Byler and Susi 1986;

Susi and Byler 1986; Surewicz and Mantsch 1988; Dong and Caughey 1994; Dong et al. 1995).

To obtain this detailed structural information, it is necessary to enhance the resolution of the protein amide I band, which usually appears as a single broad absorbance contour (see Figure 4.3). The widths of the overlapping component bands are often greater than the separation between the absorbance maxima of neighboring bands. Because the band overlapping is beyond instrumental resolution, several mathematical band-narrowing methods (i.e., resolution enhancement methods) have been developed to overcome this problem (reviewed in Dong et al. [1995]). Bands can be resolved equally well by either Fourier self-deconvolution or by obtaining the second derivative of the amide I band.

For studies of lyophilization-induced structural transitions, Fourier self-deconvolution is discouraged (see Dong et al. [1995] for further details). First, the choice of values for two parameters required for the calculations (bandwidth and enhancement factor) is arbitrary and subjective. Secondly, and more importantly, the

Figure 4.3. Comparison of infrared spectra of α-chymotrypsin in aqueous solution and dried solid state. The insert shows the second derivatives in the amide I region for the spectra in the main panel. Figure is reproduced from Dong et al. (1995).

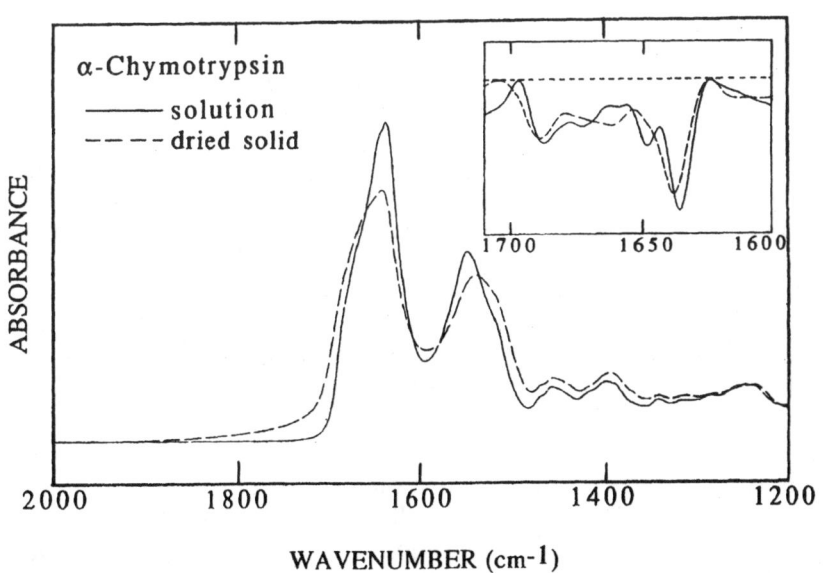

bandwidth relations are lost in the deconvoluted spectrum, as a result of arbitrary bandwidth input. In order to make a meaningful comparison between two spectra using this method, one must use the same input parameters for both spectra. However, as will be described later, the bandwidths of amide I components for a lyophilized protein are much broader than those for the native protein. Thus, it is difficult to deconvolute the spectra for a protein in the aqueous and dried states in a manner that allows meaningful and reliable comparisons to be made.

This difficulty is avoided with the second derivative method, because it is completely objective; the input of arbitrary parameters is not required. Also, alterations in component bandwidths are preserved in the second derivative spectrum. With this resolution enhancement method, it is apparent that the spectra of most unprotected proteins (i.e., lyophilized only in the presence of buffer) in the dried solid are greatly altered relative to the respective spectra for the native proteins in aqueous solutions (Prestrelski, Tedeschi, et al. 1993; Prestrelski, Arakawa, et al. 1993; Prestrelski et al. 1994; Dong et al. 1995). For example, Figure 4.3 compares the original and second derivative spectra for α-chymotrypsin in solution and in the dried solid. Second derivative spectra for aqueous and dried α-lactalbumin and LDH, which are also altered by lyophilization, and granulocyte colony stimulating factor (GCSF), which is not, are shown in Figure 4.4. For all the proteins, except GCSF, lyophilization induces shifts in band positions, the loss of some bands, and band broadening.

Dehydration-induced spectral alterations in the conformation-sensitive amide I region are due to protein unfolding and *not* simply to the loss of water from the protein. The intrinsic effects of water removal on the vibrational properties of the peptide bond, and, hence, protein infrared spectra, were found to be insignificant by Prestrelski, Tedeschi, et al. (1993). This conclusion is supported by the finding that the second-derivative spectrum of GCSF is not altered in the dried solid. The infrared spectra of all proteins should be altered in a similar fashion in the dried solid, if the direct vibrational effects of water removal were responsible for drying-induced spectral changes.

To date, GCSF is the only example from literature, or from unpublished studies on numerous proteins, of an unprotected protein that does not unfold during lyophilization. All other proteins are unfolded (nonnative, but not a random coil associated with complete denaturation) in the dried solid, but display two different behaviors during rehydration.

Figure 4.4. Second derivative amide I spectra of GCSF, α-lactalbumin, and LDH in aqueous solution (upper spectra) and dried solid (lower spectra) states. Figure is taken from Dong et al. (1995), employing data from Prestrelski, Tedeschi, et al. (1993) and Prestrelski, Arakawa, et al. (1993).

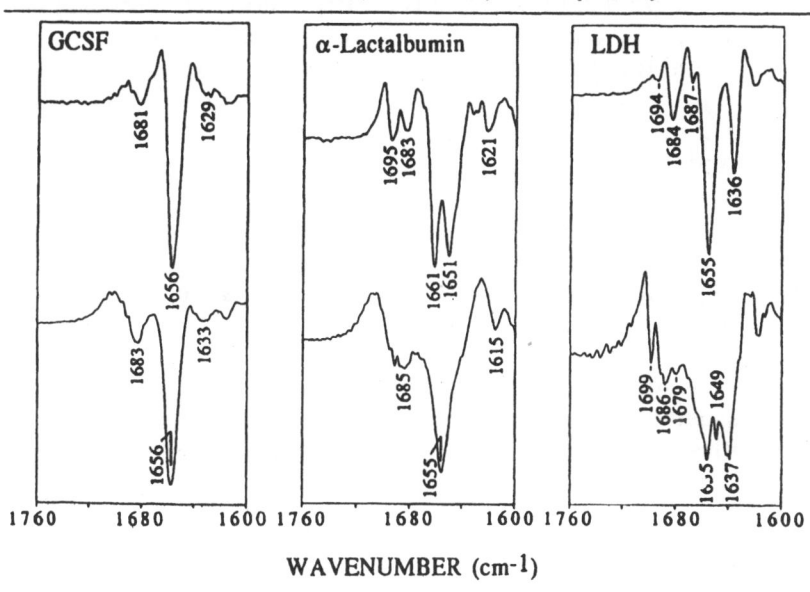

WAVENUMBER (cm⁻¹)

1. The protein regains the native conformation upon rehydration (reversible unfolding), as observed for α-lactalbumin, lysozyme, chymotrypsinogen, ribonuclease, β-lactoglobulins A and B, α-chymotrypsin, and subtilisin (Prestrelski, Tedeschi, et al. 1993a; Dong et al. 1995; Dong and Carpenter, unpublished observations).

2. The protein aggregates upon rehydration (irreversible unfolding), as noted for LDH, PFK, interferon-gamma, basic fibroblast growth factor, and interleukin-2 (Prestrelski, Tedeschi, et al. 1993; Prestrelski, Arakawa, et al. 1993; Prestrelski et al. 1995; Dong et al. 1995).

Furthermore, it has been documented with infrared spectroscopic studies of several proteins that prevention of aggregation and recovery of activity of labile proteins after rehydration correlate directly with retention of the native structure in the dried solid (reviewed in Dong et al. [1995]). That is, the mechanism by which stabilizing additives (e.g., sugars) protect proteins during lyophilization is to prevent unfolding (Prestrelski, Tedeschi, et al. 1993; Prestrelski, Arakawa, et al. 1993; Prestrelski et al. 1994). For example, the spectra for interferon-gamma dried in the presence of 1 M sucrose is very similar to that for the native aqueous protein, whereas that for the protein dried alone is greatly distorted (Figure 4.5). For analysis of these data, a baseline was fitted to the second-derivative spectra, and the data have been normalized for total area (Dong et al. 1995). This data presentation is useful because it allows visualization of the relative shifts of area from one component band to another and, hence, the redistribution of secondary structural types. After rehydration the spectra of both samples are very nativelike, indicating that the majority of nonnative molecules have refolded.

Figure 4.5. Comparisons of second derivative spectra of interferon-gamma in the dried solid and rehydrated states, with or without 1 M sucrose, with the spectrum of the native aqueous state. The spectrum of the native aqueous state is shown with the dashed line. The arrows indicate the band arising from the nonnative intermolecular β sheet. Reproduced from Dong et al. (1995).

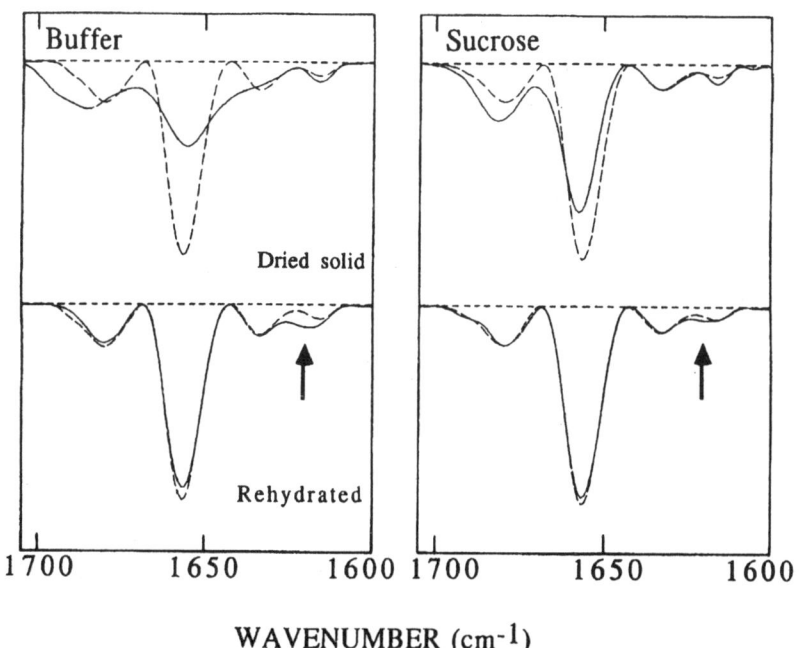

WAVENUMBER (cm^{-1})

However, in the sample lyophilized without sucrose, the appearance of a new band near 1625 cm^{-1}, which is assignable to intermolecular β-sheet structure, and the decreased intensities in vibrational bands ascribed to the α-helix (1656 cm^{-1}) and turn (1688–1665 cm^{-1}) structures indicate the formation of protein aggregate upon rehydration. (See Dong et al. [1995] for a detailed review of the study of protein aggregation with infrared spectroscopy.) In this sample 18 percent of the protein formed insoluble aggregates. In contrast, in the sample lyophilized with sucrose, only 9 percent insoluble aggregate was noted after rehydration. This reduction in aggregation is reflected in a much weaker 1625 cm^{-1} band in the spectrum of the rehydrated sample. In this case 1 M sucrose does not provide complete protection during freeze-drying, presumably because it is inadequate at preserving the protein structure during the freezing step (see later). However, these results do support the contention that minimizing aggregation upon rehydration is directly dependent on maintaining the native conformation of a protein in the dried state.

Also, unfolding of proteins that refold, if immediately rehydrated, can be inhibited by stabilizing additives (Prestrelski, Tedeschi, et al. 1993). As will be documented later, it appears crucial that even these proteins should be stabilized against acute unfolding, in order to maintain stability during long-term storage. Thus, an important criterion for a successful freeze-dried formulation of any protein is the retention of the native protein structure in the dried solid.

Although a qualitative visual comparison of second derivative spectra can be useful to assess the influence of additives on protein structure during lyophilization, a quantitative comparison is often more desirable and meaningful. For research on lyophilization-induced structural transitions, two approaches can be employed. Occasionally, there is a need to know the secondary structural content. Then the relative band areas can be determined with curve fitting (Dong et al. 1995). For example, the percentage of intermolecular β sheet can be used to calculate the percentage of aggregated protein in dried samples (see Dong et al. [1995] for further details).

However, for the general assessment of protein stabilization needed to evaluate formulations, it is adequate to make an overall global comparison between two spectra. For this analysis Prestrelski, Tedeschi, et al. (1993); and Prestrelski, Arakawa, et al. (1993) have developed a mathematical procedure to calculate the spectral correlation coefficient (similarity) between two second derivative spectra (Equation 4.2):

$$r = \frac{\sum^{N} x_i y_i}{\sqrt{\sum x_i^2 \sum y_i^2}} \qquad (4.2)$$

where x_i and y_i are the spectral absorbance values of the reference and sample spectra at the ith frequency position in the amide I region. The correlation coefficient of two spectra equals one when there is no conformational change in the protein. The larger the changes in conformation, the smaller the r value becomes.

As an example of this analysis, the spectral correlation coefficient for chymotrypsinogen's second derivative spectrum in the dried solid relative to that in the initial aqueous state is 0.664 (Figure 4.6). This result fits well with the visual impression of the gross alteration of the spectrum in the dried solid. Interestingly, quantitating the secondary structure with curve fitting demonstrates that the actual proportions of structural components are essentially unchanged (Table 4.1). This is because the bands were shifted to new positions in the dried sample, but these positions can be assigned to the same secondary structures as those noted in the aqueous protein. For example, there are several component bands under the amide I contour that are assigned to β-sheet structure (Table 4.1). Therefore, although it is sometimes useful to know the quantitative secondary structure of proteins in various states, the correlation coefficient provides a more reliable estimate for the overall degree of structural similarity to a reference state. Simply quantitating secondary structural content, without taking notice of band shifts and broadening, can be misleading.

Fourier-transform infrared spectroscopy can also be used to study the effect of solution properties that are known to have specific effects on a protein's resistance to lyophilization. In the first published example of such data, Prestrelski et al. (1995) have recently found that the spectrum for interleukin-2 lyophilized from a solution of pH 7.0 was greatly altered relative to the control aqueous spectrum ($r = 0.75$), indicating that the protein was unfolded. Furthermore, the appearance of a new strong band at 1617 cm^{-1} and a weaker band at 1690 cm^{-1} suggested that the protein was aggregated in the dried solid. Slightly less structural perturbation was noted when the protein was lyophilized from a solution of pH 6.0 ($r = 0.83$). In contrast, when pH 5.0 was employed, the dried protein's spectrum was very similar to that for the native aqueous protein ($r = 0.92$). Prior to lyophilization, altering the solution pH from 1.5 to 7.0 did not affect the protein's spectra. Thus, with interleukin-2

Figure 4.6. Curve-fitted inverted second-derivative spectra of chymotrypsinogen A in aqueous solution and dried states. Reproduced from Dong et al. (1995).

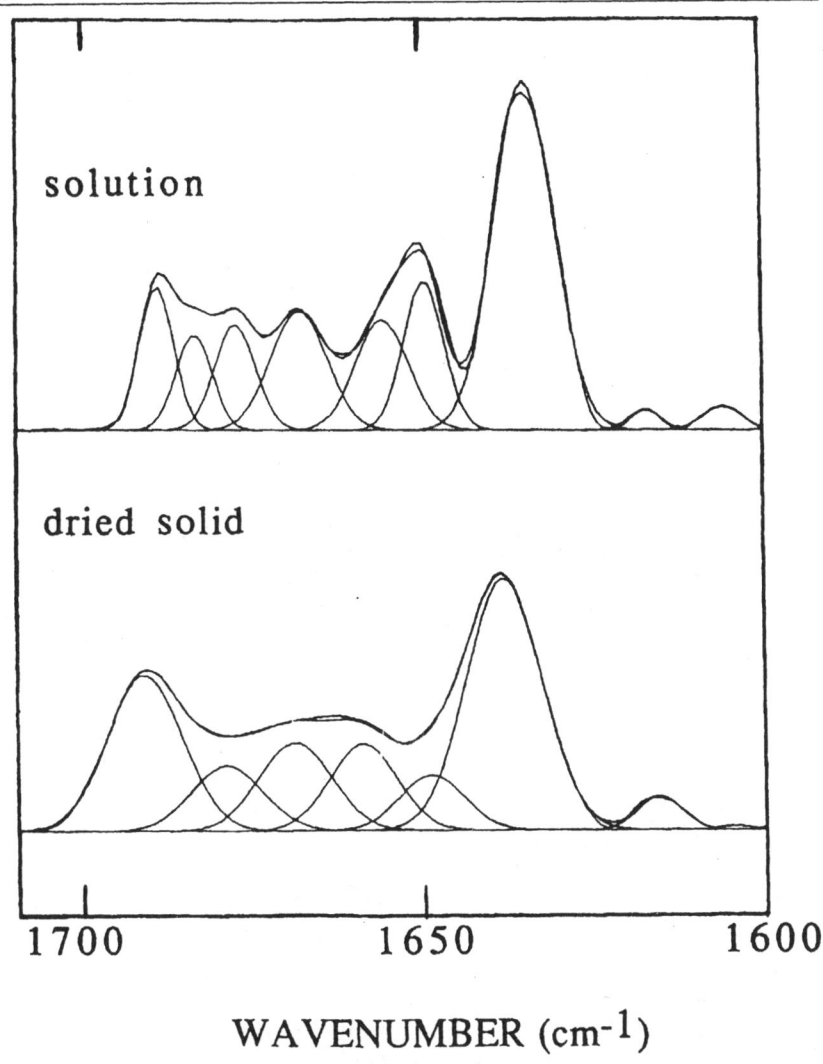

solution

dried solid

1700   1650   1600

WAVENUMBER (cm⁻¹)

it is possible to inhibit lyophilization-induced unfolding to a great degree simply by optimizing the pH of the initial solution. Although this is a new observation for freeze-drying, it should not be surprising.

Table 4.1. Assignments and Relative Areas of Amide I Components of Chymotrypsinogen in Aqueous Solution and Dried Solid States

Aqueous Solution		Dried Solid		
v (cm^{-1})	Area (%)[a]	v (cm^{-1})	Area (%)[a]	Assignment
1616[b]	—	1615	1.2	Intermol. β sheet
1635	40.3	1638	36.6	Intramol. β sheet
1649	11.5	1649	7.0	Unordered
1656	11.3	1659	11.3	α-helix
1668	12.7	1669	12.3	Turn
1677	8.3	1679	9.0	Turn
1683	6.6	—	—	Turn
1689	9.4	1691	22.6	Intramol. β sheet

[a]Relative areas determined by curve-fitting analysis of spectra shown in Figure 4.6.

[b]The weak 1616 cm^{-1} band in the aqueous native state arises from side chain vibrations and is included in the secondary structure estimation. It has also been subtracted from the overlapping band at 1615 cm^{-1}, which is due to intermolecular beta sheet in the dried protein.

The resistance of many proteins to stresses imposed in solution is known to show a strong pH dependence. It is not known whether the influence of pH manifests itself during freezing, drying, or both.

Prestrelski et al. (1995) also took advantage of the acute instability of interleukin-2 at pH 7.0 during lyophilization to compare the capacity of carbohydrates of increasing molecular weight to stabilize the protein. This study provides the most recent insight into the mechanisms for solute-induced stabilization during dehydration. As molecular weight increased, the capacity of the carbohydrate to inhibit unfolding decreased, and the level of protein aggregation after rehydration increased. Also, it was clear that acute protection of the protein did not correlate directly with the formation of a glass (all samples were found to be amorphous) or with the T_g of the sample (the T_g increased as carbohydrate molecular weight increased). Rather, as was the case with the experiments of Tanaka et al. (1991)

described above, there was a negative correlation of stabilization with molecular weight, which supports the water replacement mechanism concept for stabilization.

It is obvious from the infrared studies to date that the effect of a given additive may vary depending on the protein (e.g., Prestrelski, Tedeschi, et al. 1993), the presence of other additives, and other specific solution conditions (e.g., pH). Therefore, the structure of each dried protein in each formulation should be studied with infrared spectroscopy. Unfortunately, this will not be possible with certain formulations. If albumin is used, then, as is the case with any physical measurement, it will not be possible to separate the albumin contribution to the data from that of the protein drug. If other compounds (e.g., PVP and arginine), which absorb strongly in the amide I region, are used in large excess relative to the protein, then they may interfere with the protein spectrum. However, if relatively low concentrations of such additives are used, it may be possible to subtract quantitatively their specific absorbances from the protein spectra in both aqueous solutions and dried solids.

There should be few barriers to implementing infrared spectroscopic analysis, at least in industrial laboratories. The instrumentation is available commercially at relatively modest costs. Considering the wealth of information obtained, an investment of as little as $30,000 is reasonable. Also, high quality spectra can be acquired in less than five minutes and with minimal sample preparation. The main disadvantage of the technique is that a minimum protein concentration of 15 mg/mL is needed to obtain quality spectra of proteins in H_2O solutions. The absolute mass of protein needed is not great, since usually less than 50 μL of solution is required to load the sample cell. If solubility is limited, then the protein can be studied at much lower concentrations ($\approx$ 1 mg/mL) in D_2O. However, the researcher must then be aware of the potential difficulties of data interpretation due to the direct effects of H-D exchange on the vibrational frequencies of amide I component bands (Dong et al. In press). In some cases, deuteration of the protein makes assignment of bands to different secondary structural types uncertain. This can be a problem if quantitation of secondary structural content is needed. However, if all that is required is a global comparison between a spectrum for an aqueous control sample and that for a freeze-dried protein, then proteins can be studied reliably in D_2O. The only caveat is that sufficient time for H-D exchange must be allowed prior to lyophilization, so that additional exchange does not arise during freezing and drying.

Finally, in our opinion, infrared spectroscopy could have more industrial applications than simply for structural studies during development of lyophilized formulations. First, the analysis of protein structure in each new lot of lyophilized protein product could be valuable for routine quality assurance assessment. Secondly, infrared spectroscopy provides a rapid method for determining the quantitative structural effects of mutations or posttranslational modifications (Dong et al. In press). And, if needed, the valuable protein can be recovered undamaged.

Evidence for Freezing-Induced Unfolding During Lyophilization

If a protein is not adequately protected during freezing, the protein will be unfolded in the final dried solid, no matter how effective the stabilization is during the dehydration step (Carpenter et al. 1993; Prestrelski, Arakawa, et al. 1993). There is considerable evidence documenting the freezing sensitivity of proteins. First, many proteins are irreversibly denatured by freeze-thawing (Carpenter and Crowe 1988a). Since this damage is due primarily to freezing, then similar damage should also arise during the freezing step of lyophilization. Secondly, the capacity of an additive to protect during freeze-drying is often directly related to its initial bulk concentration and not to the final mass ratio of additive to protein. For example, the data in Figure 4.7 show that the recovery of PFK activity after lyophilization and rehydration increases as the prefreeze concentration of trehalose increases, even though the same mass ratio of trehalose to protein was used for all the samples. As will be explained later, freezing protection is governed by the initial concentration of the additive, whereas drying protection is related primarily to the mass ratio between the additive and protein.

Thirdly, Carpenter et al. (1993) recently have tested more rigorously the suggestion that freezing damage can play an important role in the overall damage to a protein during lyophilization. The impetus for this research was the observation that the disaccharide trehalose was effective at protecting labile enzymes, whereas the constituent monosaccharide, glucose, was not. For example, when PFK is freeze-dried in the presence of 0.2–0.4 M trehalose, over 60 percent of the initial activity is recovered after rehydration (Carpenter et al. 1987). In contrast, when similar amounts of glucose are used, the recovery is less than 5 percent. When considering only the effect of the sugar on the protein during dehydration, these results present a dilemma. If hydrogen bonding of the sugar to dried protein in the place of water was all that was needed for stabilization,

Figure 4.7. The effect of varying the concentration of trehalose, while maintaining a constant sugar to protein mass ratio, on recovery of PFK activity after freeze-drying and rehydration. Data taken from Carpenter and Crowe (1988b). The protein concentration was adjusted concomitantly with the sugar concentration to maintain a constant sugar to protein mass ratio of 945.

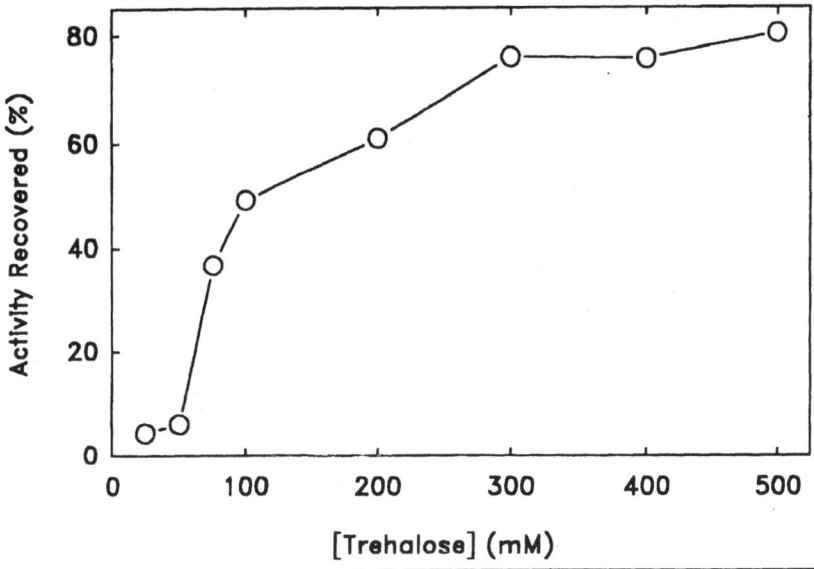

then mono- and disaccharides should provide similar protection. Glucose does not protect during freeze-drying because it provides minimal stabilization during freezing (based on freeze-thawing results), whereas trehalose is effective at protecting the protein during both freezing and dehydration (Carpenter et al. 1986, 1987).

To examine the separate roles of protein damage and stabilization by freezing and dehydration, Carpenter et al. (1993) developed a two-component system for stress-specific stabilization during lyophilization. In this stabilization scheme polyethylene glycol (PEG) is used as a cryoprotectant and various carbohydrates can be used to protect during dehydration. Polyethylene glycol alone completely stabilizes either LDH or PFK during freeze-thawing. However, it provides little or no protection during dehydration, because it crystallizes during lyophilization. When small amounts (e.g, 10–100 m*M* initial concentration) of trehalose or glucose are added, which alone at the concentrations tested are ineffective at protecting these enzymes during freeze-thawing or freeze-drying, excellent stabilization is noted during freeze-drying. Under conditions where cryoprotection is provided by PEG, glucose is as effective as trehalose in stabilizing dried enzymes (i.e., LDH and PFK).

In a complementary structural study of stress-specific stabilization using FT-IR spectroscopy, Prestrelski, Arakawa, et al. (1993) found that the recovery of activity after rehydration correlated directly with the ability of the additives to preserve the native structure of the enzymes in the dried state. Full activity recovery and maintenance of an essentially aqueous structure in dried samples are only noted when a combination of PEG and sugar is employed. Based on these results Prestrelski, Arakawa, et al. (1993) have proposed a model of the conformational events during lyophilization, which is shown in Figure 4.8. Briefly, this model proposes that, in order to recover structure and function after rehydration, the native structure of labile proteins must be retained, both upon freezing and during subsequent dehydration. The appropriate cryoprotectant is required for the initial structural preservation and a specific stabilizer against drying is needed for the terminal stress during lyophilization. In some instances (e.g., with disaccharides) a single additive can serve both protective functions.

Finally, preliminary FT-IR spectroscopic investigations have provided direct evidence for freezing-induced perturbation of protein secondary structure (Kendrick, Dong, Krielgard, and Carpenter, unpublished observations). For example, it was found that the structure of lysozyme was slightly perturbed in the frozen state and that the protein refolded upon thawing. In contrast, recombinant Factor XIII dimer was irreversibly unfolded by freezing. In all cases the degree of structural perturbation noted in the frozen state was intermediate to that noted in the dried solid, indicating that freezing-induced unfolding contributes partly to the total protein damage noted during lyophilization. This FT-IR method will be valuable for assessing the relative contributions of excipients to stabilization during the freezing and drying steps and, hence, for testing the model presented in Figure 4.8. The only caveat is that at the concentrations necessary (i.e., > 15 mg/mL) to obtain high quality protein infrared spectra in aqueous solution and in the frozen state, many proteins, which are known to be denatured at lower concentrations (e.g., catalase), are not unfolded during freezing.

Practical Approaches to Minimizing Freezing-Induced Damage

An important question that must be addressed when one is designing a formulation for protein lyophilization is as follows: To what

Figure 4.8. Schematic representation of a model for conformational changes during freezing, drying, and rehydration. Key: N = native; U = unfolded; K_1 = conformation equilibrium upon freezing, which shifts toward the native state in the presence of a cryoprotectant; k_1 = rate constant for refolding; k_2 = rate constant for formation of irreversibly denatured (aggregated) forms. Reproduced from Prestrelski, Arakawa, et al. (1993).

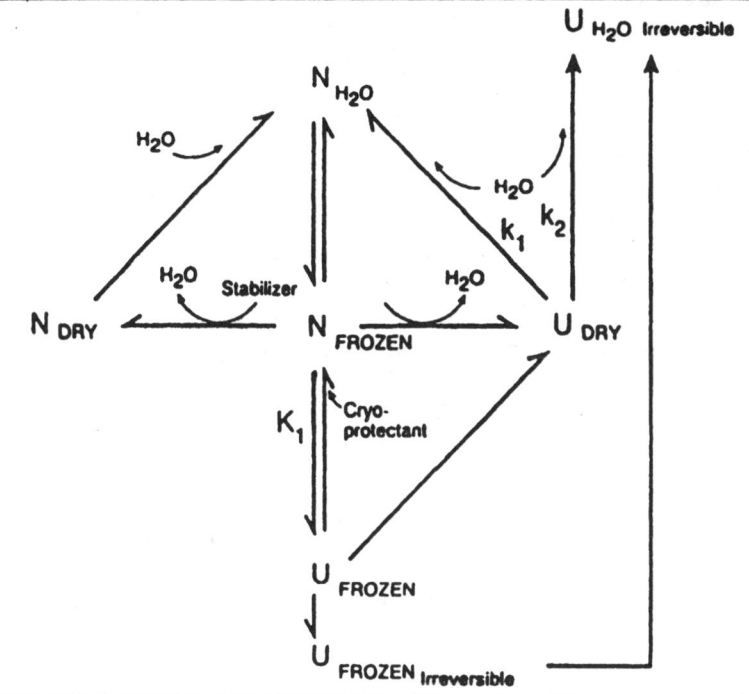

degree does freezing damage contribute to the overall unfolding noted during lyophilization? The approaches outlined above can be employed to answer this question, with direct examination of the protein in the frozen state, with FT-IR spectroscopy being the most informative. However, even without this information, since it appears that most proteins are freeze-labile, it will probably be necessary to add a stabilizer or stabilizers to prevent damage at this step.

Before discussing how to prevent protein unfolding during freezing, it is useful to review briefly the reasons why this process damages proteins. The most damaging stresses to which proteins are exposed to during freezing are low temperature and the formation of ice. Cold denaturation has been documented for many proteins, and by itself may be sufficient to account for at least some of the damage noted during freezing (Brandts et al. 1970, 189–212; Becktel and Schellman 1987; Privalov 1990). Also, the protein, which partitions into the nonice phase, is exposed to extremely high solute concentrations as the sample is frozen. If solutes that are destabilizing to the protein are present, then this concentrating effect can contribute to protein denaturation. Finally, as noted above, there can be dramatic pH changes during freezing. For example, the dibasic form of sodium phosphate crystallizes in frozen solution, which results in a system that only contains the monobasic salt and has a very low pH (van den Berg and Rose 1959; van den Berg 1959). Other components in a formulation may inhibit the crystallization of dibasic sodium phosphate (Chang and Randall 1992). However, such inhibition is not predictable and must be investigated for each formulation, with methods such as calorimetry or direct pH measurement of the frozen systems. pH measurements of frozen systems can be made easily with pH-sensitive dyes, which are available commercially. To minimize problems associated with pH changes sodium phosphate buffer should be avoided whenever possible. Also, although somewhat obvious, it is important to realize that a sodium phosphate system will be present if one starts with potassium phosphate buffer salts and NaCl, as is the case with phosphate-buffered saline.

Fortunately, to prevent freezing-induced damage to proteins, it is not necessary to discern which stresses are responsible for the damage or to target selectively each of these specific stresses. Rather, the most efficient approach is to design a formulation that provides the greatest overall resistance of the protein to denaturing forces. One exception to this generalization is the apparently specific protection against surface denaturation afforded by low levels of surfactants during freeze-thawing (Chang, Kendrick, and Carpenter, unpublished observations). As noted above, the first step in any stabilization process is to choose the specific conditions (pH or ligand) that maximize the stability of the given protein. These specific conditions, or adding a cryoprotectant solute such as sucrose, will protect the protein during freezing, whether the ultimate cause of denaturation is low temperature, high solute, or some combination of stresses.

A wide variety of compounds have been found to provide non-specific cryoprotection to proteins. These include sugars, amino acids, polyols, salting-out salts, methylamines, alcohols, other proteins, and synthetic polymers. During the initial screening of compounds as cryoprotectants, it is important that a relatively wide range of concentrations be tested for each compound. The range to be tested will be dictated by other formulation concerns (e.g., total excipient mass and tonicity of final rehydrated product) and the effectiveness of the cryoprotectant. The most potent cryoprotectants are polymers, such as PEG, PVP, and other proteins (e.g., albumins). Especially for proteins that must be formulated at low concentration, polymers can be useful as protectants and to minimize loss of active protein on the walls of the vial. Also, if high excipient mass is a concern, polymers are good candidates for cryoprotectants, because they are effective at relatively low concentrations (i.e., < 1 percent wt/vol). For some proteins sufficient freezing protection can be obtained by using a disaccharide (e.g., sucrose), which has the added benefit of also protecting the protein during subsequent drying. However, much higher concentrations (e.g., > 30 percent wt/vol) of such low molecular weight solutes are often needed to confer adequate protection during freezing.

The choice of compound to be used may also be influenced by other concerns with the freeze-drying process. For example, the common bulking agents, mannitol and glycine, are modestly effective as stabilizing proteins during freeze-thawing (Carpenter and Crowe 1988a). Although their effects during the freezing step of lyophilization have not been assessed, it is likely that they would contribute to protein stabilization at this point. The amount used may be dictated by the desired final cake properties. Even if another compound must be added to augment cryoprotection, the stabilization conferred by the bulking agent can be viewed as a "bonus."

This brings up the important point that it may be advantageous to employ a mixture of stabilizers to maximize protection during freezing and subsequent drying. Such an approach may be necessary if, for example, a high concentration of a low molecular weight cryoprotectant is needed for protein stabilization, which is detrimental because it lowers the $T_{g'}$ of the formulation too much. This formulation would be very difficult to lyophilize rapidly. In such a case, if the low molecular weight compound (e.g., sucrose) was needed for protection during drying, then a relatively low initial solution concentration could be used, if a polymer was added to aid in cryoprotection. It is not too difficult to envision a formulation in which at least three different agents confer freezing protection and also augment other favorable properties. For example, glycine could be used as a bulking agent, a polymer could be used to increase both $T_{g'}$ of the frozen solution and the T_g of the dried solid, and a disaccharide could be used to protect during dehydration.

Thermodynamic Mechanism for Cryoprotection of Proteins

Since many more classes of compounds will protect proteins during freezing than during drying, it appears that the mechanisms for protection from these stresses are different. Based on the results of freeze-thawing experiments with LDH and PFK and a review of the literature on protein freezing, Carpenter and Crowe (1988a) have determined that protein cryopreservation can be explained by the same universal mechanism that Timasheff (1992, 265–285) and Arakawa et al. (1993) have defined for solute-induced protein stabilization in nonfrozen, aqueous solution (see also Carpenter et al. 1994). And as will be described later, this single mechanism can also explain the observed differences in the relative potencies of cryoprotectants.

Prior to examining the specifics of the Timasheff mechanism, it is instructive to consider the general effects of ligand binding on protein stabilization. Here, a simplified, qualitative description of the most salient aspects of this relationship will be provided, which is referred to as the Wyman linkage function (i.e. in this case, the link between ligand binding and stability of protein states binding to the ligand). Rigorous explanations can be found in Wyman (1964) and Wyman and Gill (1990). Here a two-state model will be considered, in which there is an equilibrium between native and denatured states of the protein (N $\leftrightarrow$ D). At room temperature and in nonperturbing solvent environments, the native state is favored because it has a lower free energy than the denatured state. The magnitude of the difference in free energy between the two states (i.e., the free energy of denaturation) dictates the relative stability of the native state. Any alteration in a system that decreases this difference will reduce stability (e.g., reduce the melting temperature of the protein). Conversely, increasing this free energy difference will increase native state stability.

Binding of a ligand to either state will reduce the free energy (chemical potential) of that state, because thermodynamically binding can only occur if the free energy of the protein-ligand complex is lower than that for the protein alone. The effect of ligand binding on protein stability depends on the difference in binding between the two states. The state that binds the most ligand will have the greatest reduction in free energy. Consequently, if more ligand binds to the native state than to the denatured state, then the free energy of denaturation will be increased, and the native state will be stabilized. The opposite will be seen if more ligand binds to the denatured state. If binding to the denatured state is sufficiently greater than that to the native state, then the denatured state will have the lowest free energy and will predominate.

Now consider how this general ligand binding argument relates specifically to the Timasheff mechanism for solute-induced protein stabilization and destabilization. Detailed, rigorous reviews of the Timasheff mechanism can be found elsewhere (e.g., Timasheff 1992; Arakawa et al. 1993). For the purpose of the current review, a brief summary, which purposely provides only a simplified explanation, will suffice. First, a descriptive overview will be given and then an examination in more detail of the most relevant thermodynamic equations. This latter analysis is necessary for an understanding of the relative potencies of cryoprotectants.

In protein cryoprotection, and stabilization and denaturation in nonfrozen aqueous solution, by nonspecific compounds, usually relatively high concentrations ($\approx > 0.5\ M$) of ligand (solute) are needed to affect protein stability. This is because the interactions of the solute with the protein are relatively weak. These weak interactions are determined by equilibrium dialysis experiments, in which ligand binding is determined by the difference in the ligand concentration in the dialysis bag with the protein and that outside the bag. Binding measured by this method is actually a measure of the relative affinities of the protein for water and ligand. Therefore, the ligand interaction is referred to as preferential.

Ligand-induced destabilization by denaturants will be considered first, because logically it is the easiest to understand in the context of the general ligand binding effects noted above. Timasheff (1992) found that denaturants (e.g., urea and guanidine HCl) are bound preferentially to proteins and that the degree of binding is greatest for the denatured state. The free energy (chemical potential) of the denatured state is decreased more than that for the native state, because more surface area for binding is exposed to the solvent as the protein unfolds. Therefore, the free energy barrier between the two states is reduced. Consequently, the native state's resistance to stress is reduced (e.g., the melting point of the protein is lowered). If this effect is great enough, the protein will be denatured at room temperature.

Conversely, Timasheff and Arakawa and colleagues observed experimentally that there is a deficiency of stabilizing solutes (e.g., sugars and polyols) in the presence of the protein relative to that seen outside the dialysis bag. That is, the solutes are preferentially excluded from contact with the surface of the protein. Preferential exclusion, in a thermodynamic sense, means that the solute (ligand) has negative binding to the protein. Thus, there is an increase in the free energy (chemical potential) of the protein. In the presence of preferentially excluded solutes, the native state is stabilized. This is because denaturation leads to a greater surface area of contact between the protein and the solvent and greater preferential solute exclusion. Thus, even though there is an increase in the free energy of the native state, this effect is offset by the greater increase in the free energy of the denatured state.

Timasheff's preferential interaction mechanism also explains the influence of solutes on the degree of assembly of multimeric proteins. Preferentially excluded solutes tend to induce polymerization and stabilize oligomers, since the formation of contact sites between constituent monomers serves to reduce the surface area of the protein exposed to the solvent. Polymerization reduces the thermodynamically unfavorable effect of preferential solute exclusion. Conversely, preferential binding of solute induces depolymerization, since there is greater solute binding to monomers than to polymers.

Now the key thermodynamic aspects of this mechanism (reviewed in Timasheff [1992] and Arakawa et al. [1993]) will be examined in more detail. Setting component 1 = principal solvent (here water), component 2 = protein, and component 3 = solute (e.g., sucrose or PEG), the preferential interaction of component 3 with a protein is expressed, within close approximation, by the parameter, $(\delta m_3/\delta m_2)_{\mu_1,\mu_3}$, at constant temperature and pressure, where μ_i and m_i are the chemical potential and molal concentration of component i, respectively. A positive value of this interaction parameter indicates an excess of component 3 in the vicinity of the protein over the bulk concentration (i.e., preferential binding of the solute). A negative value for this parameter indicates a deficiency of component 3 in the protein domain. Component 3 (the solute) is preferentially excluded and component 1 (water) is in excess in the protein domain.

The preferential interaction parameter is a direct expression of changes in the free energy of the system induced by component 3, and has the following relation:

$$(\delta\mu_2/\delta m_3)_{m_2} = -(\delta m_3/\delta m_2)_{\mu_1,\mu_3}(\delta\mu_3/\delta m_3)_{m_2} \qquad (4.3)$$

The term on the left-hand side of the equation defines the change in protein chemical potential as a function of solute concentration. The first term on the right-hand side of the equation is the preferential interaction parameter, which was defined earlier. The second term is the solute self-interaction parameter, which will be described in detail later. Equation 4.3 indicates that those compounds that are excluded (i.e., $(\delta m_3/\delta m_2)_{\mu_1,\mu_3} < 0$) from the surface of the protein will have positive values of $(\delta\mu_2/\delta m_3)_{m_2}$; they will increase the chemical potential (free energy) of the protein, rendering the system more thermodynamically unfavorable. In the presence of excluded solutes, the exclusion will be greater for the denatured form of the protein than for the native form because the former has a larger surface area, as indicated by

$$(\delta m_3/\delta m_2)^D < (\delta m_3/\delta m_2)^N < 0$$

Consequently, the increase in chemical potential is greater for the denatured form than for the native form in the presence of a preferentially excluded solute, as indicated by

$$(\delta\mu_2/\delta m_3)_{m_2}{}^D > (\delta\mu_2/\delta m_3)_{m_2}{}^N > 0$$

There is an increase in the free energy difference between the native and denatured forms, thus stabilizing the native state.

The opposite is seen for potent protein denaturants, such as urea and guanidine HCl. These solutes bind preferentially to both the native and the denatured form of the protein (reviewed in Timasheff [1992] and Arakawa et al. [1993]) and, hence, decrease the chemical potential of the protein. Since the number of available binding sites is increased on unfolding of the protein, an increase in preferential solute binding occurs, as indicated by

$$(\delta m_3/\delta m_2)^D > (\delta m_3/\delta m_2)^N > 0$$

There is a concomitant decrease in protein chemical potential, which is greater for the denatured state:

$$(\delta\mu_2/\delta m_3)_{m_2}{}^D < (\delta\mu_2/\delta m_3)_{m_2}{}^N < 0$$

This serves to lower the free energy difference between the two states, and when the native state becomes the higher energy state, protein denaturation should result.

In more general terms, so long as $(\delta m_3/\delta m_2)^D < (\delta m_3/\delta m_2)^N$, then the native state will be stabilized. Thus, stabilization could also arise if the solute bound preferentially to the native state and was excluded from the denatured state, or if the solute was preferentially bound to both states, but binding was less for the denatured state. Conversely, in any situation in which $(\delta m_3/\delta m_2)^D > (\delta m_3/\delta m_2)^N$, the native state will be destabilized.

It is not possible to measure preferential interactions between solutes and proteins in frozen samples. Therefore, it is not known if cryoprotectants are actually preferentially excluded from frozen proteins. However, preferential interactions of solutes with proteins in nonfrozen, aqueous solutions can be used to explain the relative cryoprotective capacity of solute. The data for two cases, which are shown in Figure 4.9 and Table 4.2, illustrate this point. Figure 4.9 compares cryoprotection of LDH by PEG 8000 (MW 8000), PEG 400 (MW 400), and sucrose (MW 342). Lactate dehydrogenase is completely protected during freeze-thawing by PEG 8000 at concentrations of ≥ 0.01 percent (wt/vol). In contrast, full protection in the presence of PEG 400 is not realized until the concentration is at least 2.5 percent (wt/vol). On a weight percentage basis PEG 8000 is 250-fold more potent as a cryoprotectant. On a molar basis PEG 8000 is 5000-fold more potent. Sucrose is much less effective than even PEG 400. Even at sucrose concentrations as high as 10 percent (wt/vol), the protein is not fully protected.

The basis for these differences in protein stabilization can be realized by examining Timasheff's thermodynamic data in Table 4.2. The only protein for which the needed thermodynamic parameters have been measured in the presence of all three cryoprotectants is chymotrypsinogen. Although, these data are not directly applicable to LDH, the general trends shown should be relevant to any protein.

Figure 4.9. Effects of PEG and sucrose on LDH stability during freeze-thawing. Data taken from Carpenter et al. (1994) and Carpenter and Crowe (1988a).

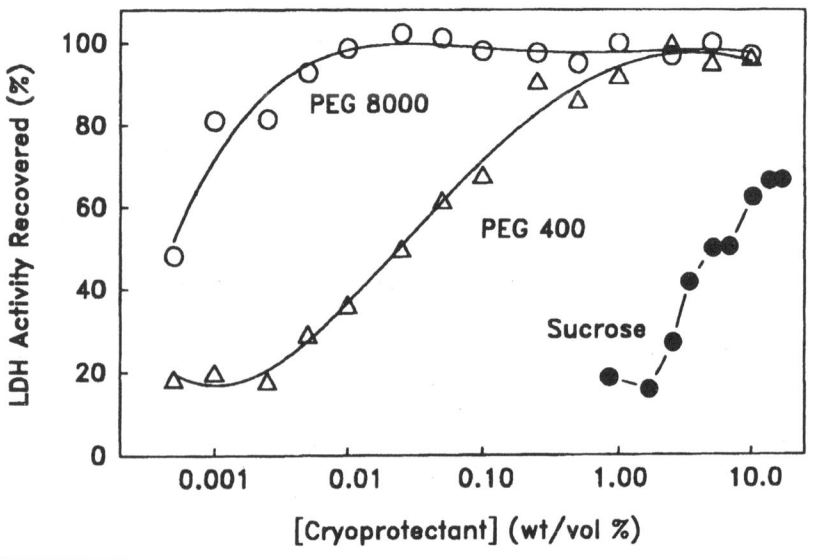

Table 4.2. Parameters for Solute Interactions with Chymotrypsinogen

Solute	Conc.	$(\delta m_3/\delta m_2)_{\mu_1,\mu_3}$	$(\delta\mu_3/\delta m_3)_{m_2}$ [a]	$(\delta\mu_2/\delta m_3)_{m_2}$ [b]
Sucrose[c]	1.27 mol	–10.35	0.56	5.7
PEG 400[d] (0.27 mol)	10% w/v	–6.87	2.42	16.6
PEG 6000[d] (0.0017 mol)	1% w/v	–0.62	480.00	297.6

[a]kcal (mol of solute)$^{-1}$ (mol of solute in 1000 kg $H_2O)^{-1}$

[b]kcal (mol of protein)$^{-1}$ (mol of solute)$^{-1}$

[c]Data taken from Lee and Timasheff (1981)

[d]Data taken and calculated from Bhat and Timasheff (1992)

The increase in chymotrypsinogen chemical potential, $(\delta\mu_2/\delta m_3)_{m_2}$, in the presence of either of two different molecular weights of PEG (e.g., MW = 400 or 6000), is greater than that noted in the presence of the sucrose, even though the PEGs are excluded to a lesser degree on a per mole of solute basis. Comparing the two PEG molecules indicates that the larger the PEG, the less it is excluded on a mole basis, but the more that it increases protein chemical potential.

The basis for these observations can be explained by examining Equation 4.3. The other major component in determining the effect of solute on protein chemical potential is the self-interaction parameter for the solute, $(\delta\mu_3/\delta m_3)_{m_2}$. The value for this parameter is several-fold greater for PEG 400, and almost three orders of magnitude greater for PEG 6000, than that for sucrose. The self-interaction parameter is given as follows:

$$(\delta\mu_3/\delta m_3)_{m_2} = [(RT/m_3) + RT(\delta\ln\gamma_3/\delta m_3)_{m_2}] \tag{4.4}$$

where γ_3 is the activity coefficient of the solute and R is the universal gas constant (Timasheff 1992, 265–285; Arakawa et al. 1993). The molal concentrations needed for preferential exclusion of PEG are very small, and the activity coefficient of PEG is quite large, relative to values for sucrose. Therefore, the self-interaction parameter for PEG is very large compared to that for sucrose. In addition, as the size of PEG increases, there is a great increase in such nonideality (Table 4.2).

Since degree of stabilization correlates directly with increase in protein chemical potential in the presence of a solute, it is not surprising that PEG is much more effective than sugars at protecting labile enzymes during freezing. Interestingly, this correlation does not hold for high temperature denaturation experiments. Sugars increase the melting temperature for proteins, but PEG decreases protein stability at high temperature. This effect has been ascribed to increased hydrophobic interaction of PEG with proteins as temperature is increased, which leads to preferential binding to the denatured state (Arakawa et al. 1993).

OPTIMIZING FORMULATIONS FOR LONG–TERM STORAGE STABILITY

Several review papers have been published to describe the physical (e.g., aggregation and precipitation) and chemical (i.e., covalent alterations) degradation pathways of proteins during storage in aqueous solution (Wang and Hanson 1988; Manning et al. 1989; Wang and Pearlman 1993; Cleland et al. 1993; Manning et al. 1995). Very little published information is available about the effect of lyophilization on the rate of individual degradation pathways in protein formulations. However, it is important to understand the major degradation pathways arising during storage in the dried solid and to develop the appropriate analytical methods before attempting to optimize the formulation. This is especially important if the protein undergoes chemical degradation (e.g., deamidation), for which very specific formulation adjustments (e.g., reduced pH) are needed to prevent protein damage. To develop the analytical methods needed and to identify the types of degradation products with which one might have to deal, degradation can be accelerated. The protein is lyophilized in the absence of stabilizers and stored at relatively high temperatures (e.g., > 50°C). The protein is then rehydrated and analyzed for changes, such as aggregation and specific chemical alterations. Since this analysis is performed in solution, the approaches outlined in reviews on solution stability can be used. Detailed accounts can be found in Manning and Ahern (1992) and Manning et al. (1989, 1995).

Ideally, the damage noted during accelerated degradation will be obviated by optimizing the formulation for general protein stability, as described below. It may not be necessary to perform separate accelerated degradation studies. However, in practice, the most expedient approach is to run accelerated degradation studies and formulation optimization in parallel. Then, if damage is still noted in a formulation in which general stabilization has been optimized, the specific degradation pathway(s) will most likely have already been identified and can be inhibited by the appropriate measures, in a rational manner.

As noted at the beginning of this chapter, during the process of formulation optimization for long-term storage stability, it appears that only four criteria must be met:

1. Acute lyophilization-induced unfolding must be minimized and, ideally, the protein should be native in the dried solid.

2. The dried powder must have a glass transition temperature that is higher than the desired storage temperature.

3. The residual moisture must be relatively low (i.e., $\approx$ < 0.01 g H_2O per g dried solid).

4. Specific formulation conditions (e.g., pH) must be developed to inhibit chemical degradation pathways, which might arise even in native proteins.

All but the final criterion has already been discussed. A brief consideration is now given as to how inhibition of chemical degradation can be achieved during lyophilization and storage, and then how each of the other criteria, which can be considered physical factors, affect storage stability.

Inhibition of Chemical Degradation of Lyophilized Proteins

The types and pathways of the chemical degradation of proteins, and specific methods to inhibit degradation, have been extensively reviewed in the literature of storage stability of liquid formulations (e.g., Manning et al. 1989, 1995; Manning and Ahern 1992; Cleland et al. 1993), to which the reader is referred for more details. The most common types of degradation are deamidation and oxidation, which can occur even under relatively "mild conditions" (e.g., low temperature). Other chemical degradation reactions include racemization, beta elimination, and hydrolysis, which generally occur under extreme conditions of temperature and pH (Manning et al. 1989, 1995). For lyophilized formulations these types of degradative reactions might be inhibited sufficiently by maintaining the protein in a native conformation, keeping the formulation below its T_g, and obtaining a low residual moisture (see below). However, as has been the case with liquid formulations, these general approaches of increasing physical stability may not be sufficient to inhibit certain pathways of chemical degradation. Due to the paucity of published information on specific approaches to minimize the chemical degradation of lyophilized proteins, the best approach currently used is to test methods previously found to be effective in solution. For example, Hageman et al. (1992) found that the deamidation rate of lyophilized recombinant bovine somatotropin could be decreased by almost an order of magnitude when the prelyophilization pH was decreased from 9.6 to 4.7. The loss of protein due to the other degradation pathway, dimerization, was independent of pH. Chang et al. (in press) found that deamidation of interleukin-1 receptor antagonist during storage in the dried solid was also inhibited by lowering the initial formulation pH and by avoiding phosphate buffers. However, in this case, the trade-off was that if pH was too low (i.e., < 6.0), the protein became physically unstable and aggregated upon rehydration. Such compromises between chemical and physical protein stability must be considered in the optimization of lyophilized formulations of many proteins.

Finally, it is important to note many of the commonly used excipients contain contaminants that could reduce protein stability.

For chemical degradation the most prominent contaminants are transition metals, which are found in most preparations of sugars and in many polyols (e.g., Carpenter et al. 1986, 1987, 1990). Also, peroxides can be found in surfactants (e.g., Hora et al. 1990). Such contaminants might greatly accelerate protein oxidation during storage and could catalyze other degradative reactions (e.g., the Maillard reaction [Ellis 1959]).

Effect of Physical Factors on the Storage Stability of Dried Proteins

It has been proposed that all that is needed to assure the long-term stability of dried proteins is to maintain the formulation below its T_g (Franks 1990; Franks et al. 1991). In the dried powder the protein is a component of a glassy phase that includes amorphous excipients and residual water. If this phase is held below its characteristic T_g, which can be determined with DSC or other thermal scanning methods (Nail and Gatlin 1993), the rate of diffusion-controlled reactions, including protein unfolding and chemical degradative processes, should be greatly reduced, relative to the rates noted above the transition temperature (Franks 1990; Franks et al. 1991). In such a system, rates for the various degradation pathways are proposed to fit predictions from Williams-Landel-Ferry (WLF) kinetic theory (Williams et al. 1955; Franks et al. 1991; Roy et al. 1990; Hageman 1992). This theory states that degradative reactions will be limited by sample mobility; hence, the further below the T_g a sample is stored, the greater the protein stability. Storage above the T_g, due to the greatly increased mobility, greatly accelerates reaction rates, to a much greater level than expected, based on Arrhenius kinetics. Roy et al. (1990) found that WLF kinetics explained the temperature and residual moisture–dependent changes in storage stability of a lyophilized monoclonal antibody-vinca conjugate. However, even though it is plausible, there currently is little other direct experimental evidence supporting the glass transition theory for protein storage stability.

Also, as noted above for acute stabilization during lyophilization, a protein alone will form an amorphous phase in the final dried solid. The transition temperatures of pure protein glasses are relatively high and, as with other glasses, vary inversely with sample water content. For example, dry legumin has a T_g of about 140°C, and in the presence of 10 percent water (by weight), the T_g is about 50°C (Angell 1995). Clearly, simply keeping a protein sample below its T_g is not adequate for storage stability. Proteins lyophilized without stabilizers have very poor storage stability in the dried solid, even if they are held at temperatures much below the range associated with a dried protein's T_g. As recently reviewed by Pikal (1994), this might be due, at least in part, to the fact that even below T_g there can be significant molecular mobility, which is permissive to degradative reactions. And a recent paper from Hancock et al. (1995) indicates that glasses of PVP and sucrose must be cooled to temperatures more than 50°C below T_g for molecular motions to be negligible over the normal lifetime of a typical pharmaceutical product.

In support of the role of a glassy matrix in protein stabilization, a limited number of studies have documented that, as is the case for acute stabilization, an amorphous excipient must be present with the dried protein to confer storage stability (e.g., Izutsu et al. 1991, 1994). Izutsu et al. (1991, 1994) found that damage to β-galactosidase could arise if the solute crystallized during the lyophilization process or during subsequent storage above the T_g. In the latter case, the presence of polymers (e.g., Ficoll or dextran) inhibited the crystallization of inositol and increased the storage stability of the enzyme.

In these earlier studies, the effect of additives on acute lyophilization-induced unfolding was not monitored, but can be inferred from data on the recovery of enzyme activity after rehydration. For example, in a comprehensive survey of numerous excipients, Isutzu et al. (1991) found that the storage stability of β-galactosidase at 70°C for 7 days was greatest in the presence of amorphous compounds (e.g., trehalose and sucrose). These stabilizers also led to full enzyme activity recovery in samples rehydrated immediately after lyophilization. Notable exceptions were reducing sugars, which provided acute protection and remained amorphous, but which degraded the protein via the Maillard reaction. Under the conditions employed by Isutzu and his colleagues, acute irreversible loss of activity was noted in samples lyophilized without stabilizers or with agents that crystallized. In both cases substantial additional loss of activity was noted during subsequent storage and rehydration. Taken with the current understanding that the inhibition of acute loss of activity correlates with the inhibition of unfolding during lyophilization, their data suggest strongly that a major factor in the increased storage stability by amorphous excipients is the maintenance of the native protein structure during the lyophilization process. Unfortunately, in their study the T_gs of the final dried solids were not measured. Presumably, the excipients would not have raised the T_g of the formulation above that expected for the protein alone. And it is most likely that the T_gs of the formulations were higher than the storage temperature of 70°C, and/or the duration of storage was not sufficient for the degradative processes to be manifested in samples with T_gs lower than 70°C.

To date, the most comprehensive long-term storage study of a lyophilized protein is that by Chang et al. (in preparation) on inter-leukin-1 receptor antagonist. In support of the glass transition theory, they found that for any given formulation (among more than 15 tested), storage above the T_g greatly accelerated degradation, which was due to deamidation and aggregation. However, in a series of formulations (100 mg/mL protein) with varying initial sucrose concentrations ranging from 0 percent–10 percent (wt/vol), all of which had a T_g of 66 ± 2°C, those with sucrose concentrations < 5 percent degraded rapidly (via deamidation and aggregation, which were measured after rehydration) during storage below the T_g at 50°C. In contrast, formulations with higher sucrose concentrations had less than 2 percent deamidation and no detectable aggregation after 14 months at 50°C. Infrared spectroscopy indicated that these stable formulations contained native protein in the dried solid, whereas the protein was unfolded in the unstable formulations. Thus, it appears that storage of a dried formulation below the T_g is necessary but not sufficient for stability. It is also necessary to obtain a native protein during the lyophilization cycle. Similarly, Prestrelski et al. (1995) found the greatest storage stability of lyophilized interleukin-2 in formulations that provided a high T_g and also prevented acute unfolding.

In the storage study with interleukin-1 receptor antagonist, it appears that, in addition to an environment permissive to chemical degradation, the glassy state also allowed sufficient mobility for further structural alterations in, and intermolecular interactions between, unfolded protein molecules. In samples prepared with ≤ 1 percent sucrose, the infrared spectra after 6 months of storage at 50°C were greatly altered relative to those for the protein immediately after lyophilization (Chang et al. in press). The appearance of bands at 1620 cm^{-1} and 1695 cm^{-1}, which are due to the intermolecular beta sheet, indicate that protein aggregation was arising during storage in the dried solid. These interactions were not seen in the preparations containing 5 percent and 10 percent sucrose, in which the initial lyophilization-induced protein unfolding was inhibited.

Finally, storage stability of dried proteins can be reduced if the residual moisture in the dried cake is too high (e.g., ≈ > 1 percent by weight). This is because water can participate directly in reactions that degrade the protein (e.g., hydrolysis). In addition, water has a very low T_g (-135°C) and will serve as a plasticizer of other glasses. Therefore, increasing the water content of a dried powder will decrease the T_g of the sample (Franks et al. 1991; Roy et al. 1990; Hageman 1992).

ACKNOWLEDGMENTS

We gratefully acknowledge support by grants to John F. Carpenter from the Office of Naval Research (N00014-94-1-0402), the National Science Foundation (NSFBES9505301 and NSFBES9520288), the Whitaker Foundation, Boehringer-Mannheim Therapeutics, Genetics Institute, Zymogenetics, and Genentech, Inc. We also thank the American Foundation for Pharmaceutical Education for providing a predoctoral fellowship to S. Dean Allison in Carpenter's lab. We thank Michael Pikal and Steve Nail for their helpful comments on the manuscript; and Steve Prestrelski, Kathy Pikal, and Tsutomu Arakawa for providing us with a copy of their paper on interleukin-2 stabilization prior to publication.

REFERENCES

Angell, C. A. 1995. Formation of glasses from liquids and biopolymers. *Science* 267:1924–1935.

Arakawa, T., S. Prestrelski, W. Kinney, and J. F. Carpenter. 1993. Factors affecting short-term and long-term stabilities of proteins. *Adv. Drug Delivery Rev.* 10:1–28.

Becktel, W. J., and J. A. Schellman. 1987. Protein stability curves. *Biopolymers* 26:1859–1877.

Bell, L. N., M. J. Hageman, and L. M. Muroaka. 1995. Thermally induced denaturation of lyophilized bovine somatotropin and lysozyme as impacted by moisture and excipients. *J. Pharm. Sci.* 84:707–712.

Bhat, R., and S. N. Timasheff. 1992. Steric exclusion is the principal source of the preferential hydration of proteins in the presence of polyethylene glycols. *Protein Science* 1:1133–1143.

Bock, P. E., and C. Frieden. 1978. Another look at the cold lability of enzymes. *Trends Biochem. Sci.* 3:100–103.

Brandts, J. F., J. Fu, and J. F. Nordin. 1970. The low temperature denaturation of chymotrypsinogen in aqueous solution and in frozen aqueous solution. In *The frozen cell,* edited by G. E. W. Wolstenholme, and M. O'Conner. London: Churchhill.

Brostreaux, J., and I-B. Ericksson-Quensel. 1935. Etude sur la dessication des proteines. *Archive de Physique Biologique* 23 (4): 209–226.

Byler, D. M., and H. Susi. 1986. Examination of the secondary structure of proteins by deconvoluted FT-IR spectra. *Biopolymers* 25:469–487.

Carpenter, J. F., and J. H. Crowe. 1988a. The mechanism of cryoprotection of proteins by solutes. *Cryobiology* 25:244–255.

Carpenter, J. F., and J. H. Crowe. 1988b. Modes of stabilization of a protein by organic solutes during desiccation. *Cryobiology* 25:459–470.

Carpenter, J. F., and J. H. Crowe. 1989. Infrared spectroscopic studies on the interaction of carbohydrates with dried proteins. *Biochemistry* 28:3916–3922.

Carpenter, J. F., T. Arakawa, and J. H. Crowe. 1990. Interactions of stabilizing additives with proteins during freeze-thawing and freeze-drying. *Dev. Biol. Standard.* 74:225–239.

Carpenter, J. F., L. M. Crowe, and J. H. Crowe. 1987. Stabilization of phosphofructokinase with sugars during freeze-drying: Characterization of enhanced protection in the presence of divalent cations. *Biochim. Biophys. Acta* 923:109–115.

Carpenter, J. F., S. Prestrelski, and T. Arakawa. 1993. Separation of freezing- and drying-induced denaturation of lyophilized proteins by stress-specific stabilization: I. Enzyme activity and calorimetric studies. *Arch. Biochem. Biophys.* 303:456–464.

Carpenter, J. F., S. C. Hand, L. M. Crowe, and J. H. Crowe. 1986. Cryoprotection of phosphofructokinase with organic solutes: Characterization of enhanced protection in the presence of divalent cations. *Arch. Biochem. Biophys.* 250:505–512.

Carpenter, J. F., S. J. Prestrelski, T. J. Anchordoguy, and T. Arakawa. 1994. Interactions of stabilizers with proteins during freezing and drying. In *Formulation and delivery of proteins and peptides.*

Symposium Series No. 567. Washington, DC: American Chemical Society.

Chang, B. S., and N. L. Fischer. 1995. Development of an efficient single-step freeze-drying cycle for protein formulations. *Pharm. Res.* 12:831–837.

Chang, B. S., and C. S. Randall. 1992. Use of subambient thermal analysis to optimize protein lyophilization. *Cryobiology* 29:632–656.

Chang, B. S., G. Reeder, and J. F. Carpenter. In press. Development of a stable freeze-dried formulation of recombinant human interleukin-1 receptor antagonist. To be published in *Pharm. Res.*

Chang, B. S., R. Beauvais, and J. F. Carpenter. In preparation. The role of protein structure and glassy state in the long-term stability of lyophilized interleukin-1 receptor antagonist.

Chen, B-L., T. Arakawa, E. Hsu, L. Narhi, T. J. Tressel, and S. L. Chen. 1994. Strategies to suppress aggregation of recombinant keratinocyte growth factor during liquid formulation development. *J. Pharm Sci.* 83:1657–1661.

Chilson, O. P., L. A. Costello, and N. O. Kaplan. 1965. Effects of freezing on enzymes. *Fed. Proc.* 24 (2): S55–S65.

Cleland, J. L., M. F. Powell, and S. J. Shire. 1993. The development of stable protein formulations: A close look at protein aggregation, deamidation, and oxidation. *Crit. Rev. Therapeutic Drug Carrier Systems* 10 (4):307–377.

Dong, A., and W. S. Caughey. 1994. Infrared methods for study of hemoglobin reactions and structures. *Meth. Enzymol.* 232:139–175.

Dong, A., J. Matsuura, S. D. Allison, E. Chrisman, M. C. Manning, and J. F. Carpenter. In press. Infrared and circular dichroism spectroscopic characterization between β-lactoglobulins A and B. To be published in *Biochemistry.*

Dong, A., S. J. Prestrelski, S. D. Allison, and J. F. Carpenter. 1995. Infrared spectroscopic studies of lyophilization- and temperature-induced protein aggregation. *J. Pharm. Sci.* 84:415–424.

Edsall, J. T., and H. A. McKenzie. 1983. Water and proteins II. The location and dynamics of water in protein systems and its relation to their stability and properties. *Adv. Biophys.* 16:53–183.

Ellis, G. P. 1959. The Maillard reaction. *Adv. Carb. Chem.* 14:63–134.

Franks, F. 1990. Freeze drying: From empiricism to predictability. *Cryoletters* 11: 93–110.

Franks, F., R. H. M. Hatley, and S. F. Mathias. 1991. Material science and the production of shelf stable biologicals. *BioPharm* 4 (9): 38–55.

Geisow, M. J. 1992. Aching for approval, hoping for harmony— biotechnology product regulation. *Trends Biotech.* 10 (4): 107–108.

Hageman, M. 1992. Water sorption and solid state stability of proteins. In *Stability of protein pharmaceuticals. Part A. Chemical and physical pathways of protein degradation,* edited by T. Ahern, and M. C. Manning. New York: Plenum Press.

Hageman, M. J., J. M. Bauer, P. L. Possert, and R. T. Darrington. 1992. Preformulation studies oriented toward sustained delivery of recombinant somatotropins. *J. Agric. Food Chem.* 40:348–355.

Hancock, B. C., S. L. Shamblin, and G. Zografi. 1995. Molecular mobility of amorphous pharmaceutical solids below their glass transition temperature. *Pharm. Res.* 12:799–806.

Hellman, K., D. S. Miller, and R. A. Cammack. 1983. The effect of freeze-drying on the quaternary structure of L-asparaginase from *Erwinia carotovora. Biochim. Biophys. Acta* 749:133–142.

Her, L.-M., and S. L. Nail. 1994. Measurement of glass transition temperatures of freeze-concentrated solutes by differential scanning calorimetry. *Pharm. Res.* 11:54–59.

Her, L.-M., R. P. Jeffries, L. A. Gatlin, B. Braxton, and S. L. Nail. 1994. Measurement of glass transition temperatures in freeze concentrated solutions of nonelectrolytes by electrical thermal analysis. *Pharm. Res.* 11:1023–1029.

Hora, M. S., R. K. Rana, C. L. Wilcox, N. V. Katre, S. N. Hirtzzer, S. N. Wolfe, and J. W. Thomson. 1990. Development of a lyophilized formulation of interleukin-2. *Dev. Biol. Standard.* 74:295–306.

Izutsu, K., S. Yoshioka, and S. Kojima. 1994. Physical stability and protein stability of freeze-dried cakes during storage at elevated temperatures. *Pharm. Res.* 11:995–999.

Izutsu, K., S. Yoshioka, and S. Kojima. 1995. Increased stabilizing effects of amphiphilic excipients on freeze-drying of lactate dehydrogenase (LDH) by dispersion into sugar matrices. *Pharm. Res.* 12:838–843.

Izutsu, K., S. Yoshioka, and Y. Takeda. 1991. The effects of additives on the stability of freeze-dried β-galactosidase stored at elevated temperatures. *Int. J. Pharm.* 71:137–146.

Izutsu, K., S. Yoshioka, and T. Teroa. 1993. Decreased protein-stabilizing effects of cryoprotectants due to crystallization. *Pharm. Res.* 10:1232–1237.

Jaenicke, R. 1991. Protein folding: Local structures, domains, subunits, and assemblies. *Biochemistry* 30:3147–3161.

Knight, C. A., and J. G. Duman. 1986. Inhibition of ice recrystallization by insect thermal hysteresis proteins: A possible cryoprotective role. *Cryobiology* 23:256–262.

Knight, C. A., A. L. DeVries, and L. D. Oolman. 1984. Fish antifreeze protein and the freezing and recrystallization of ice. *Nature* 308:95–296.

Knight, C. A., J. Hallett, and A. L. DeVries. 1988. Solute effects on ice recrystallization: An assessment technique. *Cryobiology* 25:55–60.

Krimm, S., and J. Bandekar. 1986. Vibrational spectroscopy and conformation of peptides, polypeptides and proteins. *Adv. Protein Chem.* 38:181–364.

Kuntz, I. D., and W. Kauzman. 1974. Hydration of proteins and polypeptides. *Adv. Protein Chem.* 28:239–345.

Lee, J. C., and S. N. Timasheff. 1981. The stabilization of proteins by sucrose. *J. Biol. Chem.* 259:7193–7201.

Levine, H., and L. Slade. 1988a. Principles of "cryostabilization" technology from structure/property relationships of carbohydrate/water systems—a review. *Cryoletters* 9:21–63.

Levine, H., and L. Slade. 1988b. Thermomechanical properties of small-carbohydrate-water glasses and "rubbers": Kinetically metastable systems at subzero temperatures. *J. Chem. Soc. Faraday Trans.* 1 (84):2619–2633.

Levine, H., and L. Slade. 1992. Glass transitions in foods. In *Physical chemistry of foods*, edited by H. S. Shartzberg, and R. W. Hartel. New York: Marcel Dekker.

MacFarlane, D. R. 1987. Physical aspects of vitrification in aqueous solutions. *Cryobiology* 24:181–195.

MacKenzie, A. P. 1975. Collapse during freeze-drying–qualitative and quantitative aspects. In *Freeze-drying & advanced food technology,* edited by S. A. Goldblith, L. Rey, and W. W. Rothmayr. New York: Academic Press.

MacKenzie, A. P. 1976. The physicochemical basis of the freeze-drying process. *Dev. Biol. Standard.* 36:51–67.

Manning, M. C., and T. J. Ahern. 1992. *Stability of protein pharmaceuticals: Part A. Chemical and physical pathways of protein degradation.* New York: Plenum Press.

Manning, M. C., K. Patel, and R. T. Borchardt. 1989. Stability of protein pharmaceuticals. *Pharm. Res.* 6:903–918.

Manning, M. C., E. Shefter, and J. F. Carpenter. In press. Rational approach to the preformulation and formulation of protein pharmaceuticals. In *Peptide and protein drug delivery,* 2nd ed., edited by V. Lee.

Nail, S. L. 1980. The effect of chamber pressure on heat transfer in the freeze drying of parenteral solutions. *J. Parent. Drug. Assoc.* 34:358–368.

Nail, S. L., and L. A. Gatlin. 1993. Freeze-drying: Principles and practice. In *Pharmaceutical dosage forms: Parenteral medications,* vol. 2, edited by K. E. Avis, H. A. Lieberman, and L. Lachman. New York: Marcel Dekker.

Pikal, M. J. 1985. Use of laboratory data in freeze drying process design: Heat and mass transfer coefficients and the computer simulation of freeze-drying. *J. Parent. Drug Assoc.* 39:115–138.

Pikal, M. J. 1990a. Freeze-drying of proteins. Part I: Process design. *BioPharm* 3 (8):18–27.

Pikal, M. J. 1990b. Freeze-drying of proteins. Part II: Formulation selection. *BioPharm* 3 (9):26–30.

Pikal, M. J. 1994. Freeze-drying of proteins. In *Formulation and delivery of proteins and peptides,* edited by J. L. Cleland, and R. Langer. Symposium Series 567. Washington DC: American Chemical Society.

Pikal, M. J., and S. Shah. 1990. The collapse temperature in freeze drying: Dependence on measurement methodology and rate of water removal from the glassy phase. *Int. J. Pharm.* 62:165–186.

Pikal, M. J., M. L. Roy, and S. Shah. 1984. Mass and heat transfer in vial freeze-drying of pharmaceuticals: Role of the vial. *J. Pharm. Sci.* 73:1224–1237.

Pikal, M. J., S. Shah, M. L. Roy, and R. Putman. 1990. The secondary drying stage of freeze-drying: Drying kinetics as a function of temperature and chamber pressure. *Int. J. Pharm.* 60:203–217.

Pikal, M. J., S. Shah, D. Senior, and J. E. Lang. 1983. Physical chemistry of freeze-drying: Measurement of sublimation rates for frozen aqueous solutions by a microbalance technique. *J. Pharm. Sci.* 72:635–650.

Pikal, M. J., K. M. Dellerman, M. L. Roy, and R. M. Riggin. 1991. The effects of formulation variables on the stability of freeze-dried human growth hormone. *Pharm. Res.* 8:427–436.

Prestrelski, S. J., T. Arakawa, and J. F. Carpenter. 1993. Separation of freezing- and drying-induced denaturation of lyophilized proteins by stress-specific stabilization: II. Structural studies using infrared spectroscopy. *Arch. Biochem. Biophys.* 303:465–473.

Prestrelski, S. J., T. Arakawa, and J. F. Carpenter. 1994. The structure of proteins in lyophilized formulations using Fourier-transform infrared spectroscopy. In *Formulation and delivery of proteins and peptides.* Symposium Series No. 567. Washington, DC: American Chemical Society.

Prestrelski, S. J., K. A. Pikal, and T. Arakawa. 1995. Optimization of lyophilization conditions for recombinant human interleukin-2 by dried-state conformational analysis using Fourier-transform infrared spectroscopy. *Pharm. Res.* 12:1250–1259.

Prestrelski, S. J., N. Tedeschi, T. Arakawa, and J. F. Carpenter, 1993. Dehydration-induced conformational changes in proteins and their inhibition by stabilizers. *Biophysi. J.* 65:661–671.

Privalov, P. L. 1990. Cold denaturation of proteins. *Crit. Rev. Biochem. Mol. Biol.* 25:281–305.

Roy, M. L., M. J. Pikal, E. C. Rickard, and A. M. Maloney. 1990. The effects of formulation and moisture on the stability of a freeze-dried monoclonal antibody-vinca conjugate: A test of the WLF glass transition theory. *Dev. Biol. Standard.* 74:323–340.

Rupley, J. A., and G. Careri. 1991. Protein hydration and function. *Adv. Protein Chem.* 41:37–172.

Surewicz, W. K., and H. H. Mantsch. 1988. New insights into protein conformation from infrared spectroscopy. *Biochim. Biophys. Acta* 953:115–130.

Susi, H., and D. M. Byler. 1986. Resolution enhanced Fourier-transform infrared spectroscopy of enzymes. *Meth. Enzymol.* 130: 290–311.

Talmadge, J. E. 1993. The pharmaceutics and delivery of therapeutic polypeptides and proteins. *Adv. Drug Delivery Rev.* 10:247–299.

Tanaka, T., T. Takeda, and R. Miyajama. 1991. Cryoprotective effect of saccharides on denaturation of catalase during freeze-drying. *Chem. Pharm. Bull.* 39:1091–1094.

Thornton, C. A., and M. Ballow. 1993. Safety of intravenous immunoglobulin. *Arch. Neurol.* 50:135–136.

Timasheff, S. N. 1992. Stabilization of protein structure by solvent additives. In *Stability of protein pharmaceuticals. Part B. In vivo pathways of degradation and strategies for protein stabilization,* edited by T. Ahern, and M .C. Manning. New York: Plenum Press.

van den Berg, L. 1959. The effect of addition of sodium and potassium chloride to the reciprocal system: $KH_2-PO_4-Na_2HPO_4-H_2O$ on pH and composition during freezing. *Arch. Biochem. Biophys.* 84:305–315.

van den Berg, L., and D. Rose. 1959. The effect of freezing on the pH and composition of sodium and potassium solutions: The reciprocal system $KH_2-PO_4-Na_2HPO_4-H_2O$. *Arch. Biochem. Biophys.* 81:319–329.

Wang, Y. J., and M. A. Hanson. 1988. Parenteral formulations of proteins and peptides: Stability and stabilizers. *J. Parent. Sci. Technol.* 42:2–26.

Wang, Y. J., and R. Pearlman. 1993. Stability and characterization of protein and peptide drugs: Case histories. *Pharm. Biotechnol.* Volume 5.

Williams, M. L., R. F. Landel, and J. D. Ferry. 1955. The temperature dependence of relaxation mechanisms in amorphous polymers and other glass forming liquids. *J. Am. Chem. Soc.* 77:3701–3707.

Wyman, J. 1964. Linked functions and reciprocal effects in hemoglobin: A second look. *Adv. Protein Chem.* 19:223–286.

Wyman, J., and S. J. Gill. 1990. *Binding and linkage: Functional chemistry of biological molecules.* Mill Valley, CA: University Science Books.

5

ADVANCES IN BLOW/FILL/SEAL TECHNOLOGY: A CASE STUDY IN THE QUALIFICATION OF A BIOPHARMACEUTICAL PRODUCT

Vincent L. Wu

Genentech, Inc.

Frank N. Leo

Automatic Liquid Packaging, Inc.

Aseptic filling and packaging by blow/fill/seal (b/f/s) technology has gained wide acceptance for a variety of products in recent years. Applications have included the filling of respiratory drugs, ophthalmics, terminally sterilized and heat-sensitive small-volume parenterals (SVPs) and large-volume parenterals (LVPs), and, more recently, a human biological product.

There are many desirable advantages offered by b/f/s technology, when compared with conventional aseptic processing, that are consistent with the current thinking in the pharmaceutical industry. This includes minimizing personnel in the fill room, through automation and by implementing a barrier system for the aseptic filling process, and decreasing product cost through streamlined manufacturing operations.

In addition, b/f/s has other advantages that address key issues currently affecting pharmaceutical manufacturing. Most important of these is the move toward packaging drug products in single-dose units, obviating the need for preservatives and antimicrobials. It also facilitates the replacement of glass containers with safer alternatives, and its inherent flexibility allows a variety of user-friendly containers to be produced (Forrester-Coles 1995).

In recent years studies have been conducted to prove the high sterility assurance levels (SALs) obtained by the b/f/s process. Since b/f/s is a completely automated technology that is designed for remote operation, it is an ideal system for examining the relationship between the extent of contamination by airborne microorganisms during media fill studies and the level of airborne microorganisms in the environment. A series of airborne microbial challenges have suggested that the equipment tested may achieve SALs equal to that demanded of terminal sterilization.

Over the last 20 years b/f/s systems have undergone significant design changes to accommodate the increasing requirements of scrutinizing regulatory agencies. One recent design for a b/f/s system utilizes an enclosure with a Class 100 HEPA–filtered air shower surrounding the filling assembly area, which protects the product from extraneous sources of contamination during the filling operation.

This chapter reviews issues concerning facility design, sterility assurance, validation, and the operational performance of a b/f/s system developed for the manufacture of a sterile, liquid-packaged biopharmaceutical product. However, many of the same process development and operational concerns are applicable to b/f/s processes in general, and to many products. Specific concerns for filling a sensitive protein product include assessment of heat imparted to the product via plastic extrusion, extractables from plastic resin, and product stability.

For this specialized product, Genentech has implemented the proprietary technology of Automatic Liquid Packaging, Inc. (ALP), Woodstock, IL, for the sterile packaging of Pulmozyme®. Pulmozyme®, or recombinant human DNase, was approved by the Food and Drug Administration (Center of Biologics Evaluation and Research) and the Medicines Control Agency in December 1993 for the respiratory treatment of cystic fibrosis. The dosage form is a

3 mL, low density polyethylene (LDPE) ampoule produced by b/f/s technology using ALP's Model 624 B/F/S Machine.. An LDPE ampoule was chosen since it was a convenient dosage container for dispensing the single-use, preservative-free product into a nebulizer. From a product stability standpoint, the LDPE container offered improved pH control for the nonbuffered, low pH formulation when compared to storage in glass vials. pH change of unbuffered aqueous solutions in borosilicate glass vials has been well studied, and its cause has been identified as an ion-exchange process occurring between hydrogen ions in the product solution and sodium ions from the glass vial (Borchert et al. 1989). Since ions are not a constituent of LDPE containers, b/f/s packaging offered a good alternative to glass vials in improving the product's pH stability.

From a manufacturing and quality control standpoint, the plastic ampoule offered significant advantages over a rubber-stoppered glass vial, including freedom from potential stopper extractables, contamination by foreign matter derived from glass and stopper processing, elimination of the problem of container breakage, and allowed contact of product with only one material since stoppers and silicone were not required.

The b/f/s process enables a container to be formed, filled, and sealed in one continuous, integrated operation within a single automated machine. The process has been well described elsewhere by industry experts (Sharp 1987, 1988; Leo 1989). The major attributes of the b/f/s equipment and the process sequence for the production of Genentech's 3 mL LDPE ampoules is given as a review in Figure 5.1. (1) LDPE resin pellets are fed by a vacuum system to the resin feed hopper. (2) Resin is continuously melted and sterilized in the extruder at high temperature and pressure. (3) Resin is formed into 4 molten plastic tubes or parisons. (4) The main molds close on the parisons, forming the containers with the aid of tiny vacuum holes in the mold, and a hot-knife cuts the parisons. (5) The containers in the chilled mold move to the filling station and are provided with Class 100 HEPA–filtered air flow. (6) The filling assembly, located in the HEPA–filtered air enclosure, moves downward and fills the containers with the sterile-filtered product. (7) The necks of the containers, still molten, are then sealed by chilled seal molds. (8) The main molds and seal molds open and release the formed, filled, and sealed containers, which are then conveyed out of the b/f/s room for deflashing, inspection, and packaging. The molds then return to the parison area where the process cycle restarts.

Figure 5.1. Side view of the B/F/S Machine for production of 24-cavity 3 mL LDPE ampoules.

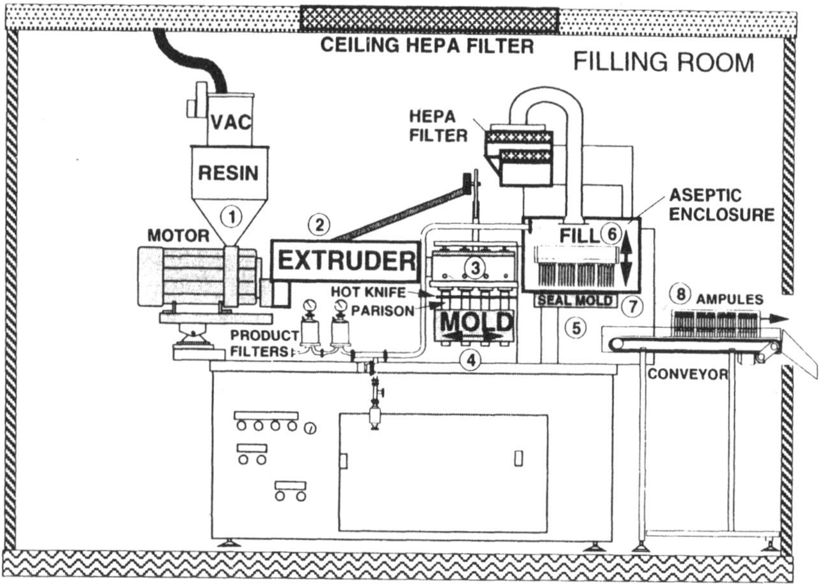

ECONOMICS

Although not all products may be suited for packaging by b/f/s technology, the cost to produce b/f/s containers is economical when compared to the production of stoppered-glass vials. The resin cost for a 3 mL LDPE ampoule, for example, is approximately 1.5¢ per ampoule (without recycling or regranulation of excess plastic generated during the b/f/s process), compared to approximately 10¢ for the components of a high quality, 3 mL stoppered-glass vial. A conservative estimate for the cost of producing a small filled, stoppered-glass vial for a parenteral drug is on the order of $2–$3 (see chapter 7). The production cost for a b/f/s container is estimated to be on the order of one-tenth the cost for the aseptic production of a stoppered-glass vial. Also, the capital cost for b/f/s equipment and facilities is significantly less than the cost for equipment and facilities necessary to clean and sterilize components, as well as to fill, stopper, and cap glass vials.

FACILITY LAYOUT AND EQUIPMENT

A facility design layout is shown in Figure 5.2 for a b/f/s operation that was suitable to European and U.S. regulatory investigators. The b/f/s room, the equipment preparation room, and the gowning room have a dedicated air handling unit. The b/f/s room is entered through a gowning room that requires personnel to gown fully with a one-piece suit, face mask, shoe covers, and gloves. (See "Environmental Monitoring" for more details.)

Figure 5.2. B/F/S facility and equipment layout.

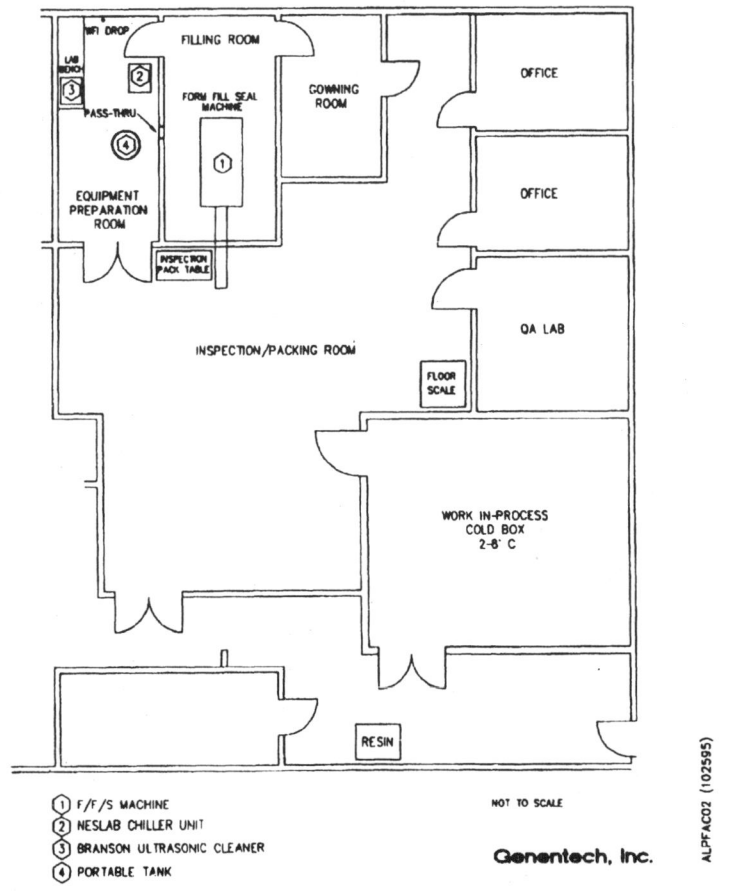

① F/F/S MACHINE
② NESLAB CHILLER UNIT
③ BRANSON ULTRASONIC CLEANER
④ PORTABLE TANK

NOT TO SCALE

Genentech, Inc.

ALPFAC02 (102595)

Adjacent to the b/f/s room there is the equipment preparation room, where a bulk feed tank is located and where cleaning procedures for the fill system are performed. A feed line is connected from the dual sterilizing product filters on the b/f/s machine to the bulk feed tank through a wall pass-through. The bulk feed tank is pressurized with inert gas at 10–15 psig for transferring and sterile filtering the product while filling.

The heat-labile protein product is maintained at 2–8°C by recirculating glycol through the jacket of the tank, using a portable chiller unit. Inspected and bulk packaged product is stored in an in-process cold room until further packaging and labeling operations are to be performed.

HEPA Air Shower for Filling Nozzles

A suitable aseptic environment must be provided to protect the product from viable and nonviable particulates during the most critical operations, which occur when the containers are open and when the product is filled. Such an environment is provided by a Class 100 HEPA–filtered air shower over the fill nozzles and opened containers. The entire filling area is designed to maintain positive pressure relative to its surroundings during filling. The Class 100 filling enclosure was provided with a differential pressure transmitter that automatically shuts down the b/f/s operation in the event of a low pressure alarm condition. Positive pressure is maintained in the fill room relative to all surrounding rooms and is monitored and alarmed during processing operations.

Figure 5.3 shows a front view of the b/f/s machine and the HEPA airflow system. Such a system can provide up to 13 air changes per minute in the enclosure that houses the filling nozzles. The HEPA air exits through a slot in the bottom of the enclosure where it is then directed over the containers during filling. A cathode ray tube (CRT) touch screen is used for controlling and monitoring fill time parameters, extrusion temperatures, and various machine speed parameters. A second CRT touch screen is located outside the fill room and allows the operator to adjust fill weights and other parameters without entering the fill room during the production run.

Peripheral Equipment

There are some recent innovations that can be adapted to the b/f/s production line to automate procedures that could only be performed manually in the past. Inspection cameras measuring fill level

Figure 5.3. Front view of the b/f/s machine illustrating the HEPA air shower.

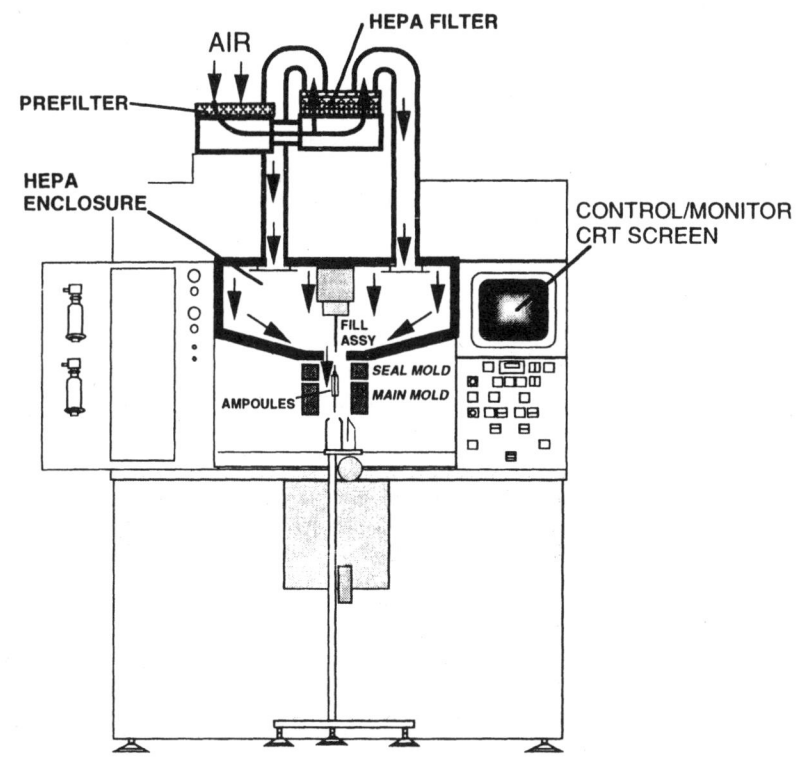

height may be adapted to the b/f/s exiting conveyor to detect containers with low fill volume. Vision systems, such as those offered by Allen-Bradley, may be designed to provide inspection of cosmetic defects of the container. Containers may then be conveyed to an automatic deflashing unit that removes excess plastic, or flashing. For some applications excess flashing may be recovered, granulated, and reused. The deflashed containers can then be conveyed to a high voltage leak detection system that automatically tests container integrity at selected potential leakage sites by measuring the electrical capacity of the container while passing it over electrodes. Containers with pinhole leaks register a high current flow and are automatically rejected. Nikka-Densok has developed such systems for glass ampoules and plastic ampoules. Filled containers may then be further inspected manually, or with a vision system, and automatically packaged in a heat-sealable pouch, for example, and then cartoned and cased for shipment.

STERILITY ASSURANCE

The high SALs achievable with the b/f/s process are attributed to the reliable automation of the process and to the fact that newly formed, clean and sterile containers, unadulterated by human contact, are filled within seconds from the time they are produced. Also, the opening of the container is small and substantially protected by the hot parison that extends from the main mold to the holding jaw that supports the molten plastic surrounding the opening of the containers. The reliability of the b/f/s process has been achieved by years of engineering refinements of the machinery's material handling systems and by attention to aseptic pharmaceutical processing needs. The reliability of the b/f/s system allows the process to go virtually unattended and has allowed critical aseptic operations to be isolated in a HEPA–filtered air shower with controls located outside the filling room.

Figure 5.4 summarizes two b/f/s airborne microbial studies conducted in the U.S. (Bradley et al. 1991; Sinclair and Tallentire 1993, 97–114). The two studies were performed using ALP Model 624 machines equipped with HEPA air showers and with identical mold tooling. Both systems were configured to provide 24 molded ampoules, each with 2 mL fill volume of tryptic soy broth. The b/f/s machine cycle time was set at 12 seconds for both studies. The air shower velocity, measured at the base of the slot of the enclosure could be varied between 1.6 m/s and 3.7 m/s. Studies were reported for the air shower on at 100 percent flow. *Bacillus subtilis* var. *niger* spores were aerosolized, dry dispersions at levels from approximately 4×10^4 to 1×10^7 spores/m^3 for study 1 (a 500-fold range of spore challenge concentration), and from 3×10^2 to 1×10^7 spores/m^3 for study 2 (a 50,000-fold range of spore challenge concentration). The authors reached the following conclusions:

- The fraction of product contaminated is determined by the microbiological quality of the b/f/s machine environment.

- Under fixed operating conditions, the relationship between the fraction contaminated and the level of airborne microorganisms is regular, highly consistent, and reproducible.

Figure 5.4. Airborne microbial studies.

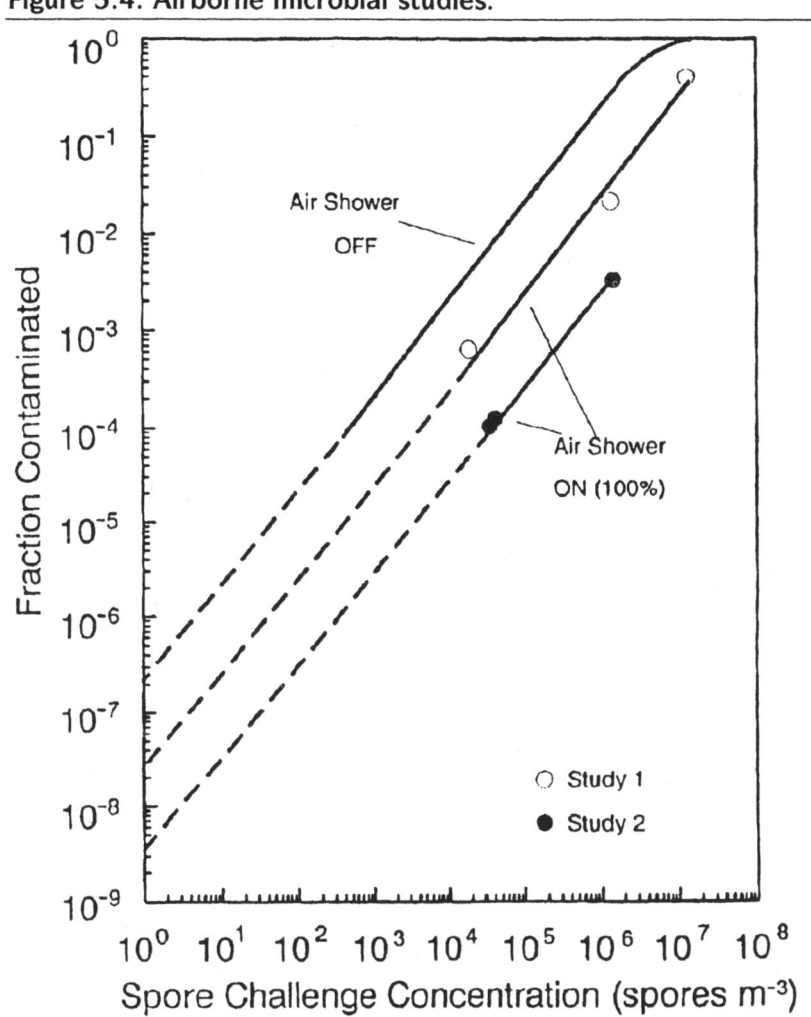

- The protective shower of air around the filling mandrels reduces the frequency of product contamination; the efficiency of local protection is dependent on air shower design and operating conditions.

- The responses to controlled microbial challenges can provide an effective approach to estimating rates of product contamination for advanced aseptic processing.

The authors suggested that since there is strong evidence that b/f/s performance under controlled conditions is highly consistent and reproducible, the linear portion of this relationship is amenable to extrapolation, providing a means for predicting the air quality under which the frequency of contamination is low and acceptable.

For those studies with the air shower off, an environmental limit of 1 CFU/m^3 is predicted to provide a rate of product contamination of 2.3 × 10^{-7}, or 1 contaminated ampoule in 4.3 × 10^6 ampoules produced. With the air shower on, an average challenge level of 1 CFU/m^3 is predicted to provide a rate of around 2.6 × 10^{-8} for study 1 and 3.5 × 10^{-9} for study 2. For study 1 with the air shower working at its maximum level, compared to the common curve derived with the air shower off, a 9-fold reduction in product contamination was observed, compared to study 2 that was observed to bring about a 70-fold reduction for maximum air shower operation. Accounting for the difference in the results for the two studies, the authors suggest that the configuration and arrangement of the air shower is critical to the efficiency of local protection. The authors note that none of the predicted contamination rates at 1 CFU/m^3 could be assessed by any practicable standard media fill study.

PROCESS TIME

Process time is an important factor for an aseptic process, since contamination is a function of the exposure time of the open containers to the environment and the actual opening size of the container. The b/f/s machine completes one cycle (or forms, fills, and seals one set of containers) in approximately 12 seconds. For a 24-cavity mold this amounts to approximately 7200 containers per hour. The approximate times for process operations for producing 3 mL LDPE ampoules using a 24-cavity b/f/s system are summarized in Table 5.1.

The time taken for the mold carriage to move from the parison area to under the fill nozzles was identified as a critical determinant of the rate of product contamination during airborne microbial challenge studies (Sinclair and Tallentire 1993). The study was performed on an ALP Model 624 b/f/s machine set up for filling 2 mL of tryptic soy broth into containers using a 24-cavity mold. The researchers performed studies comparing the machine cycle time at 12 seconds and at 14 seconds with spore concentrations in the room ranging from 3 × 10^2 to 3 × 10^6 spores/cm^3 with the HEPA shower on and with the HEPA shower off. The data indicated that there was a higher fraction of product contaminated for the 14 second cycle

Table 5.1. B/F/S Cycle Process Time

B/F/S Operation	Time (seconds)
Mold closes on parisons	0
Hot knife cuts parisons	1
Mold moves under fill nozzles	1
Mold cooling time	3
Filling	3
Sealing	1.5
Empty mold moves to parisons	2
Total Machine Cycle Time	**12**

with and without the HEPA shower, compared to the 12-second cycle. For the same air shower operating at a maximum setting, around a 70-fold reduction in product contamination was recorded at a cycle time of 12 seconds, compared to a 10-fold reduction for the 14-second cycle.

The Sinclair-Tallentire airborne microbial studies demonstrate that for the first time there is a methodology that can be used to quantify and rationalize machine design to preclude environmental contamination. For example, given the conditions of a standard media fill it would not be possible to detect the difference between a 12-second and a 14-second cycle time, because media fill validation without a challenge is not adequately sensitive.

RESIN STERILIZATION STUDIES

The sterilization of the resin occurs during the extrusion process at 170°C to 230°C depending on the type of resin, with residence times of several minutes and at pressures up to 350 atm. The process melts and heat treats the plastic granulate feed to produce a sterile, extruded tube of plastic from which the sterile container is formed. Any potential biocontamination of plastic granulate under these conditions is destroyed in the extruder.

Bacterial challenge studies that test resin sterilization on b/f/s machines have been reported (Leo 1987, 195–218; Svarnstrom et al. 1992,

132–140). The tests involved inoculation of resin feed pellets with *Bacillus subtilis* spores and performing media fills with tryptic soy broth. Filled containers with spores, seen as visible black spots in the walls of the containers, were culled and incubated at 35°C. No growth of spores after incubation was reported in either of these studies. A similar study performed at ALP tested resin spiked with various levels of endotoxin. The water-filled units were agitated on an orbital shaker and the contents were assayed using Limulus Amoebocyte Lysate. Test results showed nondetectable levels of endotoxin (Leo 1987).

ENVIRONMENTAL MONITORING

Air quality inside the HEPA–protected enclosure can be monitored for viable and nonviable particulates during the filling operation. Nonviable particle monitoring systems and a slit-to-agar system for monitoring viable particles have been successfully utilized for monitoring air quality in the aseptic enclosure. On-line monitoring of viable particulates in the aseptic enclosure during the filling operation may be performed using a slit-to-agar air sampler. An electronic particle monitoring system may be used for counting nonviable particulates. Cleaning and sanitizing with solutions of phenolic agents and with 3 percent hydrogen peroxide solution prior to filling has proven to be effective for maintaining an aseptic environment inside the aseptic enclosure.

The standard techniques for environmental monitoring have been applied to the b/f/s aseptic enclosure and outside the enclosure, including viable particulate monitoring by a slit-to agar sampler, Rodac plates, and a centrifugal air sampler. Typical environmental monitoring data during filling and at static conditions are shown in Table 5.2 for the fill room. The data were obtained during validation testing for a manufacturing facility for the production of 3 mL LDPE ampoules using an ALP 624 B/F/S machine with a 24-cavity mold. Notable are the low nonviable and viable particulate levels in the Class 100 aseptic filling area and the higher particulate levels outside the HEPA enclosure. The source of nonviable particulate counts $\geq$ 0.5 μm diameter outside the HEPA filling area has been linked to the cutting of parisons. Parison cutting is performed using a red-hot wire knife. For a 12-cavity fill system, which utilizes one parison, there are fewer nonviable particulates generated than for a 24-cavity fill system that utilizes 4 parisons. The b/f/s machine room is designated Class 100,000 when the machine is at rest. During the b/f/s operation, particulate levels ($\geq$ 0.5 μm) outside the fill assembly aseptic enclosure may approach 1.2 million particles/ft^3 for a 24-cavity fill system.

Table 5.2. Environmental Monitoring Data for a B/F/S Facility

Sample Site	Sample Type	Volume/Area Sampled	Acceptance Criteria	Count End Filling	Count End Static
Viable air	RCS	11.3 ft^3	0.5 CFU/ft^3	0	0
Floor	Rodac	25 cm^2	25 CFU/plate	1 GPR*	1 GPR
Wall	Rodac	25 cm^2	5 CFU/plate	0	0
Machine	Rodac	25 cm^2	5 CFU/plate	0	0
Air shower	STA	60 ft^3	0.1 CFU/ft^3	0	0
Air shower	Rodac	25 cm^2	5 CFU/plate	0	0
Air shower	RCS	11.3 ft^3	0.5 CFU/ft^3	0	0
Air shower	Climet	1 ft^3	100 particles	3	3
Fill room (front of machine)	Climet	1 ft^3	TREND 10^5 Static	639,106	58
Ceiling HEPA	Climet	1 ft^3	TREND 10^5 Static	0	0

*GPR: Gram-positive rod

Particulates in product produced by 12-cavity and 24-cavity fill systems have been measured by a HIAC-Royco counter. Results indicate that particulate levels for liquid product filled into b/f/s containers are well below USP requirements for small volume parenterals (see Table 5.3). These results confirm the inherent nature of the process to produce products exceeding SVP and LVP guidelines, even in the presence of high particulate levels outside the HEPA enclosure.

Although particulate levels in the product have been very acceptable, recent development efforts by machine manufacturers have focused on reducing the number of nonviable particulates in the b/f/s machine room and at the location of parison extrusion. B/f/s machines equipped with localized HEPA–filtered air around the parisons and a vacuum system to remove airborne particulates and smoke generated by the cutting of the parisons are currently being tested. However, it is evident that this new design will not only impact total room particulate levels, but will also further increase the SALs of products manufactured. New system designs are currently being analyzed using the methodology outlined by Sinclair and Tallentire.

DEVELOPMENT CONSIDERATIONS

Initial developmental work, including container compatibility and stability studies with active product and excipient formulations, may be performed using a limited number of mold cavities and smaller b/f/s equipment. Productivity is increased by scaling-up the number of mold cavities and by using larger b/f/s equipment, or, in many cases, the smaller equipment may be tooled with a greater number of mold cavities. The size and number of mold cavities also determines the size and number of parisons needed. However, during the development phase, all work should be conducted using parison extrusion systems and molds that accurately simulate the

Table 5.3. B/F/S Container Particulates

USP Particulates (per container)	Acceptance Criteria	Run #1	Run #2	Run #3
> 10 μm	6,000	11	7	23
> 25 μm	600	1	0	1

performance of b/f/s production equipment. These research and development systems have provided the necessary data for a smooth transition and scale-up to production equipment.

PACKAGING DESIGN

A variety of creative container shapes, sizes, and dispensing system designs are possible with the b/f/s process. For example, the use of an extended tab at the base of the ampoule provides Genentech's product with additional surface area for labeling in multiple languages. Containers can be embossed with the product name, the lot number, and the expiration date (see Figure 5.5). Containers may be produced and packaged in multiple attached units or offered in single units depending on the dosing regimen. For example, a daily dosage requirement may be offered as a 7-day supply, whereby a card of 7 attached ampoules may be supplied. Considerations for medical insurance reimbursement may dictate the packaging of a

Figure 5.5. B/F/S 6-ampoule card.

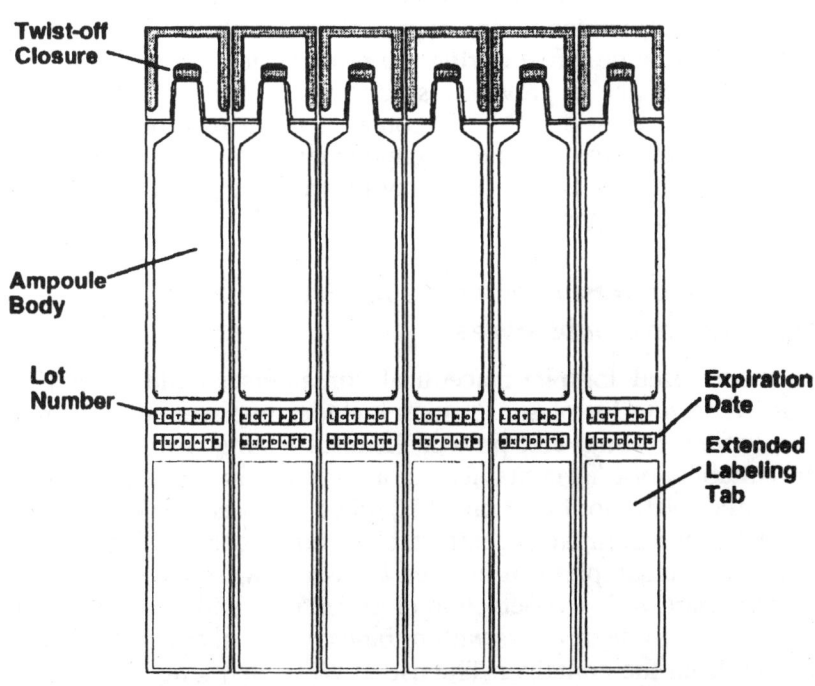

30-day supply, whereby 5 cards of 6 attached ampoules may be packaged in a carton. Many closure designs are available, including a Luer-lock design for single-use parenterals, elastomeric closures for multiuse parenterals, and a multitude of closures to meet pharmaceutical dispensing needs.

The use of a heat-sealable laminated foil pouch is a convenient method for packaging and protecting the ampoule. Pouching equipment may be installed in-line with the b/f/s machine or located in a separate facility. A horizontal pouching system works well in-line. If necessary, b/f/s containers may be packaged in pouches with an inert gas. Packages purged with helium have been used for automating leak detection of pouches using a helium leak detector.

Resin

The choice of resin for the container is a primary concern, since it contacts the product. Low density polyethylene is a popular resin due to its low level of extractables, its low permeability, and its excellent extrusion molding properties. Polypropylene resin is commonly used for applications that require terminal sterilization due to its higher melt index and density that make it more suitable for steam sterilization conditions. If possible, more than one resin supplier should be qualified during the product development and stability study phase to provide a second resin source. Clarity of the resin is also a consideration for containers that require particulate inspection. The use of random copolymer polyethylene resins, as opposed to linear LDPE resins, may provide the best transparency for inspection purposes.

Evaluation of Resin Containers for Extractable and Leachable Substances

All resins used for pharmaceutical containers should meet USP Class VI testing for plastics, which includes implantation into rabbits, extract testing, and physicochemical testing. To demonstrate the suitabilty of b/f/s containers for a given product, placebo (excipients) and Water for Injection (WFI)–filled samples may be tested to evaluate the potential for extractables and leachables. The use of placebo-filled samples can be used for assays where active product may interfere with the detection of extractives, and to determine if the active ingredient reacts with or binds potential chemical species derived from the container. The use of WFI–filled samples provides a control and enables a preliminary evaluation to determine if the formulation is reacting with the container. Studies may also compare product filled in glass vials as a control. The product-container compatibility evaluation should include a range of analytical techniques suitable to detect a broad spectrum of soluble and volatile organic and inorganic species. For Pulmozyme®, these methods included total organic carbon (TOC) analysis to measure organic extractables in placebo, thin-layer chromatography to measure organic extractables in active and placebo, ultraviolet spectrophotometry to detect the presence of UV-absorbing extractables, ion-exchange chromatography to determine anion and cation composition, and headspace gas chromatography to determine volatile organic compounds.

Long-term and accelerated stability studies should also be performed to determine the compatibility of the product in the containers for its shelf life. In addition, studies should be performed to determine if there is any significant adsorption of product to the surface of plastic containers. The studies may include storage of product in resin beads and in plastic containers, for example, at the maximum temperatures the product will be subjected to during initial filling into the newly formed container, and at normal storage conditions for extended time periods.

If the b/f/s plastic container is intended to be sealed in a heat-sealable laminated foil pouch, then the product should be evaluated in the final packaged form. Since many foil pouch structures utilize inorganic solvents, such as methyl-ethyl-ketone and ethyl acetate in adhesives used to laminate the LDPE heat sealable layer to the foil, the foil pouch should be evaluated for potential migration of volatile inorganic solvents that may permeate the plastic container.

Product Stability

Compatibility of the product with its container may be determined by monitoring the stability of the product after storage in the container for extended periods of time and at specified storage temperatures and relative humidity conditions. Important stability indicating parameters for protein products to evaluate their stability before and after storage may include determining the pH of the product, evaluating the color and clarity of the solution, and measuring the concentration of the protein by UV spectroscopy and/or enzyme-linked immunosorbent assays to determine if there is container vapor transmission. Other assays to consider include measurement of the bioactivity of the protein, determination of the presence of fragments and protein aggregates by various gel chromatography methods, and determination of the percent deamidation of the product by tryptic mapping. Studies have demonstrated that packaging nonbuffered protein products in LDPE containers can result in product with equivalent, and perhaps, improved stability compared to product stored in Type I borosilicate glass vials. For example, Figure 5.6 shows the pH stability of rhDNase when stored in ampoules manufactured from two sources of LDPE plastic (Dupont 20® and Escorene®) and Type I glass vials. Initially, the pH of the protein solution was slightly higher in the glass vials than in the plastic ampoules and increased slightly with time and temperature. These variations in pH may be caused by the extraction of silicates or other ions, such as sodium, from the glass surface by the unbuffered solution. Packaging the product in the b/f/s container eliminated this problem since ions are not expected to be a major contaminant of LDPE resins (Shire 1991).

PRODUCT TEMPERATURE

During the process development and scale-up phases, the temperature of the product immediately after filling was investigated, since subjecting the protein product to potentially high temperatures

Figure 5.6. pH stability of Pulmozyme® in glass vials versus LDPE ampoule.

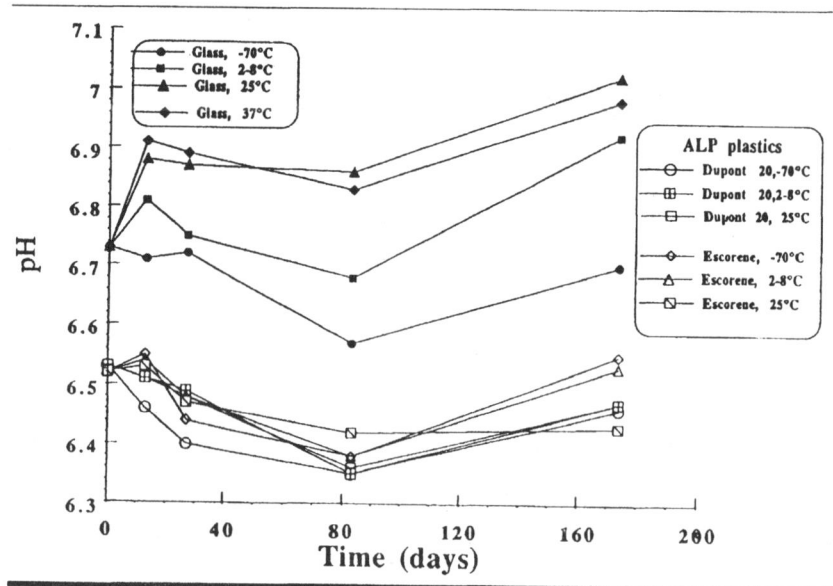

could affect its stability. A temperature survey was performed on a fill system configured for the manufacture of 3 mL ampoules using a 12-cavity mold on an ALP 624 B/F/S Machine. Product held in a jacketed feed tank was maintained at 5.9°C with recirculating glycol. The product temperature measured at the fill nozzles was 19.8°C. The temperature of the product in filled ampoules immediately after sealing averaged 27.2°C, a 7.4°C rise in product temperature. Factors that were identified that could potentially affect the temperature of the filled containers included the product feed temperature; the chilled water temperature supplied to the molds; the time for cooling the containers prior to filling, which was fixed by the cycle time; and the parison extruder temperature, which was set at 174°C. The product temperature was found to have the most affect on the product after filling. The highest product temperature after filling (32.9°C) was achieved with the product at 24.9°C at the fill nozzles (achieved by letting the product sit for several hours) and with the chilled water supply temperature for the molds elevated to 31.9°C (achieved by running chilled water through a heat exchanger). These elevated temperature conditions for product and chilled water accounted for an 8°C rise in product temperature between before and after filling. These test results indicated that the temperatures to which the product is subjected during the b/f/s process are controllable and were well within tolerable temperature parameters for the protein product.

To monitor product temperature control at 2–8°C for a sensitive protein product, the bulk feed tank was provided with a recorder and an alarm to monitor the temperature at its thermowell. As an added precaution and to provide control over the chilled water supply to the molds, a high temperature alarm limit was provided at 29.4°C (85°F) that automatically shuts down b/f/s production in the event of a chilled water temperature excursion.

OPERATIONAL QUALIFICATION

Operational parameters given in Table 5.4 show acceptance criteria and data for 3 operational qualification test runs for the manufacture of 3 mL LDPE ampoules using a 24-cavity mold for Pulmozyme®. The b/f/s filling system is based on time and pressure. Each fill nozzle has a sanitary silicone diaphragm valve that is controllable to one-hundredth of a second. Studies have demonstrated better than 2 percent accuracy for a fill target specification of 2.6 ± 0.1 g.

Table 5.4. Operational Qualification Data

	Acceptance Criteria	Run #1	Run #2	Run #3
Fill Accuracy				
Minimum (g)	2.50 g	2.53	2.55	2.56
Maximum (g)	2.70 g	2.66	2.64	2.65
Mean (g)		2.60	2.59	2.61
Standard deviation		0.02	0.02	0.02
Mean + 3 SDs	≤ 2.70 g	2.66	2.65	2.67
Mean − 3 SDs	≥ 2.50 g	2.54	2.53	2.55
Wall Thickness				
Minimum (mm)	0.45 mm	0.51	0.52	0.51
Maximum (mm)	0.67 mm	0.61	0.59	0.59
Twist Off				
Maximum (lb)	7 lb	2.4	3.0	3.6
Ampoule Integrity	No leaks	Pass	Pass	Pass

Wall thickness for the ampoule is measured and controlled by adjusting the parison thickness. Wall thickness can be maintained within 10 percent of target. The maximum twist-off force for an ampoule may be specified, with a twist-off break-seal to assure that excessive force is not required to open the ampoule.

Ampoule integrity was measured during validation studies by subjecting randomly selected samples of ampoules to the USP dye leak test. For plastic ampoules, unlike glass ampoules, the test is destructive since the dye penetrates the plastic and cannot be washed off. Therefore, 100 percent in-process testing of plastic ampoules by the USP dye leak test is not possible.

DEFECTS

According to a b/f/s production survey for Pulmozyme®, which reviewed 40 fills that produced 9.2 million ampoules, efficiency of production was better than 99 percent. A survey of manually inspected defects was conducted for the production of a 3 mL LDPE

ampoule with a twist-off closure and extended tab produced on an
ALP Model 624 B/F/S Machine with a 12-cavity mold. The survey indicated that approximately 0.9 percent were rejected due to low fill
volume or various ampoule defects. Approximately 66.8 percent of
these rejects, or 0.62 percent of total production, were attributed to
low fill level, which occurred routinely during priming of the fill system at the start of the fill, and at the end of the fill when the bulk
feed tank was empty. Container defects accounted for 0.38 percent of
the total production. In the order of frequency of occurrence, defects
included malformation of the extended labeling tab (0.11 percent),
machine rejects or machine material handling defects (0.08 percent),
product in the twist-off closure area (0.03 percent), occlusion of the
ampoule opening (0.02 percent), warpage (0.017 percent), illegible
embossed print (0.01 percent), leaks (0.0003 percent), and miscella-
neous defects (0.026 percent). The level of defects for this particular
survey are small and comparable to the level of defects for final product inspection of liquid-filled, stoppered-glass vials.

CLEANING

A typical cleaning routine begins after completion of a fill when the
fill system is rinsed in situ with WFI. After rinsing, the filling assembly, valves, and filter housings are removed and disassembled for
cleaning using an ultrasonic washer. Fixed stainless steel product
transfer piping is flushed with detergent and rinsed using a pressure
vessel. The parts are rinsed, reassembled, and then subjected to a
clean-in-place (CIP) final rinse using WFI until the conductivity of
the effluent is below a validated value.

Cleaning qualification was performed by flushing the system
with product, allowing the product to sit in the fill system for
24 hours, and then performing the cleaning routine as described.
For a soluble aqueous protein product, a sample of the effluent rinse
water will be tested for conductivity, specific protein, total protein,
endotoxin, detergent ion, and TOC. A sample of prerinse water may
be taken to provide a negative control, which demonstrates the ability of the procedure to recover protein and detergent residuals.
Swabbing studies utilizing TOC may also be performed to detect
residual protein on product contacting surfaces.

STEAM–IN–PLACE

A schematic of the typical piping configuration of a b/f/s fill system,
showing the locations of thermocouples and biological indicators

for steam sterilization validation, is illustrated in Figure 5.7. Steam-in-place (SIP) occurs within a validated time period after completion of CIP. A steam cup is attached to the fill nozzle assembly to direct steam around the outside surfaces of the nozzles and to collect condensate. Temperatures are monitored and recorded using fixed thermocouples, while an automatic cycle provides steam above 121°C for at least 30 minutes. Sterile air is supplied immediately after sterilization for drying and cooling. For systems that require parison ballooning air and blowing air, appropriate piping and filter pathways are also sterilized-in-place. Validation of SIP is performed using *Bacillus stearothermophilus* biological indicators, and additional thermocouples are inserted into the product piping for temperature monitoring. The steam cup remains in place until the start of the b/f/s operation to protect the fill nozzles, and, to ensure sterility, the blowers for the HEPA filters remain on during the sterilization process.

Figure 5.7. Steam-in-place configuration.

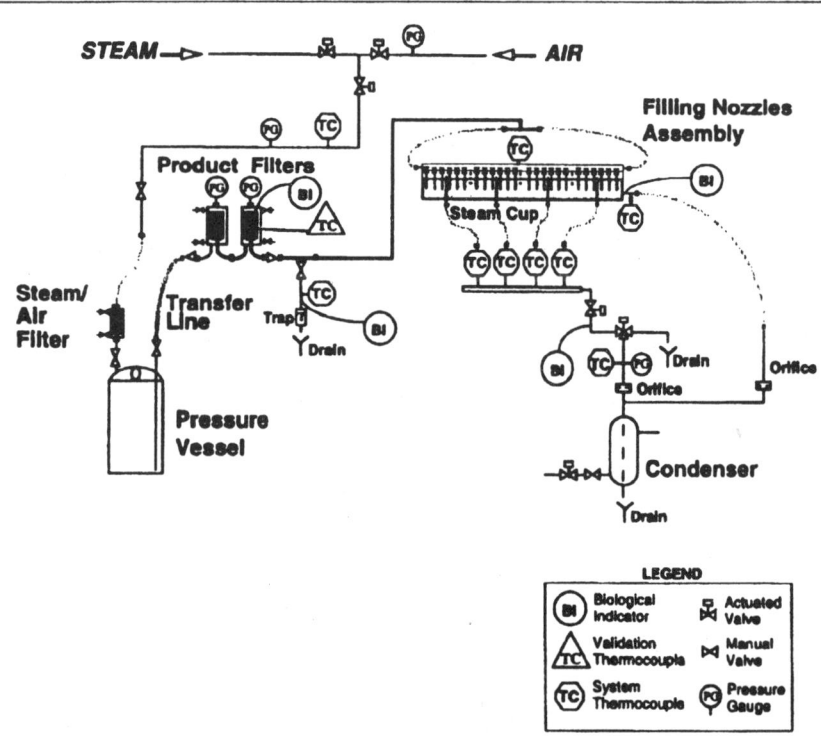

MEDIA FILLS

In total, to this date, Genentech has filled over 100,000 media-filled containers without growth positives, including media fills on a 5-cavity ALP Model 304 B/F/S machine without a HEPA–filtered air shroud, as well as media fills using 12-cavity and 24-cavity fill systems on ALP's Model 624 B/F/S machines.

Excellent media fill results have been reported by many users of b/f/s equipment under conditions that are beyond expected operating parameters. For example, Svarnstrom et al. (1992) reported for Astra Pharmaceuticals at the PDA International Congress in Basel that media fills have been performed where the system had been left filled with media overnight, and over the weekend, and then filling of media was resumed. There were no incidences of growth in these media fill studies. At ALP media fills have been routinely performed after one full week of continuous production with no growth positives.

Most recently, media fill challenges were performed at Waverly Pharmaceutical/Steripack Ltd. (Runcorn, UK) (Jones et al. 1995). The study set out to demonstrate "real-life" worst-case issues for a b/f/s machine capable of producing 3000 × 20 mL units per hour. No growth positives resulted over a 3-day media fill study involving a series of 7 fills, referred to as phases, producing approximately 44,000 units testing severe stresses to the system, including the following for day 1:

- Phase 1: running a 6000-unit media fill under normal production conditions.

- Phase 2: opening both clean room and change room doors while filling 6000 units.

- Phase 3: filling 6000 units with both clean room and change room doors open, and without clean room filtered air supply.

The machine was then cleaned and sterilized and prepared for the next day. Day 2 involved a more stressful scenario, including the following:

- Phase 4: filling 6000 units with 5–12 ungowned personnel in the b/f/s room; performing in-process controls in the room that are normally performed outside; performing inspection and packaging inside the b/f/s room; personnel performing environmental tests ungowned; and untrained personnel in the room walking, talking, sneezing, removing and putting back on factory coats, combing hair–all performed on a floor that was mopped with high bioburden water 48 hours prior to the study.

- Phase 5: 6000 units were filled under the condition of the previous study except with the air handling system turned off to the b/f/s room.

At the end of the study, the system was left filled with media overnight, without cleaning and sterilization. On day 3 phase 6 was performed with the system started without normal preparation, doors were left open, air supply to the room was off, and ungowned persons were allowed in the room, the air shower was turned off for 1 hour, and then turned on again. At the end of phase 6, normal cleaning and disinfection procedures were not carried out; however, the fill system was sterilized in preparation for phase 7, which was performed to examine the effect of the environmental conditions on production contamination during a routine machine start-up.

Simulated Interventions

Simulated interventions should be performed during media fills in order to qualify responses to routine and nonroutine physical states of the filling machine or manufacturing environment during production runs. For example, in one Genentech study, three 3000-unit media fills were performed in succession after completing a 65-hour production run. The first media fill tested the impact of opening the Class 100 aseptic enclosure door prior to starting the media fill, taking a Rodac sample, and wiping the bottom of the enclosure area with alcohol. Normally, the aseptic enclosure door is not opened after SIP has been performed. The second media fill tested the impact of intervention close to the fill nozzles, whereby the operator touched the fill nozzles with sanitized forceps prior to starting the media fill. The third successive media fill tested the impact of a 15-minute power outage for the blowers to the filling system HEPA filters prior to starting the media fill. No positive samples resulted during these media fill studies.

Intervention studies performed by Sinclair and Tallentire (1993) from the University of Manchester (Manchester, England) investigated the effects of a 5-minute and a 15-minute shutdown of the blowers to the HEPA–filtered air shower on ampoule contamination levels during airborne microbial studies. An ALP 624 B/F/S Machine was used for the study, with a 24-cavity fill system set up for filling

2 mL of tryptic soy broth in 3 mL ampoules. The study was performed with an airborne spore concentration of approximately 3×10^6 spores/m^{-3} in the fill room. The 5-minute HEPA filter shutdown indicated that when the HEPA air shower was turned off, the level of microbial contamination increased from 0.022 to 0.28 fraction of ampoules contaminated (a 13-fold increase above the mean fraction prior to intervention). For the 15-minute HEPA filter shutdown, the fraction of ampoules contaminated increased to 0.48 (a 22-fold increase). Upon restarting the blowers to the HEPA filters, the system microbial contamination levels fell and recovered to levels prior to the intervention within 5 b/f/s machine cycles or within 1 minute of processing time. During the airborne microbial studies, a control study was performed, whereby no airborne challenge was presented to the system to ensure that the machine was operating optimally and at baseline. After running repetitive airborne microbial challenge studies and obtaining data, follow-up runs without an airborne microbial challenge were performed. After contaminating the machine, the system always returned to baseline (i.e., zero positives) during these control runs.

A classification of interventions may be useful, using categories such as critical, major, and minor, based on the impact on product quality. Such a classification provides a basis for an action plan for various interventions. The concept may be applicable to b/f/s operations as well as to any sterile filling operation. An example classification program for media fill testing may include the following:

- Critical Interventions

  Critical interventions result in the termination of the fill. Critical interventions include the following:

  - Breach of product path downstream of the sterilizing filters

  - Loss of positive pressure differentials for both the nozzle shroud and the fill room for

    - Any length of time if personnel are present in the fill room

    - Greater than 15 minutes if no personnel are present in the fill room

  - Contamination of the product path from intrusion of a foreign substance

- Major Interventions

  Major interventions require manufacturing and quality control personnel to evaluate the impact on product quality, to take appropriate action to determine whether on not to continue the fill and to file an incident report. Major interventions include the following:

  - If the shroud is opened prior to the fill

  - Loss of positive pressure differential from the shroud to the fill room for less than 15 minutes if no personnel are present in the fill room (i.e., during a power loss)

  - Loss of positive pressure differential from the fill room to surrounding environments for greater than 15 minutes

  - Mechanical malfunctions occurring with the fill block assembly that necessitates contact with the fill nozzles or product path

  - Machine malfunctions that result in a change to the system as validated

  - Power losses

- Minor Interventions

  Minor interventions require manufacturing and quality control personnel to evaluate the impact on product quality and to take appropriate actions. No incident report is required. Minor interventions include the following:

  - Breach of product supply line upstream of sterilizing filters

  - Nonroutine mechanical manipulation outside the shroud in close proximity to the fill nozzles

  - Loss of HEPA–filtered air supply, which causes a zero or negative fill room pressure for less than 15 minutes

  - Spillage of material located outside the product path or nozzle shroud

- Downtime

  If intervention results in downtime, procedures that might be deemed appropriate after the downtime and prior to resuming a fill include the following:

- Additional environmental testing
- Additional room or machine surface cleaning/ disinfection
- HEPA–filtered air purge of aseptic enclosure and/or fill room for 30 minutes
- Rejection of the first 20 filled cards
- Additional product sampling for quality control testing

CONCLUSIONS

B/f/s technology has proven to be a good alternative to rubber-stoppered glass vials for the sterile packaging and filling of Pulmozyme®. The experiences reported here for this biotechnology product have shown that the b/f/s process can provide an excellent sterility assurance record and a high quality product. These experiences have been confirmed by many b/f/s users and by airborne microbial studies. Standard environmental monitoring techniques, used in traditional aseptic pharmaceutical manufacturing, have been successfully applied to the b/f/s process. The system's HEPA filter shower and reliable automation minimizes personnel contact with the product, reducing the possibility of contamination. The equipment design allows a high level of control over the process, allowing production of high quality sterile products with a low incidence of container defects (as observed for ampoule production). System controls and sterilization, cleaning, and filling operations can be validated according to traditional aseptic pharmaceutical manufacturing test methods and acceptance criteria. Simulated intervention studies during media fills have demonstrated the robustness of the system in its ability to protect the product from contamination during these challenges. The process is economical when compared to glass vial production, and the productivity of the system is high since it can be run continuously for several days. As pharmaceutical manufacturers, the biotechnology industry, and regulatory agencies become more familiar with the advantages of b/f/s technology, more sterile-packaging applications are likely to follow.

ACKNOWLEDGMENTS

The authors would like to especially acknowledge the work of those involved in the qualification of Pulmozyme®, including Jack Regan and Al Infusino from the Genentech Pharmaceutical Manufacturing Group, Steve Shire and the Pharmaceutical Research and Development Group, Dilip Parikh and Peter Rauenbuehler from the Quality Control Group, Art Blum from the Regulatory Group, and Joe Barta and Robert Baird from the Validation Group.

REFERENCES

Borchert, S. J., M. M. Ryan, and R. L. Davison. 1989. Accelerated extractable studies of borosilicate glass containers. *J. Parent. Sci. Technol.* 43 (2):67–79.

Bradley, A., S. P. Probert, C. S. Sinclair, and A. Tallentire. 1991. Airborne microbial challenges of b/f/s equipment: A case study. *J. Parent. Sci. Technol.* 45 (4):187–192.

Forrester-Coles, S. 1995. Comments on the annex of the manufacture of sterile medicinal products. Blow-Fill-Seal Operators Association.

Jones, J. J., P. Topping, and J. Sharp. 1995. Environmental microbial challenges to an aseptic blow-fill-seal process: A practical study. *J. Parent. Sci. Technol.* 49 (5):226–234.

Leo, F. 1989. B/f/s aseptic packaging technology. In *Aseptic pharmaceutical manufacturing for the 1990s,* edited by M. J. Groves and W. P. Olson. Buffalo Grove: Interpharm Press, Inc.

Sharp, J. R. 1987. Manufacture of sterile pharmaceutical products using "blow-fill-seal" technology. *Pharm J.* 239:106–108.

Sharp, J. R. 1988. Validation of a new form-fill-seal installation. *Manufact. Chem.* (Feb.):22–27, 55.

Shire, S. J. 1991. *Stability of rhDNase in plastic vials manufactured by the ALP system.* Pharmaceutical R&D Technical Report. Genentech, Inc.

Sinclair, C. S., and A. Tallentire. 1993. Predictive sterility assurance for aseptic processing. In *Sterilization of medical products.* vol VI, edited by R. F. Morrissey. Montreal: Polyscience Publication.

Svarnstrom, A. C., A. L. Ernerot, and K. Mattson. 1992. Form-fill-seal: Experience with the aseptic and terminal sterilization of SVPs. *Proceedings of the International Congress: Advanced Technologies for Manufacturing of Aseptic and Terminally Sterilized Pharmaceuticals and Biopharmaceuticals,* 17–19 February, in Basel, Switzerland.

6

MULTIPRODUCT FACILITY DESIGN: AN INTEGRATED APPROACH

Timothy Gerard Hughes

Hughes Associates

As pharmaceutical biotechnology becomes a mature manufacturing industry, several features are apparent. Most start-up organizations are pursuing several potential products simultaneously; successful biotechnology companies continue to investigate and introduce new products by building on their technology base, while many established pharmaceutical organizations are building portfolios in specific product areas by acquiring the rights or technology of potential products. In spite of all this investment in technology, however, few investigational products have progressed through clinical trials to become approved products. As a consequence, companies of all sizes increasingly are reluctant to risk large sums of capital for the construction of facilities for single, unproven products.

The current trend is, therefore, toward limiting financial exposure by the construction or use of facilities suitable for the manufacture of several products—the multiproduct facility. Several factors have added impetus and acceptability to the concept of multiprocessing, namely:

- Many potential new products are likely to have small, highly specific markets, and may not justify investment in a dedicated manufacturing facility.

- Compensation levels for therapeutics and related products are under scrutiny worldwide, spurring the search for a reduction of overall cost, of which the facility is a large component.

- New manufacturing technologies, improved equipment design, and high quality starting materials have greatly improved manufacturers' confidence in the reliability of their processes. This has allowed manufacturers to consider simultaneous manufacture of different products.

- Advances in analytical techniques have given manufacturers new tools for characterizing in-process steps, testing product quality, and determining and identifying contaminants and impurities in products and raw materials. This gives added confidence for attempting multiproduct processing.

As evidence to the increasing interest in multiproduct processing, substantial investment is being made in the construction of contract manufacturing facilities for all stages of product development (*Fifteen prime* . . . 1995), and national bodies from both industry and regulatory agencies currently are engaged in dialogue to develop guidelines for multiproduct facility design. The Pharmaceutical Manufacturers' Association (PMA) has issued a position paper (Bader et al. 1992) on multiproduct manufacturing facilities for biologicals, with the intention of initiating collaboration between industry and the Food and Drug Administration (FDA).

Any guidelines on multiproduct processing will be as applicable to the manufacture of products for human clinical trials as for approved final products; in fact, multiproduct processing probably will be more commonly encountered in the clinical manufacturing setting, where several candidate products are likely to be under development simultaneously.

A manufacturer's intention should be to build a properly designed facility accommodating equipment, processing, and staff interactions to guarantee the purest possible products consistently. Thus, facility design is an effort involving input from all functional areas of a plant, and should not be undertaken without considering and integrating all issues related to the plant's use. This chapter is intended to describe a process of the evolution of a multiproduct facility design through an integrated approach; it is not simply a description of the desirable architectural and mechanical features of a multiproduct facility.

MULTIPRODUCT PROCESSING DEFINITIONS

"Products" in the context used in this chapter may be batches of the same material or of entirely different materials. Stated simply, multiproduct processing arises when two or more products are handled in the same manufacturing space, either simultaneously or sequentially. More specifically, four main manufacturing situations are recognized when the term *multiproduct processing* applies (Hill and Beatrice 1989).

- *Same product processing:* The production of a single product in multiple lots at the same stage or different stages of manufacture in a common area. This situation would arise, for example, during simultaneous processing of subbatches of product in column steps in a purification suite.

- *Different products/same stage:* Applies to the preparation of multiple products at similar stages of manufacture in a common area. Possible scenarios include the simultaneous biosynthesis of different products in a multitrain fermentation room or the purification of several products in a suite of purification rooms.

- *Processing of infectious and noninfectious products:* Applies when a common area is used for the handling of potentially infectious and noninfectious materials. An example of this would arise in a cell culture, product purification suite where previral inactivation and postviral inactivation steps take place in the same room or equipment.

- *Campaign manufacture:* The sequential manufacture of different products in a facility. Campaign manufacture could occur at any point in a production process where common facilities and equipment are reused for multiple products, and includes, for example, filling and freeze-drying operations.

It is important for facility designers to realize that multiproduct processing under these definitions can occur at any stage of manufacture, from the preparation of fermenter seed inocula to product finishing in a packaging hall. While the risks may differ, the processing concerns apply equally at all stages.

PRINCIPAL CONCERNS OF MULTIPRODUCT PROCESSING

The principal regulatory concerns of multiproduct processing, which require special design consideration, are all related to the interaction of staff, equipment, facilities, and processes with products. The concerns fall into five main categories.

Operations Congestion

Multiple, simultaneous processes can lead to congested workspaces and confused operations, increasing the likelihood of process errors, such as loading the wrong product on a column or mixing cleaned and dirty equipment in a crowded equipment staging area. Routine quality control samples can be missed, or worse, mixed up, resulting in a compromised process or product analysis. Congestion in an analytical laboratory due to a large number of uncontrolled samples can lead to equally serious mix-ups in analysis.

Process Equipment Contamination

Reused equipment is a potential source of residues of previous products, or wash solutions which may carry over contaminants to the next use of the equipment. Cleaning cycles may vary from product to product, depending on the nature of the soiling. For example, equipment containing a solution of highly soluble salts may require only a water rinse, whereas a tank holding a protein-containing solution may require a multistep cleaning process. Control of the use of equipment and the monitoring of cleaning processes in multiproduct facilities is, therefore, essential to reducing the risk.

Airborne Contamination

Crowded and busy manufacturing facilities are difficult environments to keep clean and under control. Elevated airborne bioburden is a common result of high levels of staff activity. A dual risk may result from operations that generate aerosols: they have the potential of contaminating products, equipment, and premises; the operation may itself be prone to airborne contamination. Examples of aerosol-generating steps include equipment cleaning, column packing, dispensing raw material powders, and product sampling techniques.

Open Processing

"Open" processing is defined as a step exposed to contamination of and by the immediate environment. Some of the most critical steps in bioprocessing, such as seed bank and seed culture manipulations, collecting and pooling column eluate fractions, product final filling and lyophilization, are commonly open steps, prone to contamination by airborne routes.

Staff Activities

Staff play a key role in the success of complex processing situations; they are possibly the single, most important element in a successful multiproduct operation. Designs should take into account the interaction of process, materials, and staff. Training in process technology, current Good Manufacturing Practices (cGMP), recordkeeping, reporting, and process monitoring are key to a successful operation.

CONTRAINDICATIONS FOR MULTIPRODUCT FACILITIES

In the author's opinion, there are limits to situations in which multiproduct processing can be applied. As a basic rule, multiproduct facilities should be limited to a single technology. The following mix of technologies should not be considered for multiproduct processing.

Materials Produced by Different Biosynthetic Systems

Production by prokaryotic and eukaryotic fermentation should not be considered in the same fermenters, because the potential contaminants in these systems are so dissimilar that the downstream processes may not be capable of removing them. The process changeover requirements and respective product safety issues for these early stages of manufacture present risks too great to deal with. For example, cell cultures have the potential for containing viruses, but a bacterial product process does not have specific virus removal steps built into the purification procedure to cater for this risk.

Organic Chemical and Biosynthetic Processes

A processing area intended for organic synthesis (e.g., liposome manufacture) will not have compatible design features for it to be used simultaneously or sequentially for biosynthetic operations, without extensive compromise of one or both processes. In addition, neither process will have the specific capability of removing potential cross-contaminants from the other process. Operational staff will also have different experience backgrounds, which may not suit them for both types of operations, an important GMP consideration.

Unique Technologies

In any facility in which multiproduct processing is contemplated, all stages of processing should be carefully assessed for their potential to affect or be affected by other processes. For example, a monoclonal antibody may be produced for several uses—as a potential therapeutic, an in vivo diagnostic, or an in vitro diagnostic. Following biosynthesis, antibody destined for different final products may follow different processing steps. Careful design would be needed to ensure that the different cGMP compliance requirements of the therapeutic and diagnostic products do not compromise each other. Radiolabeling, fluorescent tagging, solvent extraction, and chemical coupling processes, for example, should invariably be dedicated processes, removing the potential for cross-contaminating other processes.

FDA AND INDUSTRY VIEWS ON MULTIPRODUCT PROCESSING

Both the FDA and industry have acknowledged the need for multiproduct facilities. The concerns elaborated above have been recognized by all parties in recent industry/regulatory forums, but there is optimism that satisfactory multiproduct facility design can be achieved, providing that adequate steps are taken in defining the risks and applying appropriate safeguards.

The regulatory consequences of the FDA rejecting an inadequate design can be severe. In an extreme case regulatory agencies may advise a manufacturer to stop all current work, condemn or quarantine all in-process and manufactured products, and order validated remedial actions to correct deficiencies, which would be subject to reinspection. If a facility was rejected during a product license filing, the consequences would be a forfeit of submission review fees, which may be as high as $100,000 for a Product License Application and $60,000 for an Establishment License Application. The FDA may also issue a Refusal to File notice, delaying the filing review and potential approval indefinitely.

INTEGRATED APPROACH TO CONCEPTUAL MULTIPRODUCT FACILITY DESIGN

Multiproduct facility operations present highly complex design problems, combining product and interproduct compatibility and safety issues, process design decisions, validation requirements, operational planning, staff management issues, provision for validated and controlled product changeover, and the application of regulatory guidelines and of cGMP.

It is standard practice to start facility designs with architectural programming (Odum 1994). While this is definitely an essential step, there is a high potential for wasted effort if expensive drafting and detail designers are contracted too early in the design phase, prior to full internal agreement on the facility design need. Overruns in design time and costs can become so severe that deadlines may eventually be set based on cost and time only, which often results in compromised designs. Even worse, the design compromises may lead to costly rework after construction, and consequent delays to operations.

The ability to influence the cost and schedule of a major construction project is greatest at the initial stages. As time and resources are consumed, this influence diminishes. Manufacturers are advised to avoid the temptation to employ architects and designers too early in the conceptual phase to draft scaled building plans embodying what is believed to be the scope of the design. Even with the best intentions, these plans are normally reworked many times as different reviewers add unique perspectives, which involves the customer in time and cost consequences. Thus, manufacturers are well advised to spend as long as necessary perfecting the design concept before committing expensive resources.

A facility design should not be undertaken without considering and integrating all issues related to its use. The following is suggested as an order of events in the facility design sequence to develop a fully integrated scope definition:

1. Gather information in-house to obtain an in-depth view of the facility requirements.

2. Write a comprehensive functional and operational description of the facility.

3. Prepare a conceptual design by the "affinity diagram" approach.

4. Review the conceptual design and make appropriate changes.

The above steps are expanded in the sections that follow.

Information Gathering

Appoint a suitably knowledgeable design team internally to solicit answers to specific questions from operational groups.

Corporate Development Plans

Building a multiproduct facility is a major corporate commitment, and as such, should form a major part of the corporate business plan. Since the lead times for the introduction of new products are long, it may be a waste of time and money building a multipurpose facility for investigational products. Expensive equipment and facilities may remain unused. Some of the factors to be considered prior to a commitment to build are as follows:

- How many products or potential products, and what volumes will be manufactured in this facility? This will aid in developing estimates of the size of the plant.

- What type of products are anticipated (diagnostic, therapeutic, preclinical, clinical, early market, or full commercial production)? This will help determine the design compliance requirements. Pilot and development facilities may not need as many features in compliance with cGMP as a plant for clinical and licensed products.

- Are any licensed biological products to be manufactured in the facility? If so, the design should include the scale at which commercial manufacturing is anticipated.

- What are the anticipated development and clinical investigation times for each product? This may assist in spreading capital expenditure by phasing the introduction of new plant or technology suites in the facility.

- How much in-house manufacturing is planned? Will products be produced from seed bank to final vial, or is some form of shared or contract manufacturing anticipated? In some instances, such as filling and lyophilization, it may be more expedient to use a contract manufacturer instead of building and staffing a final processing suite in-house.

- Will this be a new building or a renovated existing building? City architectural reviews may extend timelines on new construction, but cramming processes into an existing building can be difficult and lead to unsatisfactory compromises to process integrity through proximity to other operations.

Process Development Plan Considerations

The manufacturing processes involved will affect the facility design significantly. The following are important questions to answer in the preliminary stages:

- Which technologies are planned, and are these compatible with each other? This will help determine whether multiprocessing is feasible in the plant.

- Are the manufacturing technologies well defined? Rapidly changing technologies may require several facility and equipment changes, which may alter the compatibility of processes in the multiproduct context.

Product Quality Plan Considerations

The test laboratory needs must be included.

- Will in-process and final product testing be carried out in-house? This will help in sizing and specifying the laboratories.

- Are there animal testing requirements? To limit the chances of cross-contamination, consider contracting-out testing or locating the small animal hold or test facilities remote from the manufacturing facility.

Biosafety Issues

- Which organisms will be handled? Live viruses, spore-forming bacteria, and sensitizing organisms will probably require dedicated facilities.

- How well characterized is the cell substrate? Handling well-characterized host cells versus unknown substrate organisms could affect the facility design in the sense of the biocontainment required, and could affect the proximity of cell handling steps to other processes.

Functional and Operational Description

The functional and operational description is a team effort, involving representatives of the facility functional groups: Manufacturing, Quality Assurance, Quality Control, Regulatory Affairs, Validation, Engineering, Maintenance, and Support Services. All groups should collaborate in writing a comprehensive functional and operational description of the entire manufacturing operation.

Detailed process flow diagrams should be prepared to show the movement of products, equipment, raw materials, wastes, samples, and holding points. On an area-by-area basis, describe the process and all facilities, utilities, and equipment required, clearly stating the functions and scope of each space. Address the known regulatory and testing requirements for the processes.

Describe the plant's environmental requirements. Point out places that product or material flows intersect, the risks of open processes, and assess risks to and from the products and processes. This step leads to the identification of gowning needs, the development of operator dress codes and gowning policies, the need for biosafety and containment, and the treatment of hazardous materials.

This description should be fully comprehensive, since product quality depends as much on the immediate processing surroundings as on the support functions that monitor, test, and analyze the process and archive the results. Include all processing stages and the following support areas:

- Raw material storage
- Seed bank and seed preparation
- Main plant and process utility spaces
- Laboratory support functions
- Quality control laboratories
- Quality sample handling/storage
- Material and equipment staging areas

- Waste movement and treatment facilities
- Process automation and control rooms
- Data processing and archiving

Validation Planning

The selection of the validation effort to be applied to a bioprocessing plant can be a daunting task; however, an important element of the success of the validation program is that contingencies for validation are incorporated into the specifications and designs of equipment and facilities. Preparing a draft Validation Master Plan, which describes the validation requirements, in advance of the detailed design stage is a useful method of identifying these specifications.

Affinity Diagrams

Following the preparation of the functional and operational description and draft validation plans, add an experienced architectural designer to the team to assist in the preparation of affinity diagrams. These diagrams have more practical utility for developing and illustrating facility design concepts than the well-known architectural "bubble diagrams."

Preparation of Affinity Diagrams

Affinity diagrams are prepared in the following sequential steps:

1. Draft a basic process flow diagram (Figure 6.1).

2. Determine all of the spaces required for the manufacturing operation. Using a computer design/graphics program, construct circles with tags for all spaces, and arrange these circles adjacent to one another in relationships to the process flow. Draw connecting lines to show direct connections, avoiding any crossing over of these lines, as these signify crossed flows.

3. Continue to refine the affinity relationships, flows, the location of pass-through air locks or portals as required, and where similar spaces such as corridors and service rooms can be combined. Shapes can be adjusted to represent these common areas. Other symbols may be used to show access control points, connecting pipelines, and so on (Figure 6.2).

Figure 6.1. Affinity diagram: process flow development.

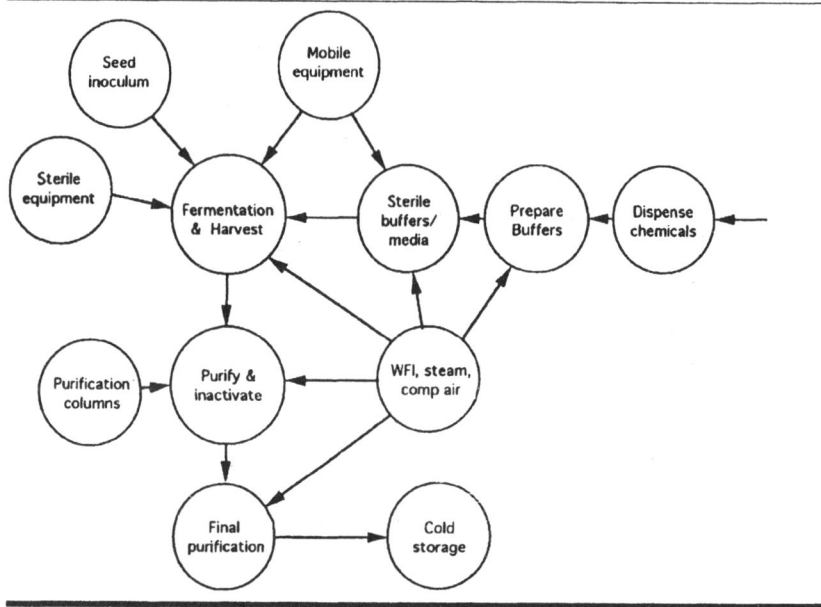

4. At this stage symbols, color shading, or patterns can be used
    to indicate areas containing related functions, different air
    quality classifications, and others with special requirements,
    such as biocontainment (Figures 6.3 and 6.4).

A series of overlays can be made to illustrate the fundamental
concepts of the affinity layout. The final family of affinity diagrams
should clearly show the movements of staff, raw materials, products,
equipment, process samples, services required, waste streams, and
how environmental and biosafety issues are addressed.

Advantages of the Affinity Diagram Approach

The affinity method provides the following advantages to the design
team:

*   Affinity diagrams present an easy method to follow the de-
    velopment and definition of the adjacency and affinity rela-
    tionship of all plant areas.

*   The concepts of flow of product, materials, staff, equipment,
    and wastes are clearly shown.

*   Environmental conditions, such as air quality, relative air
    pressures, and containment, can be readily assigned.

Figure 6.2. Affinity diagram: layout development.

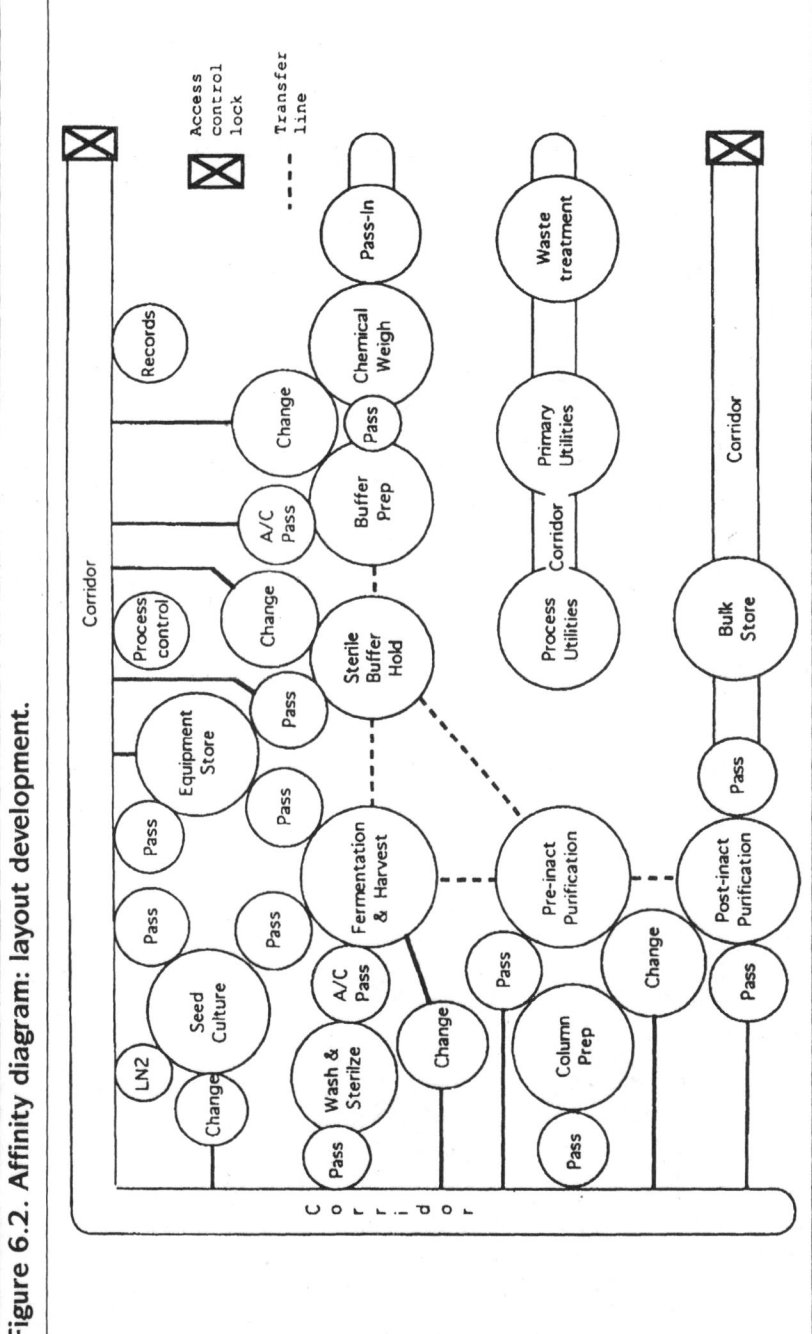

Figure 6.3. Affinity diagram: room air quality.

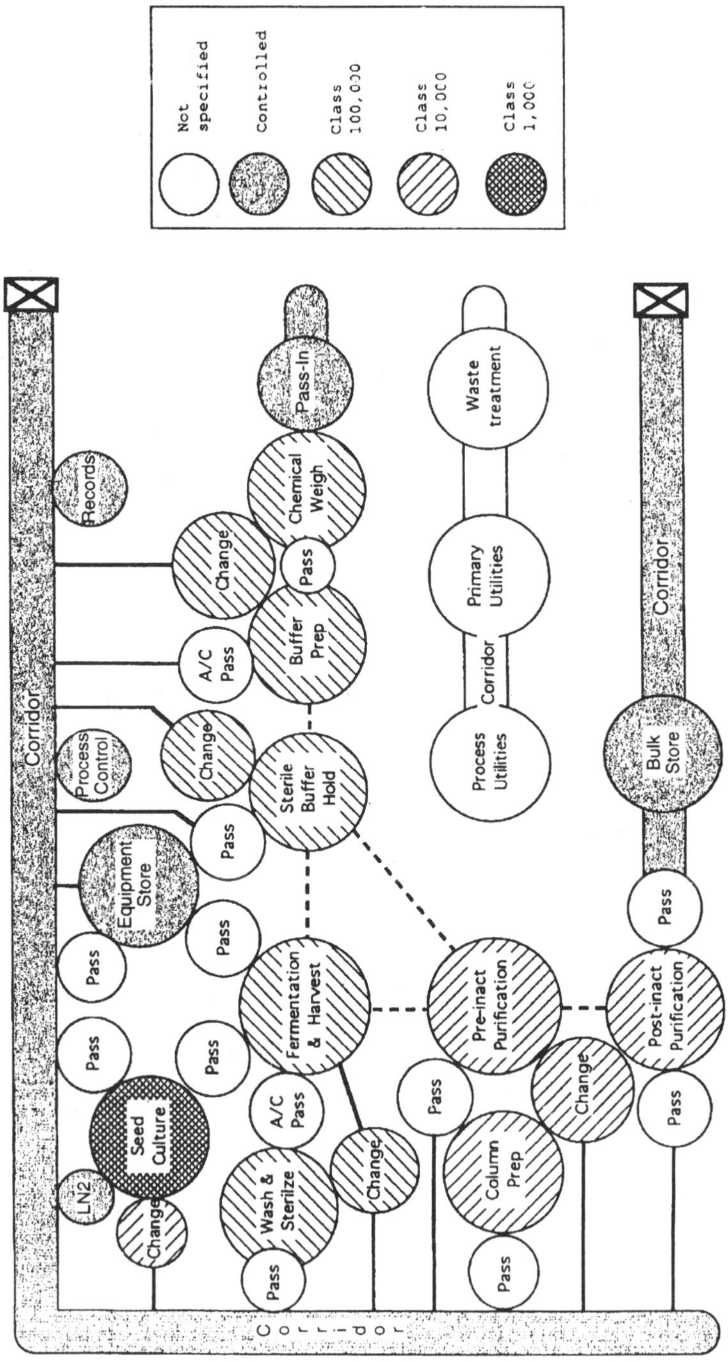

Figure 6.4. Affinity diagram: relative air pressures.

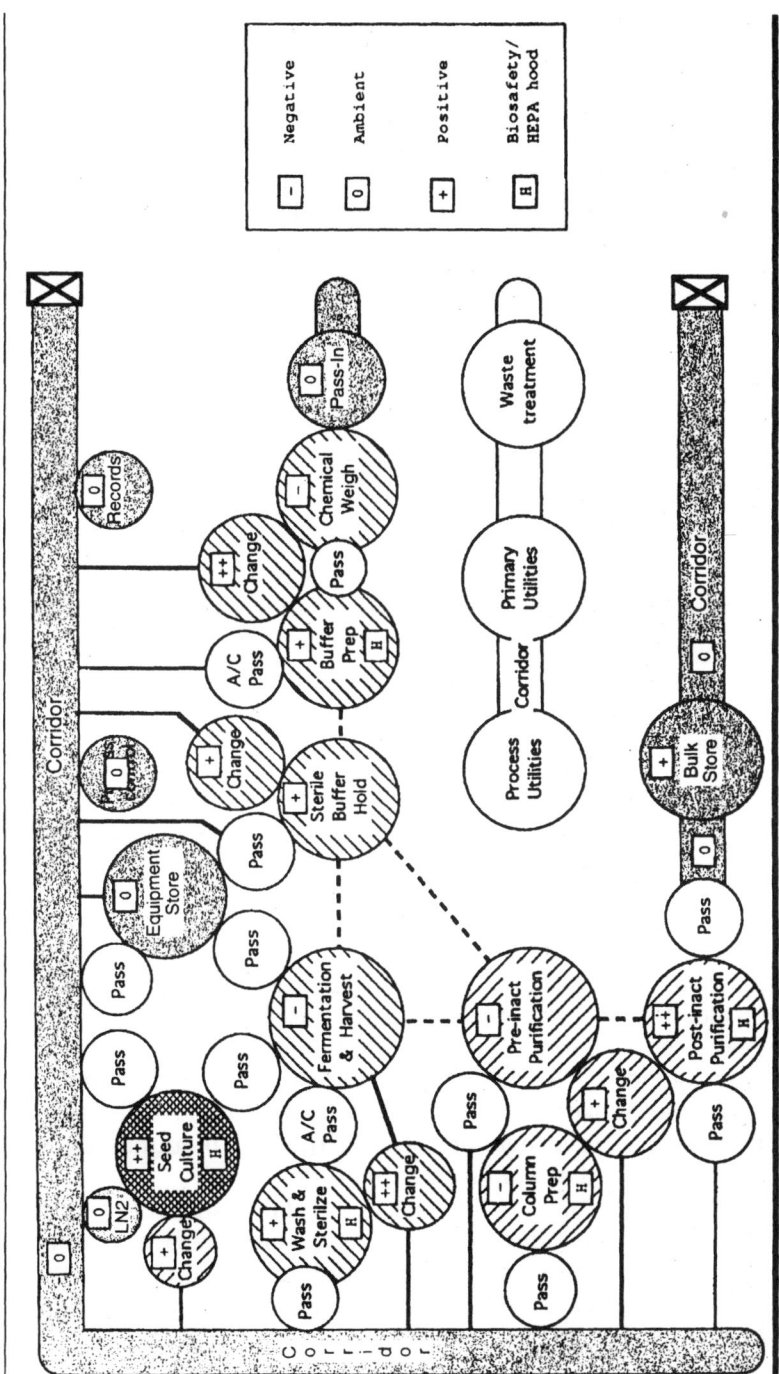

- The method imposes a discipline on all user groups to define major needs clearly at an early stage.

- The method allows quick changes to be made to concepts without incurring the significant costs that would be associated with redrafting scaled design drawings, with the side benefit of minimizing postconstruction changes due to design oversights.

- Affinity diagrams allow consultants and customers a common tool against which to check proposals and review completed work.

- Regulatory and validation specifications of the design, such as air quality and pressure, materials staging air locks, and clean/dirty corridor concepts, can be readily incorporated and reviewed.

- In instances such as a multistory building or mezzanine construction, affinity diagrams may be easier to understand and display than blueprints, since they can also be adapted to demonstrate design philosophies and intentions in three dimensions.

Predesign Scope Reviews

All participants should have the opportunity to review the functional descriptions and affinity diagrams in relation to the project goals, and comment prior to commitment to these goals. These documents serve the purpose of defining parts of the facility for more intensive design engineering and points at which more attention must be paid during validation and routine operations. Affinity diagrams are also useful as an internal reference and for use as a training aid. As a side benefit, experience has shown that these diagrams make useful presentation tools when making presentations to regulatory agencies. The documents can be used in preconstruction presentations, as part of the Chemistry Manufacturing Control (CMC) section of an Investigational New Drug (IND) submission, and as part of the Validation Master Plan descriptions.

Having established the adjacency relationships of process areas, affinity diagrams can be used to prepare architectural layouts incorporating cGMP features. These should be drafted to refine the functional, spatial, and adjacency relationships within the footprint of the facility. The next section describes the regulatory points for consideration in layout design.

REGULATORY REQUIREMENTS FOR MULTIPROCESS FACILITY DESIGN

Regulatory Design Guidelines

Manufacturers must be confident that their facility design and function are in compliance with regulatory specifications and will pass inspection, since there is the risk of the rejection of license applications through nonconformance. This implies that there is a set of regulatory standards and specifications of facility design with which manufacturers should comply. Unfortunately, there are no clear national or industry specifications on biotech facility design. There are generalities couched in the cGMP, some Codes of Federal Regulations (CFR) sections, and various FDA and National Institutes of Health (NIH) Guidelines that the manufacturer is free to interpret. However, at this time, these have not been formulated into a definitive, biotech, multiproduct facility design instrument. This is partly a recognition of the evolving nature of the industry, partly a result of historically different approaches by the separate drugs and biologics regulatory bodies, and partly an industry wish to refrain from institutional standards. Manufacturers obviously want to retain the right to keep up with the state of the art, while at the same time not rendering preexisting facilities obsolete!

The regulations for the preparation of biological products, 21 CFR 600–680 (*Biological Products* 1991) contain little information on facility design. The cGMP (1991) describes facility requirements for finished human and veterinary pharmaceuticals, but no specific reference is made to biologicals, although 21 CFR 210 states that the cGMPs are applicable to biologicals. 21 CFR 211.42 to 211.58 describe general facility requirements. In summary:

- Facilities must be adequately sized, constructed, and located for proper operation, cleaning, and maintenance.

- Process and personnel flows should be orderly to prevent mix-ups.

- There should be separate storage facilities for raw materials, components, process intermediates, and process samples.

- There should be separate processing areas for manufacturing, filling, finishing, and testing.

- General features of aseptic processing facilities, plant lighting, ventilation, plumbing, staff facilities, and maintenance are described.

The FDA *Guideline on Sterile Drug Products Produced by Aseptic Processing* (FDA 1987) should be applied to biotech processing where aseptic operations are anticipated. Process stages where the final product is exposed to the environment are classified as "critical," and the air quality is defined. "Controlled" areas, where non-sterile product and components are handled, are also defined. *The Guide to Inspection of Bulk Pharmaceutical Chemicals* (FDA 1991) also provides some general facility design and operation pointers.

Other Federal Codes Affecting Design

The prevention of accidental release to the surroundings, and the well-being of employees must be addressed in the facility design and operation, under the rules of the Environmental Protection Agency (EPA) (40 CFR) and the Occupational Health and Safety Administration (OSHA) (29 CFR). In addition, there are usually state and local government agency regulations. The President's Council on Environmental Quality regulations governs the implementation of the National Environmental Policy Act (NEPA). The EPA also has jurisdiction over certain aspects of biotech product manufacture, through the Toxic Substances Control Act (TSCA) and the Federal Insecticide, Fungicide, and Rodenticide Act (FIFRA). Applicants for product licenses for biological products must submit to the FDA either an environmental assessment under 21 CFR 25.31 or claim exemption under 21 CFR 25.24 (Environmental Impact Considerations).

Construction Codes

Building, plumbing, mechanical, and fire protection codes, such as in the Uniform Code series (1994) may need to be observed, depending on local regulations. Fire codes, particularly, may affect a biotech facility heating, ventilation, and air conditioning (HVAC) system and biosafety design through the requirements for fire protection systems and fire containment devices, smoke exhausting, and the control of chemical hazards. Expert consultation is required in these specialties.

GENERAL CONSIDERATIONS FOR MULTIPROCESS FACILITY DESIGN

Since there are no comprehensive guidelines for biotechnology facility design, facility designs have evolved by combining regulatory guidelines, biosafety considerations, industry and laboratory practices, and then matching these to the needs of their technology. Basically, multiproduct facilities require strict application of cGMP principles, which are appropriate design, reliable equipment and utilities, well-trained personnel, thorough validation programs, and appropriate routine monitoring of the whole system. The fundamental principle is to minimize at all points the potential for product mix-ups and cross-contamination. This section contains a description of standard practices and useful contingencies to consider in designing a satisfactory facility.

Facility Siting and Orientation

Determine the direction of the average prevailing wind at the site, and, if possible, locate building air intakes upwind of air exhausts to reduce the chance of drawing in contaminants and fumes from downstream processes. Waste treatment plants, animal holding facilities, engine exhausts, and boiler stacks are preferably located downwind and remote from the process facility for the same reasons.

A factor commonly overlooked in facility design is the compatibility of the planned operations with adjacent businesses or activities. A desirable rural site may be compromised by wastes and emissions from a nearby livestock farm, for example. During licensing and inspections, manufacturers may be queried as to the extent to which they have assessed the risks, assured that the known hazards are acceptable, and have developed contingency plans for emergencies. Examples of risk studies include assessing the potential impact of industrial air and wastes, the risks associated with the use of a shared access road, the quality and reliability of the water supply, and hazard assessment posed by wastes from previous tenants.

Operational Efficiency

A design providing an efficient operation would locate all building services close to the principal consumers of the services. However, this is not always an economic or practical decision. For example, materials receiving, quarantine, and released storage may be conveniently located adjacent to the principal chemical consumers—media and buffer preparation. On the other hand, process buildings are expensive to build and maintain, and a large materials storage space inside a process building may be a costly convenience. Similarly, locating upstream and downstream operations adjacent to one another may not be compatible with the HVAC design, process integrity, or staff movement.

Operational Considerations

The facility operational plan—how raw materials are processed into products that are tested to predetermined standards and released—should be well understood by the time of initial design. Intrinsic features of the plan that influence the operations and, hence, the facility layout include the following:

- Plan concurrent manufacture only in closed systems. Proving the integrity of closed, sterile systems by a series of successful sterility tests will be important corroborating evidence in allowing a manufacturer to operate a multiproduct facility. Open system processing should be considered acceptable only in campaigned production.

- Campaign production and careful scheduling of operations can provide an acceptable means of process segregation, which may reduce the need for dedicated process areas.

- Adequate time must be allowed for the validation of changeover procedures between products. This may increase the need for dedicated process areas.

Dedicated Equipment

Equipment that is difficult to clean (chromatography equipment, UF systems) or those that handle highly purified product (bulk product tanks, filling equipment) are best dedicated to single product use. Equipment used for holding low product concentrations, nonproduct containers (such as buffer tanks and equipment) that can be demonstrated to be acceptably clean, may be considered for nondedicated, common use. An important point, therefore, to avoid duplication or oversight, is to identify as early as possible the product-dedicated equipment and common equipment.

Validation Contingencies

As stated before, the installation requirements for validation identified in the functional and operational description document and Validation Master Plan should be included early in the design process.

Flow Separation

The complexity of multiproduct operations requires that "clean" or incoming materials enter process facilities by separate flow paths from "dirty" (outgoing) materials. One of the most frequently quoted reasons for regulatory citations in process areas is the lack of staging and storage space for dirty and clean materials, which, in the case of a multiprocess facility are especially important features.

Segregated process, entry, and egress flows, provided by access and return corridors, are becoming an FDA standard design requirement. Dedicated corridors may be difficult to include in designs. As an alternative, it may be acceptable to factor in separation by time, where "clean" movements take place at the beginning of the day or shift, and "dirty" movements at the end of the work period, followed by a cleaning routine prior to the next "clean" phase of use. This approach requires more detailed knowledge of the proposed operational plan, confidence that the operation can be controlled, and the use of dedicated staging space.

Materials Staging

Provide clearly separated storage areas for clean items, in-process equipment, quality control samples, used materials, wastes, and products. Do not use corridors for storage; they should be used for transit only. Clean items should be sealed and protected during storage. An effective method of storing clean tanks is to isolate and hold them under pressure using air or an inert gas.

Product Transfers

A characteristic feature of biotech processes is that products are present in very low concentrations initially, and thousands of liters of crude harvest may result in only tens of liters of formulated product. The ideal biotech process includes closed process steps from cell seed vial to product vial, with all product transfers taking place in sterile piping. However, before specifying and installing sterile pipework for product transfers, make an estimate of product losses in lengthy aseptic transfer lines, since these may be significant.

Aseptic transfers of product by piping should only be considered, therefore, where losses will constitute an acceptably small fraction of the total, or where the facility design allows convenient operation and control of the lines. Consider using mobile tanks instead of lengthy transfer lines, as these may be more convenient for facility design and less wasteful of material than transfer piping. Up to 300 L can be pushed manually in sterile mobile tanks—more using forklift trucks.

Personnel Access

A feature that will receive a great deal of regulatory scrutiny in a design is the orderly progress of clean and dirty staff, equipment, and materials in the multiproduct plant. Affinity diagrams can help in developing and testing these realities.

Staff should enter and leave by different routes (gowning/degowning air locks), maintaining a clean-to-dirty flow path, so that exiting staff do not compromise clean entry locks. This may not always be practicable, but should be rigorously applied to the most sensitive process stages, such as seed bank handling, aseptic processing areas, and where any "open" process steps are encountered.

The design should limit interaction between staff from different areas; strict parameters are required for determining which staff can work on more than one process simultaneously. Staff should be dedicated to critical steps to reduce cross-contamination risks. Staff working on multiple products require strict, documented work and gowning control in order to be acceptable to reviewers.

Separate staff entry and exit requirements imply that many gowning rooms are required. In an effort to rationalize the number of gowning rooms, it may be acceptable to implement "clean-to-dirty" access rules. Under these rules, staff may enter purification suites ("cleaner") and move without hindrance upstream to earlier process stages ("dirtier"), but may not retrace their steps without undergoing regowning or other appropriate control steps. Control of staff access is an important regulatory factor, and computerized card-key systems may be considered to provide controlled, monitored, staff access.

Gowning and Pass-Through Air Locks

Gowning-in air locks should be fitted with interlocking doors for full control of air migration. Most gowning rooms require lockers/clothing hooks, a stepover bench, wire racks (for coveralls, bootees, other clothing), covered trash bins, and a wall mirror for checking dress prior to entry. If handwashing on entry is required, a quick-drying chemical antiseptic wash from a dispenser is preferred to washing with water, since sinks, plumbing, and dryers may contribute aerosols or contaminants to the air lock. Air quality and pressurization regimes in the lock should reflect the air quality of the room to be entered. Gowning-out air locks also require interlocking doors, covered trash bins for discarding clothing, and air quality and pressurization appropriate to the adjacent rooms.

Pass through air locks should be sized and sited for use with materials and equipment. There should be minimal interaction between staff and materials streams. As far as possible, materials (such as chemicals and mobile equipment) and personnel should access via different routes to avoid unnecessary entry by delivery staff into process zones, and accidental egress by process staff into nonprocess areas. Pass-through air locks with two, three, and four interlocking doors should be considered for providing or receiving materials from more than one location.

Working Environment

Biotech plants tend to be sparse facilities, noisy from high volumes of air movement, and cut off from the outside world. Natural lighting from windows and skylights, or simply using daylight fluorescent lighting, go a long way toward softening the feeling of austerity. Windows in access corridors give the added benefit of externally showing or observing operations for quality and safety without the requirement to gown and enter the space.

DETAILED DESIGN

The following section describes, on an area-by-area basis, standard design features commonly found in biotech plants for consideration in multiproduct design.

Facility Finishes

All process rooms will be subject to vigorous routine cleaning, and, consequently, surface construction and finishes must be impervious, easily cleanable, and resistant to chemical cleaning agents.

Flooring

Floors should be sealed, impervious, and with a texture that allows for complete cleaning. In rooms where standing water is likely (and biosafety containment allows), the floor should be sloped to a floor drain. Sealed, epoxy-painted concrete or troweled epoxy-terrazzo are used on high traffic floors, such as in primary production rooms, air locks, or corridors. Nonslip texturing may be installed in appropriate locations, balancing slip resistance with cleanability. Sheet polyvinyl chloride (PVC) materials with welded seams are used on lighter-traffic floors, such as in clean rooms and downstream processes. Floor to wall joints should be coved, preferably in the same material as the flooring, and sealed sufficient to prevent build up of dirt and residual water.

Walls

Walls are commonly finished with water resistant paints, such as epoxy for process room walls and in wet or humid areas. Washable latex emulsions are used for other walls. Where walls can be damaged by the movement of equipment, impact protection (such as a wainscot of protective sheeting or a bumper) should be attached to the walls and sealed to prevent pockets or crevices that afford the opportunity for the accumulation of moisture and dirt. Stainless steel strips and flashing plates may be specified in certain locations. Users should be aware that this material is readily attacked by chlorinated solutions, and requires care to maintain an attractive finish. Plastics, epoxy-coated steel, or anodized aluminum may provide suitable alternatives.

Ceilings

Hard ceilings are preferred to suspended ceilings in process areas, owing to their ease of cleaning and integrity. If unavoidable, suspended ceiling tiles suitable for cleanroom service should be used for zones requiring cleaning and air pressurization. Cleanroom service tiles are usually made of impervious materials such as epoxy or vinyl-coated steel, and are held in place on gasketted frames by spring clips. If hard ceilings are used, the ceiling should be sealed, and access hatches should be included to service mechanical equipment in the space.

Fixed Furniture

Bench tops and equipment surfaces should be impervious and resistant to the cleaning solutions. The installation method should avoid crevices and seams between sinks, walls, and benches. Stainless steel or epoxy tops with baked epoxy-painted steel casework are preferred in processing spaces. Furniture must be installed to allow proper cleaning. Where possible, furniture should be hung off walls or from overhead supports to avoid floor joints. If floor mounted, mount on housekeeping pads or seal and cove the flooring around equipment to improve cleanability.

Design Features of Process Areas

Cell Banking

Careful design of cell bank manipulation laboratories is required, since an accidental contamination of a seed bank could have dire consequences for a potential product. Consequently, these areas will receive detailed attention from regulatory bodies. Master and working cell bank storage and handling laboratories should be dedicated, with separate entry and exit gowning locks and pass-throughs. These laboratories are best sited outside the main process areas, to allow segregation and easy access of liquid nitrogen, and so on. Only well-characterized cells should be handled in these laboratories, because of hazards from adventitious agent contaminations from uncharacterized cells.

Seed Preparation Laboratory

A similar attention to detail is required for the seed preparation laboratory as for the cell bank laboratories, for the same reasons. Seed preparation laboratories should also be dedicated, with separate entry and exit gowning locks. The segregation of different seeds is important, either by dedicated processing cubicles or separation by time with disinfection between seeds. A common seed production laboratory should be located close to the fermentation areas, using a pass-through to transfer seeds to downstream processes.

Fermentation Media Preparation

Solutions from the fermentation media preparation area should be limited to upstream operations to avoid the contamination of downstream purification processes. Media preparation is liable to generate particulates and is usually an open operation. If there is a risk of open conditions or aerosol generation, these may be prevented from spreading by negative room pressure barriers. This room usually requires washing.

Fermentation

If there is a risk of aerosol generation, a negative pressure HVAC system may be adequate to contain potential migration. Class 100,000 air quality is acceptable for totally closed operations, but bear in mind that systems defined as closed must be proven so by validation. If there are open processing steps, the design air quality may need to be higher. Fermentation suites also require frequent washing and biowaste drainage.

Biosafety regulations may require a dike around bioreactors to contain spills. The FDA recommends the capacity of waste containment to equal twice the maximum theoretical spill volume. Drains in these spaces must be capped or raised to allow the collection and decontamination of spills before release to waste treatment.

Harvest/Product Recovery

Harvest/product recovery systems should be sited close to the fermenters to reduce line losses during product transfers. These systems commonly involve centrifugation, cell disruption, and transverse flow filtration—all involving the risk of creating aerosols in the operation, cleaning, or preparation steps. Consequently, these operations are best housed in segregated areas, isolated further by negative pressure gradients.

Purification Buffer Preparation

The supply of solutions from purification buffer preparation should be limited to purification and formulation operations to avoid the contamination of upstream processes. Buffer preparation is liable to generate particulates and is usually an open operation. The spread of aerosols can be limited by negative air pressure gradients. Totally enclosed preparation operations and buffer storage would be acceptable in Class 100,000 conditions. Buffer preparation rooms usually require washing and drainage.

Purification

The potential for products of mammalian cells to contain infectious viruses is central to the design of purification facilities. Designs and operations should concentrate on limiting the dissemination of virus particles by aerosol, facility, or equipment contamination by totally enclosing these steps. Purification steps for these products contain virus-removing steps (ultrafiltration or column separation) or virus inactivation processes (low pH hold, chemical chaotropes). The design should allow the total separation of pre- and postviral removal stages. This is best achieved for open processes by using dedicated rooms with nonrecirculating Class 10,000 HVAC systems and local Class 100 laminar airflow banks. For totally closed processes it may be acceptable to use Class 100,000 rooms, but the HVAC system should nevertheless provide 100 percent extract air. Processing infectious materials in nondedicated rooms may be separated by time, with validated cleaning and decontamination between products.

Product Formulation Room

An important factor in the design of the product formulation room is to note that there are no more opportunities to remove contaminants at the formulation stage, which implies that process steps must be well defined, product contact surfaces must be high quality, equipment cleaning and sterilization processes must be appropriate and validated, and room environmental standards must be correspondingly high.

Product Filling and Lyophilization

Glassware preparation, filling, and lyophilization suite designs should conform with the industry standards for aseptic processing (21 CFR 1991). Design features should limit the dispersal of aerosols in filling and processing processes. Cleaning procedures must remove all previous product residues, such as accumulate in places like the lyophilizer condenser units, freezing trays, and so on.

Labeling and Packaging Operations

Labeling and packaging operations can be congested operations, due to the sheer volume of product or bulky packaging materials. The risks of mix-up of containers, labels, and packaging materials must be catered for when planning simultaneous or campaigned operations. The separation of product streams and the provision of secure, controlled storage for all components of these operations is critical.

Labeling and packaging operations typically create large amounts of particulates and can be quite "dirty" in the sense of the movement of materials and staff. Consider controlled air quality if the activity impacts process integrity and if the quality of adjacent areas is likely to be affected by particles.

Design of Process Support Areas

Quality Laboratories

Quality Control plays a crucial role in validating and monitoring the correct functioning of a multiproduct facility. As a consequence, these laboratories are often subject to scrutiny by regulators. The most common FDA citations to be issued in quality control laboratories are related to the potential for mix-up or spoiling of samples.

Provide designated and adequate sample receipt and storage facilities in quality control laboratories. This feature is especially important in a multiproduct situation where lost samples can result in lost material, or worse, incorrect testing.

Instrumentation Calibration

The successful changeover of rooms and equipment to different products will depend on the regular and consistent control of the process, and the retesting and monitoring of many validated parameters. Suitable space for the storage and calibration of in-process control instrumentation and validation equipment should be provided in the facility.

Routine Maintenance Workshops

Record-keeping of routine and emergency maintenance is an important part of the quality assurance of a multiproduct facility. Allow ample space for the recording and archiving of maintenance records. Adequate workshop space and tools should be provided for off-line servicing of larger equipment items.

Equipment Washing and Preparation

Allow access for bulky equipment such as tanks. Unpacking and cleaning operations may generate aerosols, and adjacent spaces should be protected from particulates by pressure gradients. These rooms may require routine wash down and drainage.

Materials Storage Rooms

Provide clearly separated storage spaces for quarantined materials on hold pending testing, tested items released following testing, and rejected goods for disposal. There should be no possibility of mixing these different items. Provide recording thermographs for routine monitoring of temperatures in controlled temperature rooms.

Solid Waste Decontamination

Decontamination and disposal of solid waste will generate aerosols, and adjacent areas should be protected by negative pressure gradients. Waste decontamination rooms may require wash down and drainage capabilities.

Liquid Waste Disposal

Standard designs provide separate waste handling streams for biowaste (for infectious or potentially infected wastes) and general waste. Backflow prevention devices are used to limit accidental reverse dispersal of infectious waste, especially to noninfected areas. Generally speaking, biowaste is collected and decontaminated in a contained system, within the biocontainment boundary of the production plant.

Staff Washing and Sanitation

Unless specifically required by biosafety regulations, staff washing and sanitation areas are best located outside the process room. If inside, restrooms pose additional cleaning and contamination risks, and process areas should be protected from potential contamination by air pressure gradients, air locks, and staff sanitation procedures.

Offices

As far as possible, limit the location of offices inside process facilities, since these provide additional cleaning and sanitation risks. Internal offices should be limited to shift activities, with the minimal passage of papers between different process stages. If data entry is required, use electronic systems wherever possible to reduce paper flow.

Food and Recreation Areas

Do not locate food and recreation areas inside process areas. Require staff to exit from the facility for these activities.

Design of Utility and Mechanical Spaces

Process Utility Rooms

Machine spaces for process utility generators, such as reverse osmosis (RO) water systems, WFI, and clean steam evaporators, are not required to be scrupulously clean, but the design of the rooms and systems themselves should take into account that the utilities must meet high standards of purity and are routinely monitored to assure these standards are maintained. Such monitoring requires clean sampling locations.

Mechanical Spaces

The designs for mechanical spaces should take into account that access will be required to sampling and recording devices on HVAC systems and main plant utilities.

Mezzanine Spaces

If accessible ceilings are not possible, the ideal (but costly) alternative is to build mezzanine floors. These provide segregated, stable spaces for installing mechanical equipment. Since mezzanines may be completely sealed from process spaces, some issues regarding the cleanliness and integrity of operations may be avoided.

Walkable ceilings made of coated, laminated steel/foam panels, commonly used in the semiconductor industry, are an alternative to permanent construction, since these provide several advantages. Here, a cleanable, sealed ceiling with some of the load-bearing potential of a mezzanine floor is combined with the convenience of being easy to modify and cut for pipe chases, light fittings, and so on.

MECHANICAL SYSTEMS, UTILITIES, AND PROCESS EQUIPMENT

Standard design features of mechanical systems, utilities, and process equipment commonly in use in biotech plants are described in this section.

General Requirements for Process and Plant Utilities

Utilities are widely distributed and circulate throughout a facility and, sometimes, between adjacent, unrelated buildings. Consequently, loops may traverse "clean" and "dirty" zones repeatedly and have the potential to act as conduits for cross-contamination between processes. These risks are sometimes addressed by designing loops to enter the most product-critical areas first, with the idea that if contaminants do enter the utility loop, there will be less risk of compromising the critical steps. The efficacy of this in the event of a real intrusion is, however, questionable. Preferably, separate loops are dedicated to "clean" and "dirty" areas. The loop designs should also include appropriate sample ports, instruments, and locations for the measurement of flow rates and temperatures where required for validation measurements and routine maintenance.

Designers frequently locate utility service generators remote from process facilities for reasons of noise, heat, and humidity. However, as process utilities are expensive both to install and to run, consider locating the generators as close as feasible to the principal consumers. It is probably cheaper to pipe and run the main plant utilities to the process utility generators than to pipe and operate the high quality process utilities in long loops to the process users. For example, in upstream processes (media and buffer preparation and fermentation), where large amounts of high purity steam and water are used, the utility generators are best located in an adjacent plant room, with remote main utilities. Smaller users of process utilities may warrant dedicated supply loops or smaller utility generators located nearby.

Biohazard Considerations

The biohazards presented by microorganisms used in manufacturing and testing, and the recombinant organisms and products prepared, must be assessed and factored into the facility design. Formal guidelines address the issues concerning the handling of microorganisms, based on their potential for causing disease in healthy adults (U.S. DHHS 1988) and for work involving the use of organisms containing rDNA molecules (*NIH Guidelines* 1986). Containment levels for large-scale operations, somewhat arbitrarily defined as culture volumes greater than 10 liters, are addressed in the Good Large-Scale Practice (GLSP) guidelines for the handling of recombinant organisms (NIH 1991). The lowest of the four large-scale containment levels is GLSP, with containment requirements assigned according to increasing biohazard in Biosafety Levels 1, 2, and 3 (BL1-LS, BL2-LS, and BL3-LS).

Principles of Biocontainment

Physical containment has two interrelated elements that should be included in designs: primary containment and secondary containment. Primary containment is the protection of equipment, operators, and the immediate working environment by using closed containers, for example, fermenters with gas filters and steam lock addition ports, or handling open cultures in biosafety cabinets or containment hoods with HEPA filters on the exhaust air.

Secondary containment involves the protection of the wider environment by surrounding primary containers with facility designs and procedures to limit exposure. Examples of designs and procedures to limit exposure include spill protection, biowaste inactivation, personnel access control systems, HEPA filtration of room exhaust air, and fail-safe design of air locks.

Process Host Cells

Most host cells used in biotechnology are benign (*Escherichia coli*, mammalian cells, yeast species, etc.) and fall into the categories GLSP or BL1-LS. In spite of this, however, the trend in biotechnology is to design facilities conservatively with features corresponding to BL2-LS. There is no regulatory requirement for this, but since these provisions concentrate on process containment and provide product protection, BL2-LS is in accordance with multiproduct design intentions.

A facility designed to BL2-LS standards requires the following:

- Physical separation from the environment by solid walls and airlocks

- HEPA filtering of or incineration of exhaust gases to prevent the release of viable organisms

- Contained sample collection procedures that prevent the release of viable organisms

- Inactivation of all cultures and effluents using validated methods before removal from the facility

- Protective clothing for personnel

- The availability of personnel decontamination (washing) facilities

- Enforcement of access restrictions and posting of biohazard signs

- Mechanical seals and other potential process leak sites to be designed to prevent leakage or to vent safely

GMP Design for a HVAC System for Multiproduct Facilities

Biosafety Considerations

Heating, ventilation, and air conditioning systems require a great deal of planning to satisfy the requirements of biosafety and to limit the risks of cross-contamination. Good manufacturing practices recommend that air-flows cascade from the cleanest (process) zones outward to nonprocess zones. With a biosafety risk, however, the design of the biocontainment zone may operate better at a negative pressure relative to surrounding spaces, or with a negative pressure barrier in an air lock between process and nonprocess areas. These balances reduce the spread of organisms in case of primary containment failure.

Room exhaust air may be HEPA filtered as appropriate for biosafety containment. Air pressure requirements are not specified in the guidelines for BL2-LS biohazard level, but a differential pressure of 0.05 inches water gauge is commonly used for containment between different spaces.

The final affinity diagrams can be helpful in the design. Divide the facility into air handling zones—areas of common activity or containment. Avoid mixing air from process stages of different product purity, or where there is a chance of spreading aerosols between areas. Air pressure cascading in linked and adjacent rooms can be used to provide stagewise incremental cleanliness and to prevent air migration from dirty areas. Air locks may provide further segregation. All penetrations through containment boundaries should be sealed.

The greatest assurance of limiting airborne cross-contamination is by providing separate HVAC systems for different processing stages using dedicated air handling units with 100 percent exhaust, and reinforcing this by supplying the appropriate quality of air to the process stages. Recirculation of air is acceptable in noncritical or nonprocess areas, and this return air is often HEPA filtered. Some room air, such as from upstream processes where host organisms are handled or at stages prior to viral inactivation, should not be recycled because of the risk of airborne, hazards such as aerosols of viable organisms. HEPA filters used on exhaust air systems may be hazardous to handle, since they will retain viable organisms and chemical dusts; bag-in/bag-out installations should be specified for safe handling.

Air Quality

Acceptable standards of facility air quality are as follows:

- Class 100,000 for closed processes (fermenters, media and buffer storage, some column processes)
- Class 10,000 for downstream operations where process quality is higher
- Class 10,000 plus local Class 100 laminar flow over critical open processes (cell seed and cell bank manipulations, column fraction collection, process sample handling)
- Class 1000/100 nonlaminar flow plus local Class 100 laminar flow for bulk product open manipulations
- Class 100 laminar flow over product filling and lyophilizer load/offload areas

Terminal Filter Testing

HEPA filters and ducts should have access ports for the introduction of dioctyl phthalate (DOP) for the in situ integrity testing of the filters. Injection ports are required upstream of filters, and sampling ports for the upstream and downstream sampling of airstreams.

Biocontainment Isolator Units

Biocontainment isolators provide a high degree of security for critical steps. They are being used increasingly for small-scale, manual operations such as cell bank manipulations or the handling of biohazardous organisms.

Isolators have several positive features for consideration for use in multiproduct facilities:

- Isolators are cost-effective: It may be possible to reduce complicated and expensive facility, HVAC, and biosafety designs. Since the product or organisms may be handled in complete isolation from the surroundings, several units may be located in proximity to one another, and air quality of Class 100,000 for the room will probably suffice.

- The chambers can be provided with 100 percent HEPA inlet and exhaust air and be run at net positive or negative air pressure relative to the room. If desired, they can be supplied with HEPA laminar flow.

- The units may be fumigated or sterilized between uses, providing additional assurance for the handling of several products.

Miscellaneous Factors

Humidity control is critical in order to reduce mold growth on surfaces; low humidities (30–50 percent RH) are commonly used. Where rehumidification is required, clean steam is used to reduce the chances of introducing contaminants into the airstream. Some areas (e.g., fermentation) have high intermittent water vapor loads evolved from steam condensate, which poses humidity control problems.

Energy conservation by air-to-air heat exchange is possible, but can be a biosafety risk as well as costly and cumbersome to install. HVAC systems are sometimes run at reduced speed when spaces are unoccupied, maintaining air gradients while conserving energy. Noise from HVAC can become a problem that requires expensive remediation unless it is taken into account at the outset of design.

Control Systems

A busy plant, where the movement of staff and materials results in constantly opening doors and where extractor fans, hoods, and so on are in use, maintaining air pressure differentials can pose control problems. Local industrial air control systems are not efficient or precise enough for this duty; thus, HVAC control requirements benefit greatly from plantwide distributed control and monitoring systems. If a distributed control system is combined with real-time displays and central data logging of flows, pressures, temperature, humidity, and (where needed) particulate levels, the data captured can be a useful addition to HVAC system validation and for trend analysis of system operation over time. Air pressure manometers indicating the pressure differential between spaces are a useful addition to biosafety control. If located externally to the process core, routine maintenance checks can be made without entering an area, and operators can check prior to entry whether or not a space is safe to enter or work in.

Liquid Waste Containment and Treatment

Errors made in the installation of liquid waste containment systems can be extremely costly to remedy. Care is required in the design phase. The following are some points for consideration.

- The industry trend is toward the concept of "double containment." Drains are comprised of double-walled leakproof construction to contain any leaks from the primary drain. Both primary and secondary systems must be proven to be leak free by validated testing. The secondary containment installation should be designed to monitor for leaks. Avoid cast iron drains because of their poor corrosion resistance against high purity water, clean steam, and salt solutions. If plastic piping is used, care must be taken to cool hot wastes (such as steam condensate) to prevent damage to the pipes.

- Gravity-fed drain systems are prone to flooding and backup due to their inability to handle large volumes of waste. This can be a serious breach of GMP and containment, and discharges to these systems must be controlled or backflow preventers must be used to prevent backups in drains from other rooms.

- The pumping or pressurization of biowaste systems should be avoided until after inactivation, since a leak may result in the release of waste to the environment.

- Water-filled drain *P* traps are prone to drying out, especially in negative air pressure zones. This could cause an influx of air and odors from the drains and other areas, resulting in a serious breach of integrity and GMP. Traps can be fitted with water primers to keep them flooded.

- Biowaste inactivation installations should include contained sampling points to test streams before and after treatment and recording devices for monitoring the inactivation process. Some local authorities will require access to these systems for periodic inspections.

- Some authorities will not allow in-ground waste tanks, for fear of leaks contaminating groundwater.

Process Utilities

High Quality Process Water Systems

When designing process water systems, divide the facility into product purity zones. Different qualities of water may be appropriate for different stages of the process. For example, low-pyrogen water may not be required for all processes and all products.

Chilled Water Service

Before specifying an ethylene glycol cooling system, check the local waste disposal regulations associated with this coolant. Disposal can be difficult in some locations.

Clean Steam

In general, clean steam condensate should not be reclaimed from process areas, due to the potential for the carryover of contaminants to generator and distribution loops. The condensate from many locations must be disposed of through a biowaste system, as it may be contaminated with host organisms.

Clean-in-Place Systems

A careful design effort is required for clean-in-place (CIP) systems. Dedicated CIP systems should be used for different stages of the process, to avoid contaminating process equipment with wastes from another process stage. Commonly, fermentation and media will share a single system, a second CIP unit will be dedicated to purification buffers and process tanks, and a third unit is provided for formulation and final process stages.

Care is required in estimating water and waste capacity in a biotech facility. Clean-in-place systems typically create demands for large volumes of high quality WFI and purified water. The volume needed is often underestimated, since the CIP cycles cannot be developed until plant installation is completed. For the same reasons, the volumes of CIP rinse and waste solutions may be underestimated. Substantial volumes of waste can be expected, and a large portion must be treated as biohazardous, requiring large treatment and holding capacities. Note that satisfactory plant operations can become bottlenecked as easily by a lack of water as by undercapacity in the waste treatment system.

Clean-in-place fluids are pumped at high velocities, frequently at elevated temperatures and pressures. Under these conditions water hammer is common, which can create momentary hydraulic pressures of several hundred pounds per square inch, sufficient to present risks to operators, equipment, and processes. Pressure damping devices and installation safety features, such as double-block-and-bleed valve assemblies, are recommended to prevent the acci- dental leakage of cleaning solutions into process equipment.

Process Equipment

Suitable access ports should be fitted on all equipment that is steamed-in-place: sterile transfer lines, sterilizing ovens and autoclaves, hot rooms, incubators, cold rooms, and refrigerators for connecting validation instruments. Access ports should also be available for taking physical samples and for introducing thermocouples for thermal mapping studies or routine monitoring.

Sterile Piping Systems

The sterile piping design and installation should precede all other facility designs, since this system is the most difficult and costly to modify in case of clashes with other services. Piping requires care in fabrication and installation; it must be sloped adequately for draining during CIP and steam-in-place (SIP) operations. Sloping can lead to substantial height changes in long runs, which can result in unforeseen design problems. Allow sufficient space in piping racks and chases to account for piping slopes.

Horizontal piping runs and racks of piping clusters provide the potential for the collection of dust and are difficult to clean. Thus, avoid exposed horizontal piping runs in process areas. Enclose piping runs in a mezzanine or chase space where possible, or, if unavoidable around process equipment, design piping runs for easy accessibility and cleaning.

DESIGN REVIEWS

A series of reviews is recommended after considering the regulatory guidelines and code requirements of building location, construction, finishes, air handling, personnel and material flows, water quality, environmental protection, biosafety, and so on, and after completing preliminary design drawings.

Internal Reviews

Thorough reviews of the design are recommended by groups representing all functional departments, with the objective of determining the suitability of the designs to the process, the operability of the plant, whether all support systems and validation needs have been included, and the ease of maintenance and accessibility to serviced equipment.

Local Authority Reviews

City, county, fire department, state, OSHA, and EPA authorities must be included in the facility review process. It is important to communicate clearly the fundamentals of the process and the biocontainment precautions designed, since local authorities often have little experience in biotechnology and may react unpredictably to the terms *biohazard* and *recombinant organisms*. For example, fire departments may respond to the word *hazard* by insisting on the installation of fire or chemical hazard precautions, which may interfere with multiproduct design intentions.

FDA Reviews

The FDA offers informal reviews of facility plans at various stages of the development (FDA 1983), and it is beneficial to take advantage of this review process. The FDA will probably have fewer questions about a new facility at the time of application for an establishment license if the agency has previewed the design during development.

Contact the FDA early in the conceptual design process. Before breaking ground, submit a design package and request a review meeting. The package should consist of affinity diagrams, well-developed layout drawings, and written operations descriptions that include product and personnel flows, types of finishes, air and water quality, material balances, and validation strategies. Adjacent premises should be identified and the potential impact of any activities should be discussed.

Environmental Assessment Review

The FDA will also consider the environmental impact of a proposal before making any final decision. It requires an environmental assessment statement from manufacturers as part of the establishment license application (CFR 21, Part 25, 1982).

SUMMARY

Multiproduct facilities for use in the biotechnology industry are becoming more commonplace as industry and regulatory authorities recognize the technical feasibility of building and operating these units, and the clear economic benefits provided by spreading the cost of facilities and equipment over several product development projects.

This chapter has sought to clarify the principal concerns of multiproduct processing, to present the prevailing industry and regulatory viewpoints, to suggest an integrated, facility design development strategy, and to review general biotech facility design requirements with an emphasis on desirable features to include in a multiproduct context. Above all, integrated teamwork cannot be emphasized enough in the development of the design. All functional groups in the facility must collaborate with designers to ensure a satisfactory design. Regulatory and local authorities must also be included in the design evolution.

ACKNOWLEDGMENTS

The author is indebted to Bruce Moon of Biotech Australia Pty., Ltd., Roseville, New South Wales, Australia; and John Moore and Emile Jansen of Moore and Cashell Architects Pty., Ltd., Greenwich, New South Wales, Australia for information on the innovative affinity diagram approach to multiproduct facility design.

Many of the details described in this chapter have been developed and expounded by eminent regulatory and industry spokespersons at public forums in recent years, and the author wishes to acknowledge their leadership in this area.

REFERENCES

Bader, F. G., A. Blum, B. D. Garfinkle, D. MacFarlane, T. Massa, and T. L. Copmann. 1992. Multiuse manufacturing facilities for biologicals. *Biopharm* 5 (11).

Biological products. 1991. Code of Federal Regulations, Title 21 Parts 600–680. Washington, DC: U.S. Government Printing Office.

Code of Federal Regulations, Title 29. Washington DC: Occupational Safety and Health Administration, U.S. Government Printing Office.

Code of Federal Regulations, Title 40. Washington, DC: Environmental Protection Agency, U.S. Government Printing Office.

Current good manufacturing practice for finished pharmaceuticals. 1991. Code of Federal Regulations, Title 21, Parts 210–211. Washington DC: U.S. Government Printing Office.

Environmental impact considerations. 1982. Code of Federal Regulations, Title 21, Part 25. Washington, DC: U.S. Government Printing Office.

FDA. 1983. *Pre-operational reviews of manufacturing facilities.* Field management directive. Rockville, MD: Food and Drug Administration.

FDA. 1987. *Guideline on sterile drug products produced by aseptic processing.* Washington, DC: Center for Drugs and Biologics and Office of Regulatory Affairs, U.S. Government Printing Office.

FDA. 1991. *FDA guide to inspection of bulk pharmaceutical chemicals.* Washington, DC: Center for Drugs and Biologics and Office of Regulatory Affairs, U.S. Government Printing Office.

Fifteen prime areas for biotech commercialization. 1995. *Genetic Eng. News* 15 (1):8–9.

Hill, D., and M. Beatrice. 1989, Biotechnology facility requirements, Part 1: Facility and systems design. *BioPharm* 2 (12).

NIH. 1991. Recombinant DNA research: Actions under the guidelines; notice. *Federal Register* Part III, 56, (138):33174–33183.

NIH guidelines for research involving recombinant DNA molecules. 1986. Washington, DC: U.S. Government Printing Office.

Odum, J. N. 1994. Developing a program for biopharmaceutical facility design. *Biopharm* 7 (7).

Uniform fire/mechanical/plumbing/building codes. 1994. Whittier, CA.: International Conference of Building Officials.

U.S. DHHS. 1988. *Biosafety in microbiological and biomedical laboratories.* Publication 88-8395. Washington, DC: U.S. Dept. of Health and Human Services, U.S. Government Printing Office.

7

ECONOMIC AND COST FACTORS OF BIOPROCESS ENGINEERING

Scott M. Wheelwright

Scios Nova Inc.

One of the major goals of any business venture is to provide a return on investment to shareholders. Because shareholders enjoy economic freedom and can choose where they invest their capital, the evaluation of alternative investments and the generation of an attractive return is crucial to the success of biotechnology companies. Bioprocess engineering is a particularly resource intensive part of biological drug development, requiring long-term investment in specialized capital equipment. This chapter addresses the economic and cost factors of bioprocess engineering, with a focus on three main areas: development, facilities, and operations. The interplay between these areas, especially the impact of development decisions on operating costs, will also be explored.

First, it is necessary to define the goal and understand why costs must be considered. In the global sense, biotechnology, just as any other business enterprise, must provide a return that is attractive to investors or there will be no capital available for product development. Thus, tools must be provided by which our return can be evaluated and how it can be maximized for the shareholder. These same tools, by which a global analysis is performed, will provide the ability to dig into the details and uncover those small factors that when accumulated, have significant impact on the global picture. In the recent past the cost of production did not prevent new biotech products from succeeding in the market. However, in the future one can anticipate that biotech drugs that must vie with existing synthetic products will be required to compete on a cost basis. The current emphasis on pharmacoeconomics (the quantitative evaluation of the quality of life and the value added by any treatment) suggests that the cost of production may be of concern not only to company accountants but also to regulatory agencies. Economic analysis may guide and support manufacturing and development strategies for both cash-flush and cash-poor companies.

Because of the interactions between the many variables, the goal of maximizing the return to investors is complex and cannot be defined by a simple objective function. In the simple view one maximizes return through minimum investment and maximum sales. But how does one achieve minimum investment? One can try to minimize the resources for development, but then one risks a delay in market entry. Increasing process development may lead to lower operating costs, but will it be justified? Similarly, an increase in facility construction cost may produce a substantial savings in operating costs. Each of these alternatives must be investigated separately and weighed together to determine the mutual impact on the overall return.

In addition to financial measures, government and corporate regulations impose constraints that are also part of the equation. These constraints work to restrict the product (including the process by which it is developed and produced) to fit standards of usefulness and performance, or, in other words, to define quality. On the corporate side these constraints include a desire to be a good neighbor and protect the safety and environment of those outside the company who contact the product, waste materials, and the facility, and to protect the well-being of company employees. Governments require compliance with regulatory agencies, such as the Food and Drug Administration (FDA), the Environmental Protection Agency (EPA), the Occupational Safety and Health Administration (OSHA), and so on. The challenge is to keep the broad view of how all these complex factors interact together while focusing on the details–it is the details that can be controlled. The big picture is the integral over time of these details.

This chapter is divided into four main areas:

1. A review of background and definitions

2. A discussion of the costs associated with development, including how development impacts later costs

3. A description of facilities costs, including design and construction

4. A presentation of operating costs

FOUNDATION

The fundamental reason for economic evaluation is that a choice exists between investment alternatives. But comparison requires measures of performance. The nebulous goal "maximize return" is too vague to keep a team of people focused: a more complete product specification (it could be called a mission statement) that covers the major constraints can serve to channel the activities of a cooperative team.

Time Value of Money

One of the main underlying principles is the time value of money, as illustrated in Figure 7.1, which shows how the quantitative worth (as measured in dollars) of an investment decreases as the time required to realize it increases. This concept forms the basis for present worth calculations, which convert the worth of future income streams to today's dollars. Consider that an alternative is to put the

Figure 7.1. The value of an investment decreases as the time required to realize it increases.

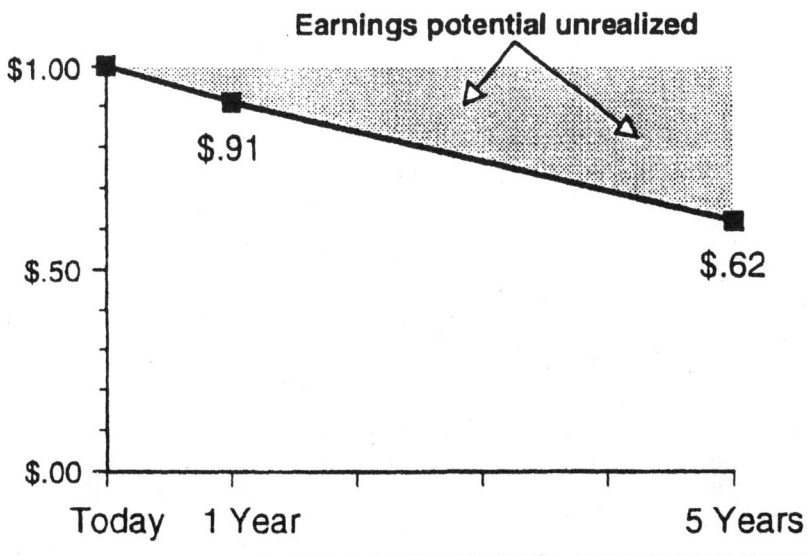

money in the bank where it accrues interest. Then every dollar invested today has greater worth later. Similarly, if one wishes to withdraw one dollar later, one needs only invest less than one dollar today. The longer one waits before making the withdrawal, the less one needs to invest. In other words, a dollar in hand today is worth more than a dollar returned in the future, not just because inflation decreases its purchasing power, but because it could have been invested somewhere else for a return of more than one dollar. Thus, if investors' money is to be attracted, a dollar in the future must be offered for less than a dollar invested today. And the farther in the future at which the dollar is returned, the less it is worth today.

A simple example will illustrate this point. If one desires a return of $1 in 5 years and can expect a 15 percent rate of return (assuming interest is compounded annually), then one needs only to invest 50¢ today. That is, in 5 years at an interest rate of 15 percent one can expect an original investment to be worth twice as much. Therefore, if investors expect a 15 percent rate of return, then every dollar returned to them in 5 years is comparable today to only 50¢. (To repeat, this is independent of any inflation adjustment.) If, instead of 5 years, their dollar is not returned until 10 years from now, its value today 10 years hence is only 25¢. The impact of inflation is additive: at 5 percent inflation, an overall return of 20 percent is required to provide a net 15 percent return to the investors. Comparisons of financial alternatives that take into account this time value of money allow quantification of the value of returns that occur over different time periods.

Another fundamental principle is the lost opportunity cost, or the cost of delay to market. Because a dollar of sales today is worth more than a dollar of sales tomorrow (or next year or any later time), the cost of delay in getting the product to market can be quantified. A product of moderate success, say $365 million in annual sales, postpones $1 million dollars income every day it is delayed. The time value of money places an additional cost of $47 million lost income (assuming 15 percent interest) on a one year delay in getting this product to market. There are two costs associated with the delay to market: (1) the delay in income from sales ($1 million/day) and (2) the interest that would have accrued had this money been available for investment during the time of delay ($47 million/year). Other intangible costs are associated with delay, notably a potential loss of competitive advantage from early market entrance relative to competitors.

In the case of biological products regulated by the FDA, the cost of process change may be very high, especially if the change results in the repetition of clinical trials or in delayed market entry. Historically, process development has been delayed as long as possible as a means to postpone expenses and preserve cash. Today, the cost of change is better recognized, and process development is pursued at earlier stages to avoid product launch delays. Also, with some clinical trials costing as much as $10,000 per patient, a crossover study with 100 patients costs $1 million; a substantial reduction in operating costs is required to justify such an expense. A good initial design that eliminates the need for later changes avoids expense.

Depreciation

Governments have recognized that physical plants wear out; therefore, they provide a tax accounting method whereby the decreasing value of capital equipment over time is reflected in the company's asset list on the balance sheet. Known as depreciation, this decreasing value is allocated as a noncash expense that is deducted from company revenues prior to the calculation of taxes. Thus, the cost of the investment is spread over several years rather than being incurred completely in the year in which the money is actually spent. If the cost were considered an expense only in the year in which the plant was built, the income for that year would be unrealistically low, while profits of later years would be exaggerated. Depreciation is subtracted from revenues and shows up as an operating expense, though it does not result in an outlay of cash.

Measures of Financial Performance

Companies have many different methods by which they evaluate financial performance, but these can be represented by three basic types, as described in Table 7.1 (Wheelwright and Asenjo in press). Return on investment is a simple ratio of annual profit and total investment (including working capital). The profit is usually specified as profit after taxes, including depreciation, and total investment includes both working capital and fixed capital. A variation is the return on average investment, which is the ratio of average yearly profit to the average fixed investment. Though return on investment is a simple measure of profitability, it neglects the time value of money.

The payback period or payout time describes the length of time necessary to recover the investment cost and is calculated as the ratio of the investment to the cash flow. Fixed capital (equipment and

Table 7.1. Comparison of Measures of Profitability

Measure	Equation	Advantages	Disadvantages
return on investment	$\dfrac{\text{annual profit}}{\text{total investment}} \times 100$	simple	neglects time value of money
payback period	$\dfrac{\text{capital} + \text{start-up}}{\text{after tax profit} + \text{depreciation}}$	intuitive; shows time to recover investment value	neglects time value of money; does not compare magnitude of return
net present value or discounted cash flow	$\displaystyle\sum_{t=0}^{t=n} \left[\dfrac{c_t}{(1+i)^t} \right]$*	considers time value of money	complex; does not indicate resources required

*Where t is the year number, n is the total number of years, i is the discount (or interest) rate, and C_t is the cash flow in year t.

facilities) and start-up are included in the investment, but not the working capital, as it is recovered periodically. The cash flow is the money recovered from the project, usually considered as the profit after taxes plus depreciation. This is a simple measure to calculate and gives an intuitive feel for the project. As with the rate of return, the payback period neglects the time value of money.

The measure most commonly used is the discounted cash flow or net present value. In effect, this measure allows a comparison of the return from any project with the return one might expect from the bank. It considers the time value of money and allows a comparison of projects with different lifetimes. The first step in the analysis is to forecast the cash flow (or net profit plus depreciation) for every year of the project. Each future annual cash flow prediction is discounted back to its present value. The sum of all discounted cash flows gives the net present value of the entire project. Figure 7.2 shows the cumulative cash flow (the sum of annual cash flows) over the life of a production plant. Note that cash flows are negative until after start-up. The discount rate strongly influences the value returned by this method. Figure 7.3 illustrates the impact on the annual cash flow of different discount rates. Typically, the greater the risk in a project, the higher the discount rate applied in evaluation. At high discount rates cash flows in later years have much lower values; at a rate of over 20 percent, cash flows beyond 10 years have little impact on the total net present value. As Shupe (1984) describes, "the higher the interest rate required for an investment, the more the balance favors the present, and the more difficult it becomes to justify an investment in the future." The selection of alternatives based on net present value will maximize the future value of the company if the assumptions hold.

A variation on the discounted cash flow is to calculate the discount rate for which the net present value at the end of the project is zero. Referred to as the discounted cash flow rate of return, this gives a measure of the minimum rate the project could return and still break even at the end of its life (Coulson et al. 1983). Many firms require the use of multiple measures, such as both the payback period and the discounted cash flow.

Uncertainty and Risk

Overlying all evaluations are the notions of uncertainty and risk. In the face of complete uncertainty, practical bounds cannot be placed on the problem (Lang 1989). On the other hand, though a given outcome is not certain, if some kind of bounds can be placed on the

Figure 7.2. Cumulative cash flow over the life of a project.

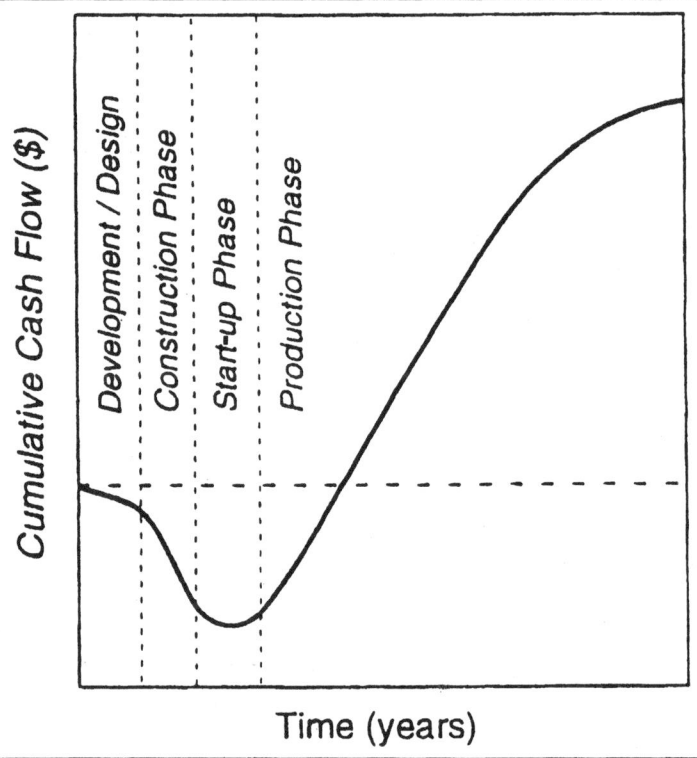

Figure 7.3. Impact of different discount rates on net annual cash flow. (From Datar and Rosen 1990. Printed with permission of Marcel Dekker, Inc.)

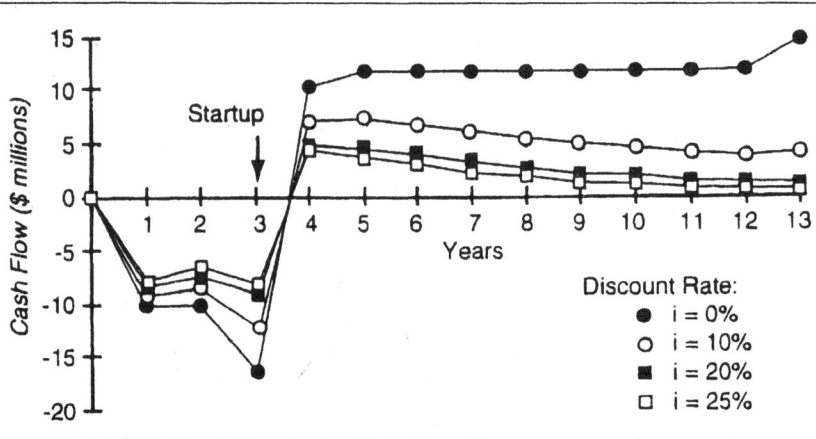

problem, a degree of risk can be assigned. Such problems as cost overruns and performance shortfalls can be assigned a distribution of probability for their occurrence and, therefore, a level of risk can be quantified. The challenge is to translate uncertainties into risks, place bounds on the problems, and assign probabilities to staying within those bounds.

Merrow (1989) describes three methods for this translation: (1) hide the uncertainties and cross one's fingers; (2) use expert judgment; or (3) rigorously assess past projects and apply the outcome to future projects. The first method is the most common, but failures can be spectacular, especially with regard to one's career. The last is difficult to apply in biotechnology, because few detailed examples are available. However, expert judgment does allow one to get a handle on risk.

The simplest incorporation of expert judgment and risk is the use of contingencies. One develops alternate scenarios in the case of failure and provides excess funds and time for unexpected overruns. The greater the risk (the less certainty in an outcome), the larger the contingency. The contingency should correlate with those factors that historically have been shown to have the greatest impact on costs.

A more sophisticated method is to use sensitivity analysis (Allen 1972). By assigning alternative values to key variables (such as an increase or decrease in raw materials costs of 15 percent), one can determine a new measure of performance for the project. Each major assumption can be tested under different scenarios to determine the consequence of changes. The value of sensitivity analysis is not restricted to plant economic return. Each development option can be evaluated to determine where development dollars are best spent. Similarly, the consequence of failure to meet a particular product specification or development goal (such as fermentation cell density) can be individually considered.

Thanks to the advent of powerful desktop computers, analysis by the Monte Carlo method is now available to everyone. Several commercial software packages allow the application of this sophisticated technique in routine studies. In the Monte Carlo method a range of values, along with a probability distribution, is assigned to each independent variable. A simulation is run many (say, 1000) times with different values of the independent variables substituted each time. The frequency at which any value is used corresponds to where that value falls in the probability distribution. Thus, more probable values are used more often. The output consists of a probability distribution for the major independent variable (for example, net present value). From this output one has some estimate of the probability the value will be within certain limits. One limitation in this method is the availability of reasonable estimates for the probability distributions of independent variables.

Value Engineering

Because of the interdependence of the variables, economic analysis is complex. There is no simple objective function for optimization. The various parts of the problem must be broken apart and evaluated separately, and then their interdependencies factored together. A powerful concept with wide applicability in economic analysis is value engineering. Usually applied to facility construction, value engineering can be used throughout the planning and development stages as well. The basic idea is to consider the value of each component separately and judge its merits against those of every other component. One begins by defining the minimum requirements (basic scope) and decides whether to add or exclude changes based on the incremental effect on the life cycle of the project. For example, in the installation of a production facility, the minimum choice of floor covering may be sealed vinyl sheet; value-added analysis will determine whether two-part trowelled epoxy or ground terrazzo is justified. The cost of each material must be considered on the basis of how one values its qualities. Those materials with a high cost that do not provide significant value beyond the minimum specifications are rejected. Value engineering can be applied to other areas, such as process development. For example, further development may reduce the consumption of sodium chloride and acetonitrile in purification steps. A substantial reduction of sodium chloride would probably have low value, but a reduction of acetonitrile could have high value.

DEVELOPMENT

Development activities influence costs in three basic ways: (1) development expenses may be high, (2) development may be on the critical path and, thus, impact the time of market entry, and (3) the process determined during development dictates the manufacturing costs, including the facility cost. For development purposes (because they require different technical skills), biological manufacturing processes are divided into three areas: (1) upstream (fermentation or cell culture), (2) downstream (recovery and purification), and (3) fill and finish (including sterilization and packaging).

Economies of Scale

Each of these areas has different major cost drivers. As a group, however, they all benefit from economies of scale; that is, as the scale of production increases, the cost of production increases at a less than proportional rate. Data are still sparse for biotechnology production, but for general chemical production the economy of scale tends to follow the six-tenths rule: the cost of a larger vessel (or system) is equal to the cost of the existing vessel times the ratio of the size of the larger vessel to the existing vessel with this ratio raised to the 0.6 power. For example, the cost of a tank that is 2 1/2 times the size of a tank that costs $100,000 is as follows:

$$\$100,000 \times (2.5/1)^{0.6} = \$173,000$$

The consequence of such economies of scale is that the cost of production on a unit basis can be reduced by employing larger equipment, which is to say, by operating at a larger scale.

Cost Drivers

Those factors that tend to control the production cost are as follows:

- In fermentation: expression, cell mass, and recovery yield
- In purification: the recovery yield at each step and the number of steps
- In fill and finish: recovery yield and packaging

The opportunity for process improvements that impact the operating cost significantly is highest in fermentation: expression levels can vary by several orders of magnitude, whereas the greatest improvement possible in purification is less than one order of magnitude (from, say, 10 percent recovery to 100 percent recovery); and possible improvements in fill and finish are even less. Note also that downstream steps cannot reduce the cost of upstream steps; a 70 percent purification yield on top of a 90 percent fermentation yield is 63 percent overall, but a 70 percent purification yield on top of a 70 percent fermentation yield is only 49 percent overall (Wheelwright 1988).

A critical factor in purification is the number of steps and the yield associated with each. Thermodynamics dictate that at each step there will be some loss of product; intuitively, the fewer the steps, the greater the yield will tend to be. But, of course, some steps have lower yields than others, so the replacement of one low-yielding step with two high-yielding steps should be carefully considered. Figure 7.4 shows the total recovery yield as a function of the number of steps and the yield of each step. Heuristics, or rules of thumb, have been developed to guide the design of purification processes (Wheelwright 1987, 1989). Listed in Table 7.2, these rules suggest the order of unit operations for purification. The dilute nature of most process streams at the early stages in a process is a key characteristic; rapid volume reduction is important in economic design (Lightfoot et al. 1987). In addition to the number of purification steps–their order and their yield–another important cost factor in purification is the throughput of chromatography steps. Though usually defined as the mass or unit volume processed per unit time,

Figure 7.4. The overall yield decreases as the number of steps increases and the step yield decreases. (From Fish and Lilly 1984. Printed with permission.)

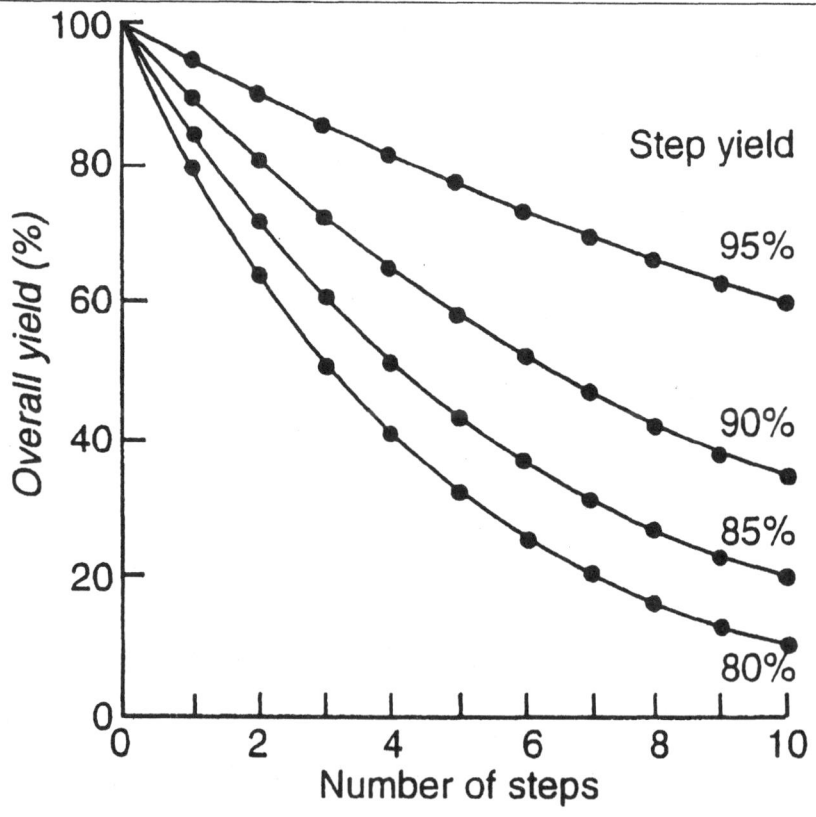

Table 7.2. Heuristics for Development of Purification Processes

Heuristic	Application	Cost Reason
Do the biggest step first.	Reduce volume or mass.	Allow smaller equipment for subsequent steps.
Do the most expensive step last.	Use gel filtration chromatography only at the end of the process.	At the end of the process, the volume will be reduced, so materials will cost less.
Choose processes that exploit the greatest differences in the physical properties of the product and the impurities.	Select step that maximizes separation.	Maximum separation should give highest yields.
Choose separations based on different physical properties.	Base subsequent separations on different methods.	Alternate physical bases should give subsequent high yields.

for cost analyses it is important to include the unit cost in the denominator. The evaluation of process steps on a mass per unit time per unit cost basis allows the direct comparison between chromatography steps, even when different sorption media and different scales are employed.

Because fill and finish plants are expensive to operate, few biotechnology companies have built them and, instead, rely on outside contractors for this operation. A fill and finish plant requires a large capital expenditure that realizes its best rate of return when it is always occupied. Since few biotech companies have enough products to keep a facility full, it is less expensive to contract this work out to a specialist. The cost of the fill and finish work, including packaging, may represent a substantial part of the total cost of goods. For example, fill and finish (with packaging) of a parenteral drug (say, under 10 mL/vial) in an efficiently operating plant may cost $2 to $3 per vial for a liquid fill and twice that for a lyophilized product.

FACILITIES

The cost of a facility includes many aspects, such as construction, validation, equipment, operation, and so forth. But all of these hinge on the intended use of the facility. The use and occupancy of any facility is referred to as the *program* for that facility, and *programming* is the activity of deciding how and what to include. Bioprocessing requires two main types of facilities: laboratories and manufacturing plants. Laboratories for process development are similar to those for biochemistry research, except that more open space is needed for large, floor-mounted equipment; as a consequence of the large equipment, the average square footage per scientist is higher than in research labs. The programming stage is another place where value engineering can be applied to assure that every component is necessary and of the proper quality. Laboratory space usually costs between $150 and $350 per square foot (including furniture, but excluding equipment).

The distribution of area in a manufacturing plant between the different functions (fermentation, purification, raw materials, etc.) will depend on the specific process. In a facility dedicated to the production of a single product, the process will dictate the programming. However, because of economies of scale, smaller-volume products will have a lower cost of goods if they are produced in a shared or multiuse facility. This requires a more flexible plan, one not overly specific for any particular product (Stark and Kurtz 1994). Also, recent failures of products in the clinic after the construction of dedicated facilities have left large plants empty, because they are not readily adapted to other products. A more flexible or generic design may be favored by the financing group, as it improves the possible resale value in the event of product failure. Figure 7.5 shows a typical distribution of building area among functional groups (these data are a composite of several sources available to the author).

Construction Alternatives

There are three basic options for construction: new or grass roots, existing shell, or renovation. Each of these alternatives offers different advantages and disadvantages (see Table 7.3). Totally new construction provides the greatest flexibility of layout, including the design of large campuses with unified architecture. New construction, however, has the longest lead time between project initiation and start-up. New construction often ends up with a larger facility than the other options; therefore, the total project cost is higher, but

Figure 7.5. Typical distribution of building area between functional groups.

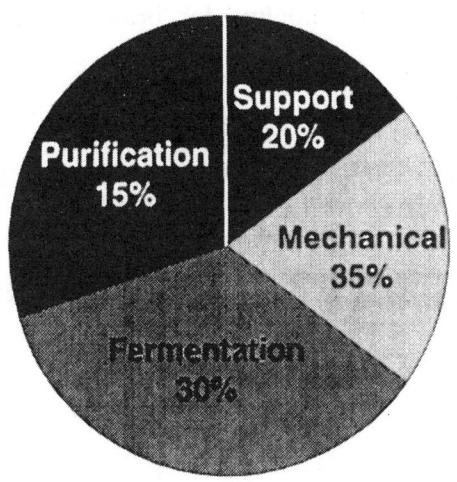

Table 7.3. Comparison of Construction Alternatives

Alternative	Advantages	Disadvantages	Cost
renovate occupied space	lower investment; convenient site	high basis cost; difficult; limited scope	high cost on square-foot basis
build out existing shell	shorter time than new construction	limited scope	similar to new
new	complete custom design; large tract possible; maximum flexibility	longest time	similar to shell

the cost on a square foot basis is not necessarily greater. Installation in an existing shell offers the advantage of quicker completion but imposes limitations on layout. Renovation of an existing occupied space is usually limited to small projects. Because of unforeseen conditions, it may be much more difficult than new or shell construction. Representative times for construction are listed in Table 7.4. In site selection the attitude of the local community is probably the most important factor (Stocker and Embree 1991). Figure 7.6 shows a representative timeline for bringing a new product to market.

Utilities

The types of utilities required depend on the use of the facility. Normal office buildings provide only tempered air, electrical power, and hot and cold water for rest rooms. Laboratories additionally may

Table 7.4. Comparison of Construction Times (in Months)

Activity	New Construction	Existing Shell	Renovation
site development	5–10	1–3	0
architectural and engineering design	6–18	6–18	4–10
construction	20–30	18–24	12–18
validation	6–10	6–10	4–6
start-up	2–3	2–3	1–2
total	39–71	33–58	21–36

Figure 7.6. Representative timeline for bringing a new product to market.

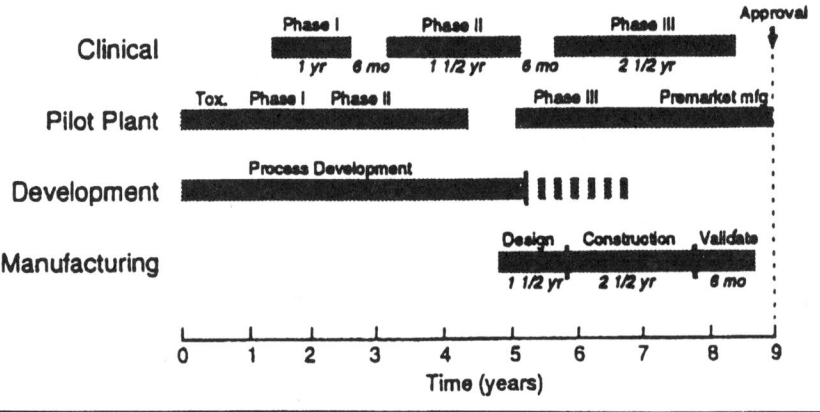

need bottled gases, piped gases (such as nitrogen and clean, dry air), purified water, vacuum, and emergency power for freezers and life safety systems (hood exhaust and alarms). Process areas may require chilled water; chilled glycol; plant steam; clean steam; a bio-waste sewer system; WFI; emergency power for operations; and strictly controlled environmental systems, including HEPA–filtered air into and out of the room, humidity control and relative pressure differentials between rooms. The environmental control of production areas requires limits on both total particles and viable particles (mold, yeast, bacteria); measurements should be conducted during dynamic (operating) conditions. Surfaces should be cleanable with sanitizing agents and should be cleaned on a regular basis. The minimum specifications for construction are defined by the current Good Manufacturing Practice (cGMP) regulations of the FDA, which are found in Title 21 of the *Code of Federal Regulations* (CFR), part 211 for human and veterinary drugs and part 820 for diagnostics.

Validation

Validation, or the verification that systems are installed properly and function as they are expected to, should be integral with construction: A validation master plan describing the overall philosophy (what gets validated and how) that is available prior to the initiation of construction can serve as a guide during construction and start-up. It is easier to validate a plant if validation is designed into the facility and begins prior to construction. Photographs during construction, for example, give evidence of the installation of equipment parts that are hidden from view during use. Validation is a major activity—one that is frequently underestimated. Six months is not an unusual amount of time for the completion of the validation of a production plant. Equipment and process validation can be scheduled with greater flexibility than utilities but should be completed before the plant begins operating; six months or longer may be required for the completion of this activity.

Containment

The containment level required depends on the activity. The facility must first be designed to provide product safety. This means that the product must be protected from possible contamination. Thus, a controlled environment is required that reduces the number of foreign particles with increasing strictness as the product moves through the process. Different products and batches must be separated by space (location) and time. The safety of workers and the environment must all be respected; and this requires containment of hazardous materials to prevent their accidental release to the external environment. The National Institutes of Health (NIH 1994) have published guidelines describing the levels of containment required for microbe, cell culture, and virus production processes. Of course, the greater the level of containment, the higher the cost. Before waste streams containing biological organisms, cells, or viruses can be discharged to a public sewer, they must be inactivated to destroy biological activity by a method such as steam injection (heat kill), pH change, or oxidation (chemical kill) (see, for example, Kossik and Miller 1994). The industry has witnessed increased emphasis on the validation of cleaning procedures, including the measurement of total organic carbon (TOC) and highly sensitive product specific assays, such as enzyme-linked immunosorbent assays (ELISA) to demonstrate cleanliness between products in equipment, especially at late stages of production.

The process equipment represents a substantial part of the total plant cost. While the specification of particular pieces of equipment depends in large measure on the details of the process, versatility considerations for other applications may also be important. The cost of building in flexibility should be scrutinized through the process of value engineering, with consideration of the degree of risk in the project and recovery scenarios in the event of product failure.

OPERATIONS

Operating expenses are those costs required for product manufacture. These include such things as raw materials, utilities, labor, royalties, depreciation, insurance, rent, and overhead. Items for which the total expense varies with production volume are called variable (or direct) expenses; items that remain constant, independent of production volume, are known as fixed (or indirect) expenses. The point at which the combined fixed and variable expenses equal revenue is called the breakeven point, as shown in Figure 7.7. Profit is represented by the area bounded by the revenue line, the total expense line, the breakeven point, and the production rate. The prime cost drivers tend to be raw materials, labor, depreciation, and other fixed costs. Generally, because of the impact of fixed costs, including depreciation, on the cost of manufacturing, and as a result of the economies of scale that are realized with larger equipment, the

Figure 7.7. Profit is represented by the area bounded by total expenses, revenue, and production level.

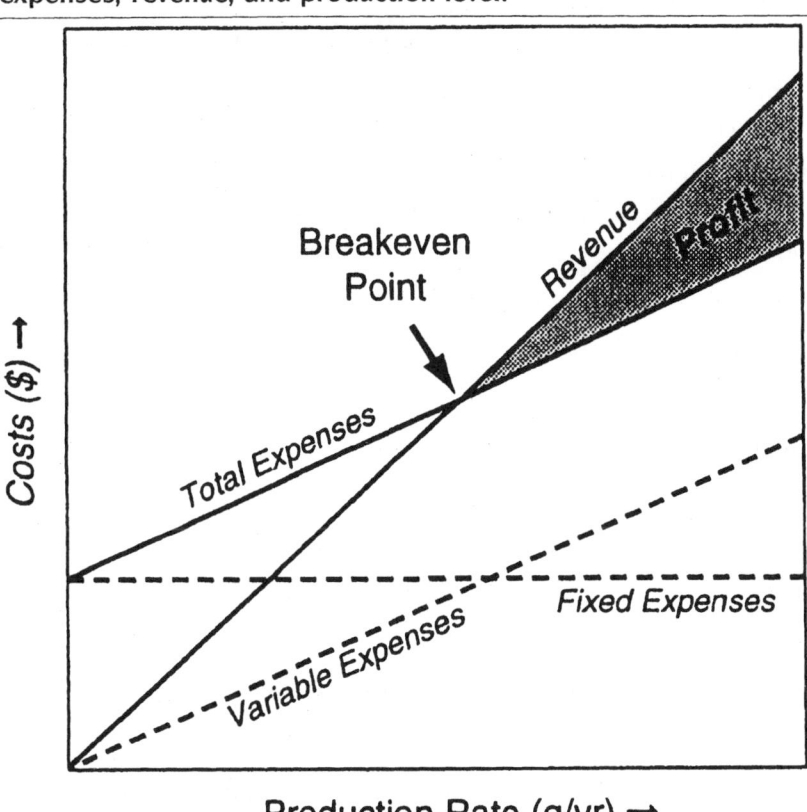

lowest unit cost is achieved with the largest volume operation. In some cases this may lead to a facility shared by multiple, small-volume products.

A study by Datar and Rosen (1990) of insulin production estimated the direct portion of the operation to be 74 percent of total annual expense (excluding general and administrative costs). A similar study (Datar et al. 1993) of tissue plasminogen activator produced in bacteria and mammalian cell culture estimated the direct expense to be 47 percent (in the case of bacteria) or 60 percent (in the case of cell culture) of the total annual expense (Table 7.5). Depending on what factors one includes in the manufacturing costs, one can expect the annual costs to fall between 3 to 10 times the

Table 7.5. Comparison of Manufacturing Expenses (Percent of Total)

Area	Insulin[1]	tPA (mammalian)[2]	tPA (bacterial)[2]
fermentation raw materials	19	33	1
purification raw materials		11	8
labor	23	9	22
utilities	14	17	20
patent/royalty		17	20
waste		10	16
other	30	3	13
overhead	14		
total	100	100	100

[1]from Datar and Rosen (1990)

[2]from Datar et al. (1993)

cost of the installed capital equipment. The total facility cost is also on the order of 3 to 6 times the cost of the installed capital equipment; to a first approximation, annual operating costs are comparable to plant capital costs. Most biotech facilities cost $500 to $600 per square foot; pilot (small-scale) facilities may range up to $1000 per square foot. Hacking (1986) gives as a general rule that pilot-plant development costs 10 times more than laboratory work, and full-scale plants cost at least 10 times more than pilot-scale work. The cost range for protein drugs manufactured at large scale is typically $50 to $5000 per gram.

OPTIMIZATION

The conclusion is that vigilant evaluation of those factors that impact costs, especially future costs, at the early stages of the development and planning process will have the greatest impact in minimizing the cost as well as minimizing the time required to bring a new product to market. A persistent review of development, facility, and operations designs yields tangible financial rewards, when folded within the framework of a guiding philosophy. Comparison of such fundamental questions as a dedicated versus a shared plant, new construction versus renovation, the number of purification steps versus the process yield, time to develop versus delay of market launch, and the acceptable risk versus the payback allows one to quantify the economic return and maximize the value to investors.

REFERENCES

Allen, D. H. 1972. *A guide to the economic evaluation of projects.* London: The Institution of Chemical Engineers.

Coulson, J. M., J. G. Richardson, and R. K. Sinnott, eds. 1983. Costing and project evaluation. In *Chemical engineering,* vol. 6. Pergamon Press.

Datar, R., and C.-G. Rosen. 1990. Downstream process economics. In *Separation processes in biotechnology,* edited by J. A. Asenjo. New York: Marcel Dekker.

Datar, R. V., T. Cartwright, and C.-G. Rosen. 1993. Process economics of animal cell and bacterial fermentations: A case study analysis of tissue plasminogen activator. *Bio/technology* 11:349–357.

Fish, N. M., and M. D. Lilly. 1984. The interactions between fermentation and protein recovery. *Bio/technology* 2:623.

Hacking, A. J. 1986. *Economic aspects of biotechnology.* Cambridge: Cambridge University Press.

Kossik, J. M., and G. Miller. 1994. Optimize cycle times for batch biokill systems. *Chem. Eng. Prog.* 90 (10):45–51.

Lang, H. J. 1989. *Cost analysis for capital investment decisions.* New York: Marcel Dekker.

Lightfoot, E. N., S. J. Gibbs, M. C. M. Cockrem, and A. M. Athalye. 1987. Scaling up protein purification. In *Protein purification: Micro to macro,* edited by R. Burgess. New York: Alan R. Liss.

Merrow, E. W. 1989. Uncertainty, new technology, and project success in the chemical industries. Paper presented at the Annual

Meeting of the American Institute of Chemical Engineers, 7 November 1989, in San Francisco.

NIH. 1994. Guidelines for research involving recombinant DNA molecules. *Federal Register* Part IV, 59 (127):1–73.

Shupe, D. S. 1984. Discounted cash flows. In *Manufacturing cost engineering handbook,* edited by E. M. Malstrom. New York: Marcel Dekker.

Stark, S., and J. Kurtz. 1994. Design and environmental considerations for the modern research laboratory. *BioPharm* 7 (1):32–39.

Stocker, A. C., and J. A. Embree. 1991. Creating cost effective biotech facilities. *Pharm. Eng.* 11 (3):37–45.

Wheelwright, S. M. 1987. Designing downstream processes for large-scale protein purification. *Bio/technology* 5:789–793.

Wheelwright, S. M. 1988. The impact of downstream recovery operations on upstream production methods: Vertical integration and process optimization. In *Biotechnology research and applications,* edited by J. Gavora, D. F. Gerson, J. Luong, A. Storer, and J. H. Woodley. New York: Elsevier Applied Science.

Wheelwright, S. M. 1989. The design of downstream processes for large-scale protein purification. *J. Biotechnol.* 11:89–102.

Wheelwright, S. M., and J. A. Asenjo. In press. Economic analysis of downstream processes. In *Handbook of downstream processing,* edited by K. H. Kroner, and N. Papamichael. New York: Wiley Interscience.

NAME INDEX

SUBJECT INDEX

Drug Manufacturing Technology Series
KEY CONCEPT CROSS-REFERENCE INDEX

Note: This key concept index is designed to reflect all of the major topics of the *Drug Manufacturing Technology Series* as they are published. It will be expanded for each volume. Volume numbers are identified by an Arabic numeral followed by a colon.

384